Do you know that the Sanford Guide is available in two larger sized print editions and electronic editions for handheld PDA devices?

The pocket-sized edition (4 x 6 in) is handy to keep in your labcoat, but if the print is becoming a challenge, consider the bigger books:
handy spiral-bound edition (5 x 8 in) and
full-sized Desk/Library edition (7.250 x 11 in)

Did you know that the Sanford Guide is updated annually?

Don't rely on outdated recommendations. Order a current edition today!

For more information, go to
www.sanfordguide.com

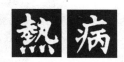

P9-BHZ-916

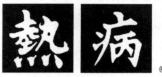

SANFORD GUIDE®

熱病®

Thirty-Eighth Edition

THE SANFORD GUIDE
TO ANTIMICROBIAL
THERAPY
2008

Editors:

David N. Gilbert, M.D.
Director of Medical Education & Earl A. Chiles Research Institute
Providence Portland Medical Center
Professor of Medicine
Oregon Health Sciences University
Portland, Oregon

Robert C. Moellering, Jr., M.D.
Shields Warren-Mallinckrodt Professor of Medical Research
Harvard Medical School
Boston, Massachusetts

George M. Eliopoulos, M.D.
Chief, James L. Tullis Firm, Beth Israel Deaconess Hospital
Professor of Medicine
Harvard Medical School
Boston, Massachusetts

Merle A. Sande, M.D. (1939-2007)
Professor of Medicine
University of Washington School of Medicine
Seattle, Washington

Contributing Editors:

Henry F. (Chip) Chambers, M.D.
Professor of Medicine
University of California at San Francisco
Chief of Infectious Diseases
San Francisco General Hospital
San Francisco, California

Michael S. Saag, M.D.
Professor of Medicine & Director, Division of Infectious Dieases
Director, UAB Center for AIDS Research
University of Alabama
Birmingham, Alabama

THE SANFORD GUIDE TO ANTIMICROBIAL THERAPY 2008
(38TH EDITION)

Jay P. Sanford, M.D.
1928-1996

Editors

David N. Gilbert, M.D.   Robert C. Moellering, Jr., M.D.
George M. Eliopoulos, M.D.   Merle A. Sande, M.D. (1939-2007)

Contributing Editors

Henry F. (Chip) Chambers, M.D.   Michael S. Saag, M.D.

The SANFORD GUIDES are updated annually and published by:

Antimicrobial Therapy, Inc.
P.O. Box 276, 11771 Lee Highway, Sperryville, VA 22740-0276 USA
Tel 540-987-9480 *Fax* 540-987-9486 *Email:* info@sanfordguide.com
www.sanfordguide.com

Acknowledgements

Thanks to Lingua Solutions, Inc., Los Angeles, CA for assistance in preparation of the manuscript; Royalty Press, Westville, NJ for printing and Fox Bindery, Quakertown, PA for finishing this edition of the Sanford Guide to Antimicrobial Therapy.

Publisher's Note to Readers

Though many readers of the SANFORD GUIDE receive their copy from a pharmaceutical company representative, please be assured that the SANFORD GUIDE has been, and continues to be, independently prepared and published since its inception in 1969. Decisions regarding the content of the SANFORD GUIDE are solely those of the editors and the publisher. We welcome your questions, comments and feedback concerning the SANFORD GUIDE. All of your feedback is reviewed and taken into account in preparing the next edition.

Every effort is made to ensure the accuracy of the content of this guide. However, current full prescribing information available in the package insert of each drug should be consulted before prescribing any product. The editors and publisher are not responsible for errors or omissions or for any consequences from application of the information in this book and make no warranty, express or implied, with respect to the currency, accuracy, or completeness of the contents of the publication. Application of this information in a particular situation remains the professional responsibility of the practitioner.

**Content-related notices are published on our website. To find such notices go to:
http://www.sanfordguide.com/notices**

Printed in the United States of America
ISBN 978-1-930808-45-4
Pocket Edition (English)

ABBREVIATIONS 2

TABLE 1   Clinical Approach to **Initial Choice** of Antimicrobial Therapy 4

TABLE 1B   Prophylaxis and Treatment of Organisms of Potential Use as **Biological Weapons** 59

TABLE 2   Recommended Antimicrobial Agents Against **Selected Bacteria** 61

TABLE 3   Suggested **Duration** of Antibiotic Therapy in Immunocompetent Patients 64

TABLE 4   Comparison of **Antimicrobial Spectra** 65

TABLE 5   Treatment Options for Selected **Highly Resistant Bacteria** 71

TABLE 6   Suggested Management of Suspected or Culture-Positive **Community-Acquired Phenotype** of Methicillin-Resistant S. Aureus (CA-MRSA) Infections 73

TABLE 7   Methods for **Penicillin Desensitization** 74

TABLE 8   **Risk Categories** of Antimicrobics in **Pregnancy** 74

TABLE 9A   Selected **Pharmacologic Features** of Antimicrobial Agents 75
      9B   Pharmacodynamics of Antibacterials 79

TABLE 10A   Selected Antibacterial Agents—**Adverse Reactions**—Overview 80
      10B   Antimicrobial Agents Associated with **Photosensitivity** 84
      10C   Summary of **Antibiotic Dosage**, Side-Effects, and Cost 85
      10D   **Aminoglycoside** Once-Daily and Multiple Daily Dosing Regimens 93

TABLE 11A   Treatment of **Fungal, Actinomycotic, and Nocardial Infections**—Antimicrobial Agents of Choice 94
      11B   **Antifungal Drugs:** Adverse Effects, Comments, Cost 105
      11C   **Summary of Suggested Antifungal Drugs Against Treatable Pathogenic Fungi** 109

TABLE 12A   Treatment of **Mycobacterial Infections** 110
      12B   **Dosage**, Price and Selected Adverse Effects of Antimycobacterial Drugs 120

TABLE 13A   Treatment of **Parasitic Infections** 123
      13B   **Dosage**, Price, and Selected Adverse Effects of Antiparasitic Drugs 132
      13C   Parasites that Cause Eosinophilia 134

TABLE 14A   **Antiviral Therapy** (Non-HIV) 135
      14B   **Antiviral Drugs** (Other Than Retroviral) 147
      14C   **Summary of Suggested Antiviral Agents Against Treatable Pathogenic Viruses** 151
      14D   **Antiretroviral Therapy** in Treatment-Naïve Adults 152
      14E   **Antiretroviral Drugs** and Adverse Effects 164

TABLE 15A   **Antimicrobial Prophylaxis** for Selected Bacterial Infections 167
      15B   **Surgical Antibiotic Prophylaxis** 168
      15C   Antimicrobial Prophylaxis for the Prevention of **Bacterial Endocarditis** in Patients with Underlying Cardiac Conditions 171
      15D   Management of **Exposure to HIV-1 and Hepatitis B and C** 172
      15E   Prevention of Opportunistic Infection in Human Stem Cell **Transplantation** (HSCT) or Solid Organ Transplantation (SOT) for Adults with Normal Renal Function 175

TABLE 16   **Pediatric Dosages** of Selected Antibacterial Agents 177

TABLE 17A   Dosages of Antimicrobial Drugs in Adult Patients with **Renal Impairment** 178
      17B   **No Dosage Adjustment** with Renal Insufficiency by Category 185

TABLE 18   Antimicrobials and **Hepatic Disease** Dosage Adjustment 185

TABLE 19   Treatment of **CAPD Peritonitis** in Adults 185

TABLE 20A   Recommended Childhood and Adolescent **Immunization Schedule**: United States (Includes Schedule for ages 7-18), 2007 186
      20B   **Catch-Up Immunization Schedule** For Persons Aged 4 Months–18 Years Who Start Late Or Who Are ≥1 Month Behind — United States, 2007 189
      20C   **Adult Immunization In The United States** 191
      20D   Anti-**Tetanus** Prophylaxis, Wound Classification, Immunization 195
      20E   **Rabies** Post-Exposure Prophylaxis 196

TABLE 21   Selected **Directory of Resources** 197

TABLE 22A   Anti-Infective **Drug-Drug Interactions** 198
      22B   Drug-Drug Interactions Between **Protease Inhibitors** 204
      22C   Drug-Drug Interactions Between **Non-Nucleoside Reverse Transcriptase Inhibitors (NNRTIS) and Protease Inhibitors** 205

TABLE 23   List of **Generic** and **Common** Trade Names 206

INDEX OF MAJOR ENTITIES 208

SUMMARY OF ABBREVIATIONS

DRUG NAME ABBREVIATIONS

Antibacterial & Antimycobacterial Drugs

AG = aminoglycoside
AMK = amikacin
AM-CL = amoxicillin-clavulanate
AM-CL-ER = amoxicillin-clavulanate extended release
Amox = amoxicillin
Amp = ampicillin
AM-SB = ampicillin-sulbactam
AP Pen = antipseudomonal penicillins
APAG = antipseudomonal aminoglycoside (tobra, gent, amikacin)
Azithro = azithromycin
BL/BLI = beta-lactam/beta-lactamase inhibitor
CARB = carbapenems (ERTA, IMP, MER)
CFB = ceftobiprole
Cfpdx = cefpodoxime proxetil
Cftaz = ceftazidime
Cftri = ceftriaxone
CIP = ciprofloxacin; CIP-ER = extended release
Clarithro = clarithromycin; ER = extended release
Clinda = clindamycin
CLO = clofazimine
Dalba = dalbavancin
Dapto = daptomycin
Dori = doripenem
Doxy = doxycycline
EES = erythromycin ethyl succinate
ERTA = ertapenem
Erythro = erythromycin
ETB = ethambutol
FQ = fluoroquinolone (CIP, Oflox, Lome, Peflox, Levo, Gati, Moxi, Gemi)
Gati = gatifloxacin
Gemi = gemifloxacin
GNB = gram-negative bacilli
IMP = imipenem-cilastatin
INH = isoniazid
IVIG = intravenous immune globulin
Levo = levofloxacin
Macrolides = azithro, clarithro, dirithro, erythro, roxithro
MER = meropenem
Metro = metronidazole
Mino = minocycline
Moxi = moxifloxacin
NF = nitrofurantoin
O Ceph 1,2,3 = oral cephalosporins—see Table 10B
Oflox = ofloxacin

P Ceph 1,2,3,4 = parenteral cephalosporins—see Table 10B
P Ceph 3 AP = parenteral cephalosporins with antipseudomonal activity—see Table 10B
PIP-TZ = piperacillin-tazobactam
PZA = pyrazinamide
Quinu-dalfo = Q-D = quinupristin-dalfopristin
RFB = rifabutin
Rifampin = rifampin
RIF = rifampin
Roxi = roxithromycin
SM = streptomycin
Sulb = sulbactam
Tazo = tazobactam
TC-CL = ticarcillin-clavulanate
Teico = teicoplanin
Telithro = telithromycin
Tetra = tetracycline
Tica = ticarcillin
TMP-SMX = trimethoprim-sulfamethoxazole
Tobra = tobramycin
Vanco = vancomycin

Antifungal Drugs

Ampho B = amphotericin B
ABCD = ampho B cholesteryl complex
ABCD = amphotericin B colloidal dispersion
ABLC = ampho B lipid complex
Clot = clotrimazole
Flu = fluconazole
Flucyt = flucytosine
Griseo = griseofulvin
Itra = itraconazole
Keto = ketoconazole
LAB = liposomal ampho B
Vori = voriconazole

Antiparasitic Drugs

AP = atovaquone proguanil
CQ = chloroquine phosphate
MQ = mefloquine

Antivirals, Anti-HIV Drugs

3TC = lamivudine
d4T = stavudine
ddC = zalcitabine
ABC = abacavir
NRTI = nucleoside reverse transcriptase inhibitor
NtRTI = nucleotide reverse transcriptase inhibitor
PI = protease inhibitor
ddl = didanosine
ATV = atazanavir
RTV = ritonavir
FTC = emtricitabine
FOS-APV = fosamprenavir
SQV = saquinavir
TDF = tenofovir
TPV = tipranavir
DLV = delavirdine

ZDV = zidovudine
EFZ = efavirenz
NVP = nevirapine

LP/R = lopinavir/ritonavir
NFR = nelfinavir

PQ = primaquine
Pyri = pyrimethamine
QS = quinine sulfate

IDV = indinavir
ENT = enfuvirtide
ADF = adefovir
IFN = interferon

DRUG DOSAGE & DRUG ADMINISTRATION

mcg = microgram
mg = milligram
gm = gram
DS = double strength
bid = twice a day
tid = 3 times a day
qid = 4 times a day
DOT = directly observed therapy

AD = after dialysis
div = divided
IA = intraarterial
IT = intrathecal
po = per os (by mouth)
subcut = subcutaneous
dc = discontinue
rx = treatment

BW = body weight
ASA = aspirin
NSAIDs = non-steroidal anti-inflammatory drugs

DRUG-RELATED

G = generic
I = investigational
IA = injectable agent
NB = name brand
NFDA-I = not FDA-approved indication
NUS = not available in the U.S.

DISEASE-ASSOCIATED

AIDS = Acquired Immune Deficiency Syndrome
ARDS = acute respiratory distress syndrome
ARF = acute rheumatic fever
CAPD = continuous ambulatory peritoneal dialysis
CRRT = continuous renal replacement therapy
CSD = cat-scratch disease
DIC = disseminated intravascular coagulation
ESRD = endstage renal disease
HEMO = hemodialysis
PEP = post-exposure prophylaxis
PTLD = post-transplant lymphoproliferative disease
RTI = respiratory tract infection
STD = sexually transmitted disease
TBc = tuberculosis
TST = tuberculin skin test
UTI = urinary tract infection

ORGANISMS

CMV = cytomegalovirus
DOT group = B. distasonis, B. ovatus, B. thetaiotaomicron
DRSP = drug-resistant S. pneumoniae
EBV = Epstein-Barr virus
gonococcus
HHV = human herpesvirus
HIV = human immunodeficiency virus
HSV = herpes simplex virus
LCM = lymphocytic choriomeningitis virus
MRSA = methicillin-resistant S. aureus
MSSA = methicillin-sensitive S. aureus
M. Tbc = Mycobacterium tuberculosis
Rick = Rickettsia
RSV = respiratory syncytial virus
VISA = vancomycin intermediately resistant S. aureus
VZV = varicella-zoster virus

ABBREVIATIONS (2)

MISCELLANEOUS

Diagnosis

CrCl = creatinine clearance
C&S = culture & sensitivity
CDC = Centers for Disease Control
CSF = cerebrospinal fluid
CXR = chest x-ray
ESBLs = extended spectrum β-lactamases
ESR = erythrocyte sedimentation rate
HLR = high-level resistance
HSCT = hematopoietic stem cell transplant
LCR = ligase chain reaction
PCR = polymerase chain reaction
TEE = transesophageal echocardiography
VL = viral load

Organizations

ACIP = Advisory Committee on Immunization Practices
ATS = American Thoracic Society
CDC = Centers for Disease Control
ICAAC = International Conference on Antimicrobial Agents & Chemotherapy
IDSA = Infectious Diseases Society of America
WHO = World Health Organization

Other

AUC = area under the curve
DBPCT = double-blind placebo-controlled trial
IOU = intraocular/unit
PRCT = Prospective randomized controlled trials
Pts = patients
R = resistant
S = potential synergy in combination with penicillin, AMP, vanco.
Sens = sensitive (susceptible)

ABBREVIATIONS OF JOURNAL TITLES

AAC: Antimicrobial Agents & Chemotherapy
Adv PID: Advances in Pediatric Infectious Diseases
AIDS Res Hum Retrovir: AIDS Research & Human Retroviruses
AJG: American Journal of Gastroenterology
AJM: American Journal of Medicine
AJRCCM: American Journal of Respiratory Critical Care Medicine
AJTMH: American Journal of Tropical Medicine & Hygiene
Aliment Pharmacol Ther: Alimentary Pharmacology & Therapeutics
Am J Hlth Pharm: American Journal of Health-System Pharmacy
AnEM: Annals of Emergency Medicine
AnIM: Annals of Internal Medicine
AnPharmacother: Annals of Pharmacotherapy
AnSurg: Annals of Surgery
ArDerm: Archives of Dermatology
ArIM: Archives of Internal Medicine
Antivir Ther: Antiviral Therapy
ARRD: American Review of Respiratory Disease
BMJ: British Medical Journal
BMTr: Bone Marrow Transplantation
Brit J Derm: British Journal of Dermatology
Can JID: Canadian Journal of Infectious Diseases
CCM: Critical Care Medicine
CID: Clinical Infectious Diseases
Clin Micro Inf: Clinical Microbiology and Infection
Clin Micro Rev: Clinical Microbiology Reviews
CMAJ: Canadian Medical Association Journal
COID: Current Opinion in Infectious Disease
Curr Med Res Opin: Current Medical Research and Opinion
Derm Ther: Dermatologic Therapy

Dig Dis Sci: Digestive Diseases and Sciences
DMID: Diagnostic Microbiology and Infectious Disease
EID: Emerging Infectious Diseases
EJCMID: European Journal of Clin. Micro. & Infectious Diseases
Eur J Neurol: European Journal of Neurology
Eur Mol Path: Experimental & Molecular Pathology
Gastro: Gastroenterology
Hpt: Hepatology
ICHE: Infection Control and Hospital Epidemiology
IDC No. Amer: Infectious Disease Clinics of North America
IDCP: Infectious Diseases in Clinical Practice
IJAA: International Journal of Antimicrobial Agents
Inf Med: Infections in Medicine
JAIDS: JAIDS Journal of Acquired Immune Deficiency Syndromes
J AIDS & HR: Journal of AIDS and Human Retrovirology
J All Clin Immun: Journal of Allergy and Clinical Immunology
Am Ger Soc: Journal of the American Geriatrics Society
JChemother: Journal of Chemotherapy
JCI: Journal of Clinical Investigation
J Clin Micro: Journal of Clinical Microbiology
J Clin Virol: Journal of Clinical Virology
J Derm Treat: Journal of Dermatological Treatment
Hpt: Journal of Hepatology
Inf: Journal of Infection
J Med Micro: Journal of Medical Microbiology
J Micro Immunol Inf: Journal of Microbiology, Immunology, & Infection
J Ped: Journal of Pediatrics

JAC: Journal of Antimicrobial Chemotherapy
JAMA: Journal of the American Medical Association
JAVMA: Journal of the Veterinary Medicine Association
JCM: Journal of Clinical Microbiology
JID: Journal of Infectious Diseases
JNS: Journal of Neurological Sciences
JTMH: Journal of Tropical Medicine and Hygiene
J Viral Hep: Journal of Viral Hepatitis
Ln: Lancet
LnID: Lancet Infectious Disease
Mayo Clin Proc: Mayo Clinic Proceedings
Med Lett: Medical Letter
Med Mycol: Medical Mycology
MMWR: Morbidity & Mortality Weekly Report
NEJM: New England Journal of Medicine
Neph Dial Transpl: Nephrology Dialysis Transplantation
Ped Ann: Pediatric Annals
Peds: Pediatrics
Pharmacother: Pharmacotherapy
PIDJ: Pediatric Infectious Disease Journal
QJM: Quarterly Journal of Medicine
Scand J Inf Dis: Scandinavian Journal of Infectious Diseases
Sem Resp Inf: Seminars in Respiratory Infections
SGO: Surgery Gynecology and Obstetrics
SMJ: Southern Medical Journal
Surg Neurol: Surgical Neurology
Transpl: Transplantation
Transpl Inf Dis: Transplant Infectious Diseases
TRSM: Transactions of the Royal Society of Medicine
West J Med: Western Journal of Medicine

TABLE 1 – CLINICAL APPROACH TO INITIAL CHOICE OF ANTIMICROBIAL THERAPY*

Treatment based on presumed site or type of infection. In selected instances, treatment and prophylaxis based on identification of pathogens *(Abbreviations on page 2)*

ANATOMIC SITE/DIAGNOSIS/ MODIFYING CIRCUMSTANCES	ETIOLOGIES (usual)	SUGGESTED REGIMENS*		ADJUNCT DIAGNOSTIC OR THERAPEUTIC MEASURES AND COMMENTS
		PRIMARY	ALTERNATIVE‡	
ABDOMEN: See Peritoneum, page 42; Gallbladder, page 14; and Pelvic Inflammatory Disease, page 23				
BONE: Osteomyelitis. Microbiologic diagnosis is essential. If blood culture negative, need culture of bone. Culture of sinus tract drainage not predictive of bone culture. Review: *Ln. 364:369, 2004*				
Hematogenous Osteomyelitis				
Empiric therapy—Collect bone and blood cultures before empiric therapy				
Newborn (<4 mos.) See Table 5 for dose	S. aureus, Gm-neg. bacilli, Group B strep.	**MRSA possible: Vanco + (Ceftaz or CFP)**	MRSA unlikely: **Naticillin or oxacillin) + (Ceftaz or CFP)**	Table 16 for dose. Severe allergy or toxicity: **Linezolid**[NAI] 10mg/kg IV/po q8h (+ **aztreonam**). Could substitute **clindamycin** for linezolid.
Children (>4 mos.)—Adult: Osteo of extremity	S. aureus, Group A strep. Gm-neg. bacilli rare	**MRSA possible: Vanco** Add **Ceftaz or CFP** if Gm-neg. bacilli on Gram stain (Doses below. In 1). Peds Doses: Table 16	MRSA unlikely: **Naticillin or oxacillin**	Severe allergy or toxicity: **Clinda** or **TMP-SMX** or **linezolid**[NAI]. Dosages in Table 16. See Table 10 for adverse reactions to drugs.
Adult (>21 yrs) Vertebral osteo ± epidural abscess; other sites (NEJM 355:2012, 2006)	S. aureus most common but variety other organisms. **Blood & bone culture essential.**	**MRSA possible: Vanco** gm IV q12h	MRSA unlikely: **Naticillin or oxacillin** 2 gm IV q4h	**Dx: MRI** early to look for epidural abscess. Allergy or toxicity: **TMP-SMX** 8–10mg/kg per day div. IV q8h or **linezolid** 600mg IV/po q12h *(AnM 138:135, 2003)*[NAI++]. See MRSA specific therapy comment. Epidural abscess ref: *AnM 164:2409, 2004.*
Specific therapy—Culture and in vitro susceptibility results known				
MSSA		**Naticillin or oxacillin** 2 gm IV q4h or **cefazolin** 2 gm IV q8h	**Vanco** 1 gm q12h IV	**Other options if susceptible in vitro and allergy/toxicity issues:** 1) **TMP-SMX** 8-10mg/kg/d IV q8h. Minimal data on treatment of osteomyelitis; 2) **Clinda** 600-900mg IV q8h – have lab check for inducible resistance especially if erythro resistant *(CID 40:280,2005)*; 3) **Clip** 750mg po bid or **levo** 750mg po q24h) + **rif** 300mg po bid, or **Daptomycin** 6mg/kg IV q24h; –clinical failure is secondary to resistance reported *(J Clin Microbiol 44:595,2006)*; 5) **Linezolid** 600mg po/IV bid – anecdotal reports of efficacy *(J Chemother 17:643,2005)*, optic & peripheral neuropathy with long-term use *(Neurology 64:926, 2005);* 6) **Fusidic acid**[NUS] 500mg IV q8h + **rif** 300mg po bid. *(CID 42:394, 2006)*.
	MRSA—See Table 6, page 73	**Vanco** 1 gm IV q12h	**Linezolid** 600 mg q12h IV/po or **RIF** 300 mg po/IV bid	
Hemoglobinopathy: Sickle cell/thalassemia	Salmonella, other Gm-neg. bacilli	**CIP** 400 mg IV q12h	**Levo** 750 mg IV q24h	Thalassemia: transfusion and iron chelation risk factors.
Contiguous Osteomyelitis Without Vascular Insufficiency				
Foot bone osteo due to nail through tennis shoe	P. aeruginosa	**CIP** 750 mg po bid or **Levo** 750 mg po q24h	**Ceftaz** 2 gm IV q8h or **CFP** 2 gm IV q12h	See Skin—Nail puncture, page 50. Need debridement to remove foreign body.
Empiric therapy: Get cultures! Long bone, post-internal fixation of fracture	S. aureus, Gm-neg. bacilli, P. aeruginosa	**Vanco** 1 gm IV q12h + (**ceftaz** or **CFP** [see footnote†]), See Comment	**Linezolid** 600 mg IV/po bid[NAI++] + (**ceftaz** or **CFP**); See Comment	Often need to remove hardware to allow bone union. May need revascularization. Regimens listed are empiric. Adjust after culture data available. If susceptible Gm-neg. bacillus, **CIP** 750mg po bid or **Levo** 750mg po q24h. For other S. aureus options: See Hem. Osteo. Specific Therapy, Table 1(1).

* **DOSAGES SUGGESTED** are for adults (unless otherwise indicated) with clinically severe (often life-threatening infections. Dosages also assume normal renal function, and not severe hepatic dysfunction.
‡ **ALTERNATIVE THERAPY INCLUDES** these considerations: allergy, pharmacology/pharmacokinetics, compliance, costs, local resistance profiles.
† Drug dosage: **ceftazidime** 2 gm IV q8h, **CFP** 2 gm IV q12h

TABLE 1 (2)

ANATOMIC SITE/DIAGNOSIS/ MODIFYING CIRCUMSTANCES	ETIOLOGIES (usual)	SUGGESTED REGIMENS*		ADJUNCT DIAGNOSTIC OR THERAPEUTIC MEASURES AND COMMENTS
		PRIMARY	ALTERNATIVE†	
BONE/Contiguous Osteomyelitis Without Vascular Insufficiency/Empiric therapy (continued)				
Osteonecrosis of the jaw	Probably rare adverse reaction to bisphosphonates	Infection is secondary to bone necrosis and loss of overlying mucosa. Treatment: minimal surgical debridement, chlorohexidine rinses, antibiotics (e.g. PIP-TZ), NEJM 355:2278, 2006.		
Prosthetic joint	See prosthetic joint, page 29			
Spinal implant infection	S. aureus, coag-neg staphylococci, gram-neg bacilli	Onset within 30 d. culture, treat & then suppress until fusion occurs	Onset after 30 d. remove implant, culture & treat	For details: CID 44:913, 2007.
Sternum, post-op	S. aureus, S. epidermidis	Vanco 1 gm IV q12h	Linezolid 600 mg po/IV^MRSA bid	Sternal debridement for cultures & removal of necrotic bone. For S. aureus options: Hem Osteo, Specific Therapy, Table 1(1).
Contiguous Osteomyelitis With Vascular Insufficiency. Ref.: CID S115-22, 2004				
Most pts are diabetics with peripheral neuropathy & infected skin ulcers (see Diabetic foot, page 14)	Polymicrobic [Gm+ cocci (to include MRSA) (aerobic & anaerobic) and Gm-neg bacilli (aerobic & anaerobic)]	Debride overlying ulcer & submit bone for histology & culture. Select antibiotic based on culture results & treat for 6 weeks. **No empiric therapy unless acutely ill.** If acutely ill, see suggestions, Diabetic foot, page 14. Revascularize if possible. Full contact cast.		**Diagnosis of osteo:** Culture of biopsied bone gold standard. Marrow edema on MRI best imaging. Probe to bone has high predictive value. Poor concordance of culture results between swab of ulcer and bone – need bone. (CID 42:57, 63, 2006) NOTE: (1) Revascularize if possible. (2) Culture bone. (3) Specific antimicrobial(s). (4) Full contact cast.
Chronic Osteomyelitis: Specific therapy By definition, implies presence of dead bone. **Need valid cultures**	S. aureus, Enterobacteriaceae, P. aeruginosa	Empiric rx not indicated. Base systemic rx on results of culture, sensitivity testing. If acute exacerbation of chronic osteo, rx as acute hematogenous osteo.		Important adjuncts: removal of orthopedic hardware, surgical debridement, vascularized muscle flaps, distraction osteogenesis (Ilizarov) techniques. Antibiotic-impregnated cement & hyperbaric oxygen adjunctive. NOTE: RIF + (vanco or β-lactam) effective in animal model and in a clinical trial of S. aureus chronic osteo (SMJ 79:947, 1986).
BREAST: Mastitis—Obtain culture, need to know if MRSA present. Review definitions: Ob & Gyn Clin No Amer 29:89, 2002				
Postpartum mastitis				
Mastitis without abscess Ref.: JAMA 289:1609, 2003	S. aureus, less often S. pyogenes (Gp A or B), E. coli, bacteroides species, maybe Corynebacterium sp. & selected coagulase-neg staphylococci (S. lugdunensis)	**NO MRSA: Outpatient:** Dicloxacillin 500mg po qid or cephalexin 500mg po qid. **Inpatient: Nafcillin/oxacillin** 2gm IV q4h	**MRSA Possible: Outpatient:** TMP-SMX-DS tabs 2 po bid or, (if susceptible, clinda 300 mg po qid. **Inpatient: Vanco** 1gm IV q12h	If no abscess, ↑ freq of nursing may hasten response; no risk to infant. Corynebacterium sp. assoc. with chronic granulomatous mastitis (CID 35:1434, 2002). Bartonella henselae infection reported (Ob & Gyn 95:1027, 2000). With abscess, d/c nursing (Am J Surg 182:117, 2007). Resume breast feeding from affected breast as soon as pain. **Value of dexamethasone** documented in children with H. influenzae & now allows.
Mastitis with abscess	S. aureus, less often Bacter. sp., peptostreptococcus & selected coagulase-neg. staphylococci	**MRSA Possible: Outpatient:** Await culture results. **Inpatient: Vanco** 1gm IV q12h		
Non-puerperal mastitis with abscess	S. aureus, less often Bacter. sp., peptostreptococcus & selected coagulase-neg. staphylococci	Acute: Vanco 1gm IV q12h pending culture results		If subareolar & adoriferous, most likely anaerobes; need to add metro 500 mg IV/po tid. If not subareolar, staph. Need pretreatment aerobic/anaerobic cultures. Surgical drainage for abscess.
Breast implant infection	Acute: S. aureus, S. pyogenes. TSS reported. Chronic: Look for rapidly growing Mycobacteria	Chronic: Await culture results. See Table 12 for mycobacteria treatment.		Lancet Infect Dis 5:94, 462, 2005

Abbreviations on page 2.   NOTE: All dosage recommendations are for adults (unless otherwise indicated) and assume normal renal function.

TABLE 1 (3)

9

ANATOMIC SITE/DIAGNOSIS/ MODIFYING CIRCUMSTANCES	ETIOLOGIES (usual)	SUGGESTED REGIMENS*		ADJUNCT DIAGNOSTIC OR THERAPEUTIC MEASURES AND COMMENTS
		PRIMARY	ALTERNATIVE§	
CENTRAL NERVOUS SYSTEM				
Brain abscess				
Primary or contiguous source Ref.: CID 25:763, 1997	Streptococci (60–70%), bacteroides (20–40%), Enterobacteriaceae (25–33%), S. aureus (10–15%). Rare: Nocardia (Table 11A, page 102) Listeria (CID 40:907, 2005)	**P Ceph 3** ([**cefotaxime** 2 gm IV q4h **or ceftriaxone** 2 gm IV q12h) + (**metro** 7.5 mg/kg q6h or 15 mg/kg IV q12h)] Duration of rx unclear; treat until response by neuroimaging (CT/MRI)	**Pen G** 3-4 million units IV q4h + **metro** 7.5 mg/kg q6h or 15 mg/kg IV q12h	If CT scan suggests cerebritis (JNS 59:972, 1983), abscesses <2.5 cm and pt neurologically stable and conscious, start antibiotics and observe. Otherwise, surgical drainage necessary. Neurologic deterioration usually mandates surgery. Experience with Pen G (HD) + metro without ceftriaxone or nafcillin/oxacillin has been good. We use ceftriaxone because of frequency of isolation of Enterobacteriaceae. **S. aureus rare without positive blood culture; if S. aureus, include vanco until susceptibility known.** Strep. milleri group esp. prone to produce abscess.
Post-surgical, post-traumatic	S. aureus, Enterobacteriaceae	For MSSA: (**Nafcillin** or **oxacillin**) 2 gm IV q4h + (**ceftriaxone** or **cefotaxime**)	For MRSA: **Vanco** 1 gm IV q12h + (**ceftriaxone** or **cefotaxime**)	
HIV-1 infected (AIDS)	Toxoplasma gondii	See Table 13A, page 127		
Subdural empyema: In adult 60–90% are extension of sinusitis or otitis media. Rx same as primary brain abscess. Surgical emergency: must drain (CID 20:372, 1995).				
Encephalitis/encephalopathy Ref.: CID 43:1565, 2006 (For Herpes see Table 14A page 140, and for rabies, Table 20E, page 196)	Herpes simplex, arboviruses, rabies, West Nile virus. Rarely: listeria, cat-scratch disease	Start IV **acyclovir** while awaiting results of CSF PCR for H. simplex.		Newly recognized strain of bat rabies. May not require a break in the skin. Eastern equine encephalitis causes focal MRI changes in basal ganglia and thalamus (NEJM 336:1867, 1997). Cat-scratch ref.: PIDJ 23:1161, 2004). Ref. on West Nile & related viruses: NEJM 351:370, 2004.
Meningitis, "Aseptic": Pleocytosis of 100s of cells, CSF glucose normal, neg. culture for bacteria (see Table 14A, page 135)	Enteroviruses, HSV-2, LCM, HIV, other viruses, drugs (NSAIDs, metronidazole, carbamazepine, TMP-SMX, IVIG), rarely leptospirosis	For all but leptospirosis, IV fluids and analgesics. D/C drugs that may be etiologic. For lepto (**doxy** 100 mg IV/po q12h) or (**Pen G** 5 million units IV q6h) or (**AMP** 0.5–1 gm IV q6h). Repeat LP if suspect partially-treated bacterial meningitis.		If available, PCR of CSF for enterovirus. HSV-2 unusual without concomitant genital herpes. Drug-induced aseptic meningitis: ArIM 159:1185, 1999. For lepto, positive epidemiologic history and concomitant hepatitis, conjunctivitis, dermatitis, nephritis.
Meningitis, Bacterial, Acute: Goal is empiric therapy, then CSF exam within 30 min. If focal neurologic deficit, give empiric therapy, then head CT, then LP. (NEJM 354:44,2006; Ln D 7:191, 2007) NOTE: In children, treatment caused CSF cultures to turn neg. in 2 hrs with meningococci & partial response with pneumococci in 4 hrs (Peds 108:1169, 2001)				
Empiric Therapy—CSF Gram stain is negative—immunocompetent				
Age: Preterm to <1 mo Ln 361:2139, 2003	Group B strep 49%, E. coli 18%, listeria 7%, misc. Gm-neg. 10%, misc. Gm-pos. 10%	**AMP + cefotaxime** Intraventricular treatment not recommended. Repeat CSF exam/culture 24–36 hr after start of therapy For dosage, see Table 16	**AMP + gentamicin**	Primary & alternative reg active vs Group B strep, most coliforms, & listeria. If premature infant with long nursery stay, S. aureus, enterococci, and resistant coliforms potential pathogens. Optional empiric regimens: [nafcillin + (ceftazidime or cefotaxime)]. If high risk of MRSA, use vanco + cefotaxime. Alter regimen after culture/sensitivity data available.

TABLE 1 (4)

ANATOMIC SITE/DIAGNOSIS/ MODIFYING CIRCUMSTANCES	ETIOLOGIES (usual)	SUGGESTED REGIMENS*		ADJUNCT DIAGNOSTIC OR THERAPEUTIC MEASURES AND COMMENTS
		PRIMARY	ALTERNATIVE†	
CENTRAL NERVOUS SYSTEM/Meningitis, Bacterial, Acute/Empiric Therapy *(continued)*				
Age: 1mo–50yrs See footnote¹ for empiric treatment rationale.	S. pneumo, meningococci, H. influenzae unlikely in very rare, **listeria unlikely if young & immuno-competent** (add **ampicillin** if suspect listeria 2 gm IV q4h)	Adult dosage: (**Cefotaxime** 2 gm IV q4-6h OR **ceftriaxone** 2 gm IV q12h,) + (**dexametha-sone**) + **vanco** (see footnote³) Peds: see footnote³ **Dexamethasone** 0.15 mg/kg IV q6h x 2-4 days. **Give with 1st just before or with 1st dose of antibiotic (see Comment).** See footnote⁴ for rest of ped. dosage	(**MER** 2 gm IV q8h) (Peds: 40 mg/kg IV q8h)) + IV **dexamethasone** + **vanco** (see footnote²) Peds: see footnote³	**For pts with severe pen. allergy: Chloro** 12.5 mg/kg IV q6h (max. 4gm/day) (for meningococci) + **TMP-SMX** 5mg/kg q6-8h (for listeria (if immunocom-promised) + **vanco**. Rare meningococcal isolates chloro-resistant (*NEJM 339:868, 1998*). The standard alternative for pts with severe pen. allergy was chloro. However, high failure rate in pts with DRSP (*Ln 339: 405, 1992; Ln 342:240, 1993*). **So far, no vanco-resistant S. pneumo.** **Value of dexamethasone** documented in children with H. influenzae & now confirmed in adults with S. pneumo (*NEJM 347:1549 & 1613, 2002; LnID 4:139, 2004*). **Give 1st dose 15–20min. prior to or con-comitant with 1st dose of antibiotic.** See **Table 20A, page 186.** **For meningococcal immunization, see Table 20A, page 186.**
Age: >50yrs or alcoholism or other debilitating assoc diseases or impaired cellular immunity	S. pneumo, listeria, Gm-neg bacilli Note absence of meningo-coccus.	(**AMP** 2 gm IV q4h) + (**ceftriaxone** 2 gm IV q12h or **cefotaxime** 2 gm IV q6h) + **vanco** + IV **dexamethasone** For vanco dose, see footnote². 1st dose before or concomitant with 1st dose of antibiotic.	**MER** 2 gm IV q8h + **vanco** + IV **dexamethasone**, see Comment. **Dexamethasone** 1gm IV q4-12h	**Severe penicillin allergy: Vanco** 500-750 mg IV q6h + **TMP-SMX** 5 mg/kg q6-8h pending culture results. Chloro has failed vs DRSP (*Ln 342:240, 1993*).
Post-neurosurgery, post-head trauma, or post-cochlear implant (*NEJM 349:435, 2003*)	S. pneumoniae most common, esp. if CSF leak. Other: S. aureus, coliforms, P. aeruginosa	**Vanco** (until known not MRSA) 500-750 mg IV q6h + (**cefepime** or **ceftazidime** 2 gm IV q8h)(see Comment)	**MER** 2 gm IV q8h + **vanco** 1gm IV q6-12h	**Vanco** alone not optimal for S. pneumo. If/when suspect S. pneumo or **cefotaxime**, quickly switch to **ceftriaxone** or **cefotaxime**. Rx of pseudomonas meningitis, some add intrathecal gentamicin (4 mg q12h into lateral ventricles). Cure of acinetobacter meningitis with intrathecal colistin (*JAC 53:290, 2004*). Intraventricular colistin for acinetobacter infections: (*JAC 58:1078, 2006*).
Ventriculitis/meningitis due to infected ventriculo-peritoneal (atrial) shunt	S. epidermidis, S. aureus, coliforms, diphtheroids (rare), P. acnes	**Vanco** 500-750 mg IV q6h + (**cefepime** or **ceftazi-dime** 2 gm IV q8h). If unable to remove shunt, consider intraventricular therapy; for dosages see footnote⁴	**Vanco** 500-750 mg IV q6h + IV timed **dexa-methasone** 0.15 mg/kg q6h x 2-4 days.	Usual care: 1st remove infected shunt & culture, external ventricular catheter for drainage/pressure control; antimicrobic x-14 days. For timing of new shunt, see *CID 39:1267, 2004.*
Empiric Therapy—Positive CSF Gram stain				
Gram-positive diplococci	S. pneumoniae	Either (**ceftriaxone** 2 gm IV q12h or **cefotaxime** 2gm IV q4-6h) + **vanco** 500-750 mg IV q6h + timed **dexa-methasone** 0.15 mg/kg q6h x 2-4 days.	**MER** 2 gm IV q8h or **Moxi** 400 mg IV q24h. **Dexamethasone** does not block penetration of vanco into CSF (*CID 44:250, 2007*).	**Alternatives: MER** 2 gm IV q8h or **Moxi** 400 mg IV q24h.
Gram-negative diplococci	N. meningitidis	(**Cefotaxime** 2 gm IV q4-6h or **ceftriaxone** 2 gm IV q12h)		**Alternatives: Pen G** 4 mill. units IV q4h or **AMP** 2 gm IV q4h or **chloro** 1 gm IV q6h.

¹ **Rationale**: Hard to get adequate CSF concentrations of anti-infectives; hence MIC criteria for in vitro susceptibility are lower for CNS infections (*AftM 161:2538, 2001*).
² Low & erratic penetration of **vanco** into the CSF (*PIDJ 16:895, 1997*). Adult dosage 15mg/kg IV q8h (2x standard adult dose). In adults, max dose of 2-3gm/day is suggested: **500–750 mg IV q6h**.
³ **Dosage of drugs used to treat children ≥1mo of age:** Cefotaxime 200mg/kg per day IV div. q6-8h; ceftriaxone 100mg/kg per day IV div. q12h; vanco 15mg/kg q6h.
⁴ Dosages for intraventricular therapy. The following are daily adult doses in mg: amikacin 30, gentamicin 4-8, polymyxin E (Colistin) 10, tobramycin 5-20, vanco 10-20. Ref. *CID 39:1267, 2004.*

Abbreviations on page 2. NOTE: All dosage recommendations are for adults (unless otherwise indicated) and assume normal renal function.

TABLE 1 (5)

ANATOMIC SITE/DIAGNOSIS/ MODIFYING CIRCUMSTANCES	ETIOLOGIES (usual)	SUGGESTED REGIMENS*		ADJUNCT DIAGNOSTIC OR THERAPEUTIC MEASURES AND COMMENTS
		PRIMARY	ALTERNATIVE†	
CENTRAL NERVOUS SYSTEM/Meningitis, Bacterial, Acute/Empiric Therapy *(continued)*				
Gram-positive bacilli or coccobacilli	Listeria monocytogenes	AMP 2 gm IV q4h ± **gentamicin** 2 mg/kg loading dose then 1.7 mg/kg q8h		If pen-allergic, use TMP-SMX 5 mg/kg q6–8h or MER 2 gm IV q8h
Gram-negative bacilli	H. influenzae, coliforms, P. aeruginosa	**Ceftazidime 2 gm IV q8h** or **cefepime** 2 gm IV q8h) + **gentamicin** 2 mg/kg 1° dose then 1.7 mg/kg q8h		**Alternatives: CIP** 400 mg IV q8–12h; **MER** 2 gm IV q8h
Specific Therapy—Positive culture of CSF with in vitro susceptibility results available. Interest in monitoring/reducing intracranial pressure: CID 38:384, 2004				
H. influenzae	β-lactamase positive	**Ceftriaxone** (peds): 50 mg/kg IV q12h		**Pen. allergic: Chloro** 12.5 mg/kg IV q6h (max. 4gm/day)
Listeria monocytogenes (CID 43:1233, 2006)		AMP 2 gm IV q4h ± **gentamicin** 2 mg/kg loading dose, then 1.7 mg/kg q8h		**Pen. allergic: TMP-SMX** 20 mg/kg per day div. q6–12h. One report of greater efficacy of AMP + TMP-SMX as compared to AMP + gentamicin (JID 33:79, 1996). **Alternative: MER** 2 gm IV q8h. Success reported with **linezolid + RIF** (CID 40:908, 2005).
N. meningitidis		**Ceftriaxone** 2 gm IV q12h x 7 days (see Comment). If pen. allergic, **chloro** 12.5 mg/kg (up to 1gm) IV q6h		**Alternatives: MER** 2 gm IV q8h or **Moxi** 400 mg q24h.
S. pneumoniae	Pen G MIC			
	<0.1mcg/mL	**Pen G** 4 million units IV q4h or **AMP** 2 gm IV q4h		**Alternatives: Ceftriaxone** 2 gm IV q12h; **chloro** 1 gm IV q6h
NOTES: 1. Assumes dexamethasone just prior to 1ˢᵗ dose & x4 days.	0.1–1mcg/mL	**Ceftriaxone** 2 gm IV q12h or **cefotaxime** 2 gm IV q4-6h		**Alternatives: Cefepime** 2 gm IV q8h or **MER** 2 gm IV q8h
	≥2mcg/mL	**Vanco** 500–750 mg IV q6h + **(ceftriaxone** or **cefotaxime** as above)		**Alternatives: Moxi** 400 mg IV q24h
2. If MIC ≥1, repeat CSF exam after 24-48h.	Ceftriaxone MIC ≥1mcg/mL	**Vanco** 500–750 mg IV q6h + **(ceftriaxone** or **cefotaxime** as above)		**Alternatives: Moxi** 400 mg IV q24h If MIC to ceftriaxone >2mcg/mL, add **RIF** 600mg 1x/day.
3. Treat for 10-14 days				
E. coli, other coliforms, or P. aeruginosa	Consultation advised— need for susceptibility results	**(Ceftazidime** or **cefepime** 2 gm IV q8h) ± **gentamicin**		**Alternatives: CIP** 400 mg IV q8–12h; **MER** 2 gm IV q8h. For discussion of intraventricular therapy: CID 39:1267, 2004
Prophylaxis for H. influenzae and N. meningitides				
Haemophilus influenzae type b (Neisseria CID on page 8) Household and/or day care contact: residing with index case or 24 hrs. Day care contact: same day care as index case for 5-7 days before onset		RIF 20 mg/kg po (not to exceed 600 mg) q24h x 4 doses. **Adults:** RIF 600 mg q24h x 4 days		**Household:** If there is one unvaccinated contact ≤4yr in the household, give RIF to all household contacts except pregnant women. **Child Care Facilities:** With 1 case, if attended by unvaccinated children ≤2yr consider prophylaxis + vaccinate susceptibles. If all contacts >2yr: no prophylaxis In 60 days & unvaccinated children attend, prophylaxis recommended for children & personnel (Am Acad Ped Red Book 2006, page 313).
Prophylaxis for Neisseria meningitidis exposure (close contact) MMWR 46(RR-5):1, 1997		**CIP** (adults) 500 mg po single dose) OR **Ceftriaxone** 250 mg IM x 1 dose (child <15yr 125mg IM x1) OR **RIF** 600 mg q12h po x 2 days. (Children >1 mo 10 mg/kg po q12h x 4 doses. <1mo 5 mg/kg q12h x 4 doses). OR **Spiramycin**ᴺᵁˢ 500 mg po q6h x 5 days. Children 10 mg/kg po q6h x 5 days.		Spread by respiratory droplets, not aerosols, hence close contact req. ↑ risk if close contact for at least 4hrs during wk before illness onset (e.g., housemates, day care contacts, cellmates) or exposure to pt's nasopharyngeal secretions (e.g. kissing, mouth-to-mouth resuscitation, intubation, nasotracheal suctioning). Since RIF-resistant N. meningitides documented post-prophylaxis(EID 11:977, 2005), prefer Cip or ceftriaxone (Cochrane, CD 004785, 2005) Primary prophylactic regimen in many European countries.
Meningitis, chronic Defined as symptoms + CSF pleocytosis for 24 wks	M. tbc 40%, cryptococcosis 7%, neoplastic 8%, Lyme, syphilis, Whipple's disease	Treatment depends on etiology. No urgent need for empiric therapy.		Long list of possibilities: bacteria, parasites, fungi, viruses, neoplasms, vasculitis, and other miscellaneous etiologies—see chapter on chronic meningitis in latest edition of Harrison's Textbook of Internal Medicine. Whipple's: JID 188:797 & 801, 2003.

Abbreviations on page 2.   *NOTE: All dosage recommendations are for adults (unless otherwise indicated) and assume normal renal function.*

TABLE 1 (6)

ANATOMIC SITE/DIAGNOSIS/ MODIFYING CIRCUMSTANCES	ETIOLOGIES (usual)	SUGGESTED REGIMENS*		ADJUNCT DIAGNOSTIC OR THERAPEUTIC MEASURES AND COMMENTS
		PRIMARY	ALTERNATIVE†	
CENTRAL NERVOUS SYSTEM *(continued)*				
Meningitis, eosinophilic *AJM 114:217, 2003*	Angiostrongyliasis, gnathostomiasis, rarely others	Corticosteroids	Not sure antihelminthic therapy works	1/3 lack peripheral eosinophilia. Need serology to confirm diagnosis. Steroid ref.: *CID 31:660, 2001. Recent outbreak: NEJM 346:668, 2002.*
Meningitis, HIV-1 Infected (AIDS) *See Table 11, Sanford Guide to HIV/AIDS Therapy*	As in adults, >50 yr, also consider cryptococci, M. tuberculosis, syphilis, HIV aseptic meningitis, Listeria monocytogenes	If etiology not identified: treat as adult >50yr + obtain CSF/serum cryptococcal antigen *(see Comments)*	For crypto tx, see Table 11A, page 96	C. neoformans most common etiology in AIDS patients. H. influenzae, pneumococc, Tbc., syphilis, viral, histoplasmos & coccidioides also need to be considered. Obtain blood cultures. L. monocytogenes risk >60x. ↑x present as meningitis *(CID 17:224, 1993).*
EAR				
External otitis				
Chronic	Usually 2° to seborrhea	Eardrops: [(polymyxin B + neomycin + hydrocortisone) qid] + **selenium sulfide shampoo**		Control seborrhea with dandruff shampoo containing selenium sulfide (Selsun) or [(ketoconazole shampoo) + (medium potency steroid solution, triamcinolone 0.1%)]
Fungal	Candida species	Fluconazole 200 mg po x 1 dose & then 100 mg po q24h x 3-5 days		
"Malignant otitis externa" Risk groups: Diabetes mellitus, AIDS, chemotherapy	Pseudomonas aeruginosa in >90%	[(IMP 0.5 gm IV q6h) or (MER 1 gm IV q8h) or (CIP 400 mg IV q12h (or 750 mg po q12h) or (ceftaz 2 gm IV q8h) or (CFP 2 gm q12h) or (PIP 4-6 gm IV q4-6h + tobra) or (TC 3 gm IV q4h + tobra (dose Table 10D)	CIP po for treatment of early disease. Debridement usually required. R/O osteomyelitis: CT or MRI scan. If bone involved, treat for 4-6 wks. Ref.: *LnID 4:34, 2004. PIP without Tazo may be hard to find: extended infusion of CIP (4 hr infusion of 3.375 gm every 8h) may improve efficacy (CID 44:357, 2007).*
"Swimmer's ear" *PIDJ 22:299, 2003*	Pseudomonas aerug., Enterobacteriaceae, Proteus sp. (Fungi rare). Acute infection usually 2° S. aureus	Eardrops: Ofloxacin 0.3% soln bid or [(polymyxin B + neomycin + hydrocortisone) qid] or (CIP + hydrocortisone bid)	For acute disease: dicloxacillin 500 mg po q6h	Rx should include gentle cleaning. Recurrences prevented (or decreased) by drying with alcohol drops (1/3 white vinegar, 2/3 rubbing alcohol) after swimming, then antibiotic drops or 2% acetic acid solution. Ointments should not be used in ear. Do not use neomycin if tympanic membrane punctured.
Otitis media—infants, children, adults				
Acute *(NEJM 347:1169, 2002; Peds 113:1451, 2004). For correlation of bacterial eradication from middle ear & clinical outcome, see LnID 2:593, 2002*				
Initial empiric therapy of acute otitis media (AOM) **NOTE:** Pending new data, **treat children <2 yr old.** If >2 yr old, afebrile, no ear pain, reliable caretaker—consider analgesic treatment without antimicrobials. Favorable results in routine febrile pts with waiting 48hrs before deciding on antibiotic use (*JAMA 296:1235, 1290, 2006*)	Overall detection in middle ear fluid: No pathogen 4% Virus 70% Bact. + virus 66% Bacteria only 92% Bacterial pathogens from middle ear: S. pneumo 49%, H. influenzae 29%, M. catarrhalis 28%. Ref. *CID 43:1417 & 1423, 2006*	**If NO antibiotics in prior month:** **Amox HD** or **AM-CL** (extrastrength) **If antibiotics in prior month:** Amox HD or AM-CL (extrastrength) or **cefdinir** or **cefpodoxime** or **cefprozil** or **cefuroxime axetil** For dosage, see footnotes 1 and 2, next page **All doses are pediatric Duration of rx:** <2 yr old x 10 days; 2 yr x 5-7 days. Approp. duration unclear. 5 days may be inadequate for severe disease (*NEJM 347:1169, 2002*) **For adult dosages, see Sinusitis, pages 44-45, and Table 10**	**If allergic to β-lactam drugs?** If history unclear or rash, effective oral ceph OK; avoid ceph if β-lactam allergy, e.g., anaphylaxis. High failure rate with **TMP-SMX** & **azithro** if etiology is DRSP or H. influenzae (*PIDJ 20:260, 2001*); **azithro x 5 days** or **clarithro x 10 days** (both have ↑ activity vs DRSP). **Up to 50% S. pneumo resistant to macrolides.** Rationale & data for single dose azithro, 30 mg per kg: *PIDJ 23:S102 & S108, 2004.* **Active vs DRSP** other agents listed. Variable bugs/resistance: **Spontaneous resolution occurred in:** 90% pts infected with M. catarrhalis, 50% with H. influenzae, 10% with S. pneumoniae; overall 80% resolve within 2-14 days (*Ln 363:465, 2004*). **Risk of DRSP ↑ if age <2 yr, antibiotics last 3 mo, &/or daycare attendance.** Selection of rx (based on (1) effectiveness against β-lactamase producing H. influenzae & M. catarrhalis & (2) effectiveness against DRSP pneumo, inc. DRSP. For **amox, cefdinir, cefpodoxime** listed. Other agents active vs DRSP but poor taste/smell by children 4-8 yrs old. *PIDJ 19 (Suppl):S174, 2000).*

¹ Amoxicillin UD or HD = amoxicillin usual dose or high dose. AM-CL HD = amoxicillin-clavulanic high dose. Data supporting amoxicillin HD: PIDJ 22:405, 2003.

Abbreviations on page 2.   NOTE: All dosage recommendations are for adults (unless otherwise indicated) and assume normal renal function.

TABLE 1 (7)

ANATOMIC SITE/DIAGNOSIS/ MODIFYING CIRCUMSTANCES	ETIOLOGIES (usual)	SUGGESTED REGIMENS* PRIMARY	ALTERNATIVE†	ADJUNCT DIAGNOSTIC OR THERAPEUTIC MEASURES AND COMMENTS
EAR/Otitis media—infants, children, adults (continued)				
Treatment for clinical failure after 3 days	Drug-resistant S. pneumoniae main concern	**NO antibiotics in month prior to last 3 days:** (change in flora unlikely) no change in Rx. After >3 days; fever, continued pain: **cefdinir** or **cefpodoxime** or **cefprozil** or **cefuroxime axetil** or IM **ceftriaxone** x 3 days.	**Antibiotics in month prior to last 3 days:** (change in flora likely) **cefuroxime axetil** (and/or **clindamycin** and/or tympanocentesis) See clindamycin Comments For dosage, see footnotes¹ and ² **All doses are pediatric** Duration of Rx as above	**Clindamycin** not active vs H. influenzae or M. catarrhalis. S. pneumo resistant to macrolides are usually also resistant to clindamycin. Cefdinir in failures: no change in flora with bulging TM or otorrhea after 3 days of therapy. Tympanocentesis will allow culture (PIDJ 23:390, 2004). **Vanco is active vs DRSP.** **Newer FQs active vs DRSP, but not approved for use in children.** Ceftriaxone IM x 3 days superior to 1-day treatment vs DRSP AOM (PIDJ 19:1040, 2000). AM-CL HD reported successful for pen-resistant S. pneumo (PIDJ 20:829, 2001).
After >48hrs of nasotracheal intubation	Pseudomonas sp., klebsiella, enterobacter	**Ceftazidime** or **CFP** or **IMP** or **MER** or **(Pip-Tz)** or **TC-CL** or **CIP** (For dosages, see Ear, Malignant otitis externa, page 9)		With nasotracheal intubation >48 hrs, about ½ pts will have otitis media with effusion.
Prophylaxis: acute otitis media PIDJ 22:10, 2003	Pneumococci, H. influenzae, M. catarrhalis, Staph. aureus, Group A strep (see **Comments**)	**Sulfisoxazole** 50 mg/kg po at bedtime or **amoxicillin** 20 mg/kg po q24h.	**Use of antibiotics to prevent otitis media is a major contributor to emergence of antibiotic-resistant S. pneumo!**	Pneumococcal protein conjugate vaccine decreases freq. AOM & due to vaccine serotypes. Adenoidectomy at time of tympanostomy tubes ↓ need for future hospitalization for AOM (NEJM 344:1188, 2001).
Mastoiditis				
Acute				
Outpatient	Strep, pneumoniae 22%, S. pyogenes 16%, **Staph. aureus** 7%, H. influenzae 4%, P. aeruginosa 4%, others <1%	Empirically, same as Acute otitis media, above; need **vanco** or **nafcillin/oxacillin** if cult + for S. aureus.		Has become a rare entity, presumably as result of the aggressive treatment of acute otitis media. Small ↑ in incidence in Netherlands where use of antibiotics limited to children with complicated course or high risk (PIDJ 20:140, 2001).
Hospitalized		**Cefotaxime** 1-2 gm IV q4-6h (depends on severity) or **ceftriaxone** 1 gm IV q24h)		
Chronic	Often polymicrobic: anaerobes, S. aureus, Enterobacteriaceae, P. aeruginosa	Treatment for acute exacerbations or perioperatively. No treatment until surgical cultures obtained. Empiric regimens: **IMP** 0.5 gm IV q6h, **PIP-TZ** 3.375 gm IV q4-6h or **TC-CL** 3.1 gm IV q6h, **MER** 1 gm IV q8h, or 4 hr infusion of 3.375 gm q8h.		May or may not be associated with chronic otitis media with drainage via ruptured tympanic membrane. Antimicrobials given in association with surgery. Mastoidectomy indications: chronic drainage and evidence of osteomyelitis by MRI or CT, evidence of spread to CNS (epidural abscess, suppurative phlebitis, brain abscess).

---

¹ **Amoxicillin UD or HD** = amoxicillin usual dose or high dose. **AM-CL HD** = amoxicillin-clavulanate high dose. **Dosages** in footnote 2. Data supporting amoxicillin HD: PIDJ 22:405, 2003

² **Drugs & peds dosage (all po unless specified) for acute otitis media: Amoxicillin UD** = 40 mg/kg per day div q12h or q8h. **Amoxicillin HD** = 90 mg/kg per day div q12h or q8h. **AM-CL HD** = 90 mg/kg per day of amox component. **Extra-strength AM-CL** oral suspension (Augmentin ES-600) available with HD AM & 42.9mg CL/ 5mL—dose 90/6.4mg/kg per day div bid. **Cefuroxime axetil** 30 mg/kg per day div q12h. **Cefdinir** 14 mg/kg per day div q12-24h. **Clindamycin** 20-30 mg/kg per day div q8h (may be effective vs DRSP but no activity vs H influenzae) **Ceftriaxone** 50 mg/kg IM x 3 days. **Other drugs suitable for drug (e.g., penicillin)-sensitive S. pneumo:** TMP-SMX 4 mg/kg of TMP q12h. Erythro-**sulfisoxazole** 50 mg/kg per day of erythro div q6-8h. **Clarithromycin** 15 mg/kg per day div q12h; **azithromycin** 10 mg/kg per day x 1 & then 5 mg/kg q24h x 4 days & 30 mg/kg per day as single dose. **Cefprozil** 15 mg/kg q12h. **Cefpodoxime proxetil** 10 mg/kg per day as single dose; **cefaclor** 40mg/kg per day div q8h; **loracarbef** 15mg/kg q12h or 14mg/kg q24h.

Abbreviations on page 2. NOTE: All dosage recommendations are for adults (unless otherwise indicated) and assume normal renal function.

TABLE 1 (8)

ANATOMIC SITE/DIAGNOSIS/ MODIFYING CIRCUMSTANCES	ETIOLOGIES (usual)	SUGGESTED REGIMENS*		ADJUNCT DIAGNOSTIC OR THERAPEUTIC MEASURES AND COMMENTS
		PRIMARY	ALTERNATIVE[1]	
EYE—General Reviews: *CID 21:479, 1995; IDCP 7:447, 1998*				
Eyelid: Little reported experience with **CA-MRSA** (*Ophthal 113:455, 2006*)				
Blepharitis	Etiol. unclear. Factors include Staph. aureus & Staph. epidermidis, seborrhea, rosacea, & dry eye			Usually topical ointments of no benefit. If associated rosacea, add doxy 100mg po bid for 2wk and then q24h.
Hordeolum (Stye)	Staph. aureus	Hot packs only. Will drain spontaneously.		Infection of superficial sebaceous gland.
External (eyelash follicle)	Staph. aureus, MSSA	Oral **dicloxacillin** + hot packs		Also called acute meibomianitis. Rarely drain spontaneously, may need I&D
Internal (Meibomian glands) Can be acute, subacute or chronic.	Staph. aureus, MRSA-CA	TMP/SMX-DS, tabs ii po bid		and culture. Role of fluoroquinolone eye drops is unclear. MRSA often resistant to lower conc.; may be susceptible to higher concentration of FQ in
	Staph. aureus, MRSA-HA	Linezolid 600 mg po possible therapy if multi-drug resistant.		ophthalmologic solutions of gati, levo or moxi.
Conjunctiva: *NEJM 343:345, 2000*				
Conjunctivitis of the newborn (**ophthalmia neonatorum**): by day of onset post-delivery—all doses pediatric				
Onset 1st day	Chemical due to silver nitrate prophylaxis	None		Usual prophylaxis is erythro ointment; hence, silver nitrate irritation rare.
Onset 2-4 days	N. gonorrhoeae	**Ceftriaxone** 25-50 mg/kg IV x 1 dose (see Comment), not to exceed 125 mg		**Treat neonate for concomitant Chlamydia trachomatis.**
Onset 3-10 days	Chlamydia trachomatis	**Erythro base or ethylsuccinate syrup** 12.5 mg/kg q6h x 14 days). No topical tx needed.		Diagnosis by antigen detection. Azithro suspension 20 mg/kg po q24h x 3 days reported efficacious (*PIDJ 17:1049, 1998*). Treat mother & sexual partner
Onset 2-16 days	Herpes simplex types 1,2	See keratitis on page 12		Consider IV acyclovir if concomitant systemic disease.
Ophthalmia neonatorum prophylaxis: **Silver nitrate** 1% x 1 or **erythro** 0.5% ointment x 1 or **tetra** 1% ointment x 1 application				
Pink eye (viral conjunctivitis) Usually unilateral	Adenovirus (types 3 & 7 in children, 8, 11 & 19 in adults)	No treatment. If symptomatic, cold artificial tears may help.		Highly contagious. Onset of ocular pain and photophobia in an adult suggests associated keratitis—rare.
Inclusion conjunctivitis (**adult**) Usually unilateral	Chlamydia trachomatis	**Doxy** 100 mg bid po x 1-3wk	**Erythro** 250 mg po qid x 1-3Wk	Oculoglandular disease. Diagnosis by culture or antigen detection or PCR—availability varies by region and institution. Treat sexual partner
Trachoma	Chlamydia trachomatis	**Azithro** 20 mg/kg po single dose—78% effective in children	**Doxy** 100 mg po bid x minimum of 21 days or **tetra-cycline** 250 mg po qid x 14 days.	Starts in childhood and can persist for years with subsequent damage to cornea. Topical therapy of marginal benefit. Avoid doxy/tetracycline in young children. Mass treatment works (*JAMA 292:721, 2004*).
Suppurative conjunctivitis: Children and Adults				
Non-gonococcal, non-chlamydial *Med Lett 46:25, 2004*	Staph. aureus, S. pneumo-niae, H. influenzae, *Moraxella sp. Outbreak due to atypical S. pneumo. NEJM 348:1112, 2003*	Ophthalmic solution. Gati 0.3%, Levo 0.5%, or Moxi 0.5%. All 1-2 gtts q2h while awake 1st 2 days, then q4-8h up to 7 days.	Polymyxin B + trimethoprim solution 1-2 gtts q3-6h x 7-10 days.	FQs best spectrum for empiric therapy but expensive: $40-50 for 5mL. High concentrations; likelihood of activity is dubious—even MRSA. Polymyxin B spectrum only Gm-neg. bacilli but no ophthal. prep of only. TMP: Most S. pneumo resistant to gent & tobra.
Gonococcal (peds/adults)	N. gonorrhoeae	**Ceftriaxone** 25-50 mg/kg IV/IM (not to exceed125mg) as one dose in children; 1gm IM/IV as one dose in adults.		1gm IM/IV as one dose in adults.

Abbreviations on page 2.   *NOTE: All dosage recommendations are for adults (unless otherwise indicated) and assume normal renal function.*

TABLE 1 (9)

ANATOMIC SITE/DIAGNOSIS/ MODIFYING CIRCUMSTANCES	ETIOLOGIES (usual)	SUGGESTED REGIMENS* PRIMARY	ALTERNATIVE†	ADJUNCT DIAGNOSTIC OR THERAPEUTIC MEASURES AND COMMENTS
EYE (continued)				
Cornea (keratitis): Usually serious and often sight-threatening. Prompt ophthalmologic consultation essential! Herpes simplex most common etiology in developed countries; bacterial and fungal infections more common in underdeveloped countries.				
Viral				
H. simplex	H. simplex, types 1 & 2	**Trifluridine**, one drop q2h, 9x/day for up to 21 days	**Vidarabine** ointment— useful in children. Use 5x/day for up to 21 days. If child fails vidarabine, try trifluridine.	Fluorescein staining shows typical dendritic figures. 30-50% rate of recurrence within 2 years, 400mg acyclovir po bid ↓ recurrences, p 0.005 (*NEJM* 339:300, 1998).
Varicella-zoster ophthalmicus	Varicella-zoster virus	**Famciclovir** 500 mg po tid or **valacyclovir** 1 gm po tid x 10 days	**Acyclovir** 800 mg po 5x/day x 10 days	Clinical diagnosis most common - dendritic figures with fluorescein staining in patient with varicella-zoster of ophthalmic branch of trigeminal nerve.
Bacterial (Med Lett 46:25, 2004) Acute: No comorbidity	S. aureus, S. pneumo, S. pyogenes, Haemophilus sp.	**All rx listed for bacterial, fungal, & protozoan is topical. Gati:** eye gtts. 1-2 gtts q2h while awake x 2 d, then q4h x 3-7 d. **Moxi:** eye gtts. 1 gtt tid x 7 d		Prefer Moxi due to enhanced lipophilicity & penetration into aqueous humor. Survey of *Ophthal* 50 (suppl 11.1, 2005. **Note** despite high conc. may fail vs MRSA.
Contact lens users	P. aeruginosa	**Tobra** or **gentamicin** (14 mg/mL) + **piperacillin** or **ticarcillin** eye drops (6-12mg/mL) q15-60 min around clock x 24-72 hrs, then slow reduction	**CiP** 0.3% or **Levo** 0.5% drops q15-60min around clock x 24-72hrs	Pain, photophobia, impaired vision. Recommend alginate swab for culture and sensitivity testing.
Dry cornea, diabetes, immunosuppression	Staph. aureus, S. epidermidis, S. pneumoniae, S. pyogenes, Enterobacteriaceae, listeria	**Cefazolin** (50 mg/mL) + **gentamicin** or **tobra** (14mg/mL) q15-60 min around clock x 24-72 hrs, then slow reduction	**Vanco** (50 mg/mL) + **ceftazidime** (50 mg/mL) q15-60 min around clock x 24-72 hrs, then slow reduction. See Comment	Specific therapy guided by results of alginate swab: culture and sensitivity. CiP 0.3% found clinically equivalent to ceftazidim + tobra; only concern was efficacy of CiP vs S. pneumoniae (*Ophthalmology* 163:1854, 1996).
Fungal	Aspergillus, fusarium, candida. No empiric therapy—see Comment	**Natamycin** (5%) drops q3-4 hrs with subsequent slow reduction	**Ampho B** (0.05-0.15%) q3-4 hrs with subsequent slow reduction	No empiric therapy. Wait for results of Gram stain or culture in Sabouraud's medium.
Mycobacteria. Post-Lasik	Mycobacterium chelonae	**Moxi** eye gtts. 1 gtt qid	**Gati** eye gtts. 1 gtt qid	Ref: *Ophthalmology* 113:950, 2006
Protozoan Soft contact lens users (overnight use)† risk 1-15 fold	Acanthamoeba, hartmannella	**Propamidine** 0.1% + **neomycin/gramicidin/polymyxin** Eyedrops q waking hour for 1wk, then slow taper	**Polyhexamethylene biguanide (PHMB)** 0.02% or **chlorhexidine** 0.02%	Uncommon. Trauma and soft contact lenses are risk factors. Corneal scrapings stained with calcofluor white show characteristic cysts with fluorescent microscopy. PHMB source: Leiter's Park Ave. Pharm. 800-292-6773. Ref: *CID* 35:434, 2002. *Cleaning solution outbreak: MMWR* 56:532, 2007
Lacrimal apparatus Canaliculitis	Actinomyces most common. Rarely, Arachnia, fusobacterium, nocardia, candida	Remove granules & irrigate with **pen G** (100,000 mg/mL) **Child: AM-CL** or **cefprozil** or **cefuroxime** (Dose—Table 16)	If fungi, irrigate with **nystatin** approx. 1 gtt tid	Digital pressure produces exudate at punctum; Gram stain confirms diagnosis. Hot packs to punctal area qid.

Abbreviations on page 2.   NOTE: All dosage recommendations are for adults (unless otherwise indicated) and assume normal renal function.

TABLE 1 (10)

ANATOMIC SITE/DIAGNOSIS/ MODIFYING CIRCUMSTANCES	ETIOLOGIES (usual)	SUGGESTED REGIMENS*		ADJUNCT DIAGNOSTIC OR THERAPEUTIC MEASURES AND COMMENTS
		PRIMARY	ALTERNATIVE†	
EYE/ Lacrimal apparatus (continued)				
Dacryocystitis (lacrimal sac)	S. pneumo, S. aureus, H. influenzae, S. pyogenes, P. aeruginosa	Often consequence of obstruction of lacrimal duct. Empiric therapy based on Gram stain of aspirate—see Comment.		Need ophthalmologic consultation. Can be acute or chronic. Culture to detect MRSA.
Endophthalmitis. For post-op endophthalmitis, see CID 38:542, 2004				
Bacterial: Haziness of vitreous key to diagnosis. Needle aspirate of both vitreous and aqueous humor for culture prior to therapy. Intravitreal administration of antimicrobials essential.				
Postocular surgery (cataracts) Early, acute onset (incidence 0.05%)	S. epidermidis 60%, Staph. aureus, streptococci & enterococci each 5–10%, Gm-neg. bacilli 6%	**Immediate ophthal. consult.** If only light perception or worse, immediate vitrectomy + intravitreal vanco 1mg & intravitreal ceftazidime 2.25 mg. No clear data on intravitreal steroid. May need to repeat intravitreal antibiotics in 2–3 days. Can usually leave lens in.		
Low grade, chronic	Propionibacterium acnes, S. epidermidis, S. aureus (rare)	May require removal of lens material. Intraocular **vanco** ± vitrectomy.		
Post filtering blebs for glaucoma	Strep. species (viridans & others), H. influenzae	Intravitreal and topical agent and consider systemic **AM-CL**, **AM-SB** or **cefprozil or cefuroxime**		
Post-penetrating trauma	S. pneumoniae, N. meningitidis, Staph. aureus	(**cefotaxime** 2 gm IV q4h or **ceftriaxone** 2 gm IV q24h) + **vanco** 1 gm IV q12h pending cultures. Intravitreal antibiotics as with early post-operative.		
None, suspect hematogenous		Intravitreal agent as above + systemic **clinda** or **vanco**. Use topical antibiotics post-surgery (tobra & cefazolin drops).		
IV heroin abuse	Bacillus cereus, Candida sp.	Intravitreal agent + (systemic **clinda** or **vanco**)		
Mycotic (fungal)	Candida sp., Aspergillus sp.	Intravitreal **ampho B** 0.005–0.01 mg in 0.1 mL. Also see Table 11A, page 96 for concomitant systemic therapy. See Comment.		With moderate/marked vitritis, options include systemic rx + vitrectomy ± intravitreal ampho B (CID 27:1130 & 1134, 1998). Report of failure of ampho B lipid complex (CID 28:1177, 1999).
Retinitis				
Acute retinal necrosis	Varicella zoster, Herpes simplex	IV **acyclovir** 10–12 mg/kg IV q8h x 5–7 days, then 800 mg po 5x/day x 6wk		Strong association of VZ virus with atypical necrotizing herpetic retinopathy (CID 24:603, 1997).
HIV (AIDS) CD4 usually <100/mm³	Cytomegalovirus	See Table 14, page 137		Occurs in 5–10% of AIDS patients
Orbital cellulitis (see page 48 for erysipelas, facial)	S. pneumoniae, H. influenzae, M. catarrhalis, S. aureus, anaerobes; occ. group A strep, occ. Gm-neg. bacilli post-trauma	**Nafcillin** 2 gm IV q4h (or if **MRSA-vanco** 1 gm IV q12h) + **ceftriaxone** 2 gm IV q24h + **metro** 1 gm q12h		**If penicillin/ceph allergy: Vanco + levo** 750 mg IV once daily + **metro** IV. Problem is frequent inability to make microbiologic diagnosis. Image orbit (CT or MRI). Risk of cavernous sinus thrombosis. If vanco intolerant, another option for s. aureus is dapto 6mg/kg IV q24h.

TABLE 1 (11)

ANATOMIC SITE/DIAGNOSIS/ MODIFYING CIRCUMSTANCES	ETIOLOGIES (usual)	SUGGESTED REGIMENS*		ADJUNCT DIAGNOSTIC OR THERAPEUTIC MEASURES AND COMMENTS
		PRIMARY	ALTERNATIVE†	
FOOT				
"Diabetic"—Two thirds of patients have triad of neuropathy, deformity and pressure-induced trauma. Refs.: Ln 366:1725, 2005; NEJM 351:48, 2004.				**General:**
Ulcer without inflammation	Colonizing skin flora	No antibacterial therapy		1. Glucose control, eliminate pressure on ulcer
Ulcer with <2 cm of superficial inflammation	S. aureus (assume MRSA), S. agalactiae (Gp B), S. pyogenes predominate	Oral therapy: (TMP-SMX-DS or minocycline plus (Pen VK or selected O Ceph 2, 3, or FQ) Dosages in footnote¹		2. Assess for peripheral vascular disease—very common (CID 39:437, 2004) **Principles of empiric antibacterial therapy:** 1. Include drug predictably active vs MRSA. If outpatient, can assume community-acquired MRSA (CA-MRSA) until culture results available. 2. As culture results dominated by S. aureus & Streptococcus species, empiric drug regimens should include strep & staph. Role of enterococci uncertain. 3. Severe limb and/or life-threatening infections require initial parenteral therapy with predictable activity vs Gm-positive cocci, coliforms & other aerobic Gm-neg. rods, & anaerobic Gm-neg. bacilli. 4. **NOTE:** The regimens listed are suggestions consistent with above principles. Other alternatives exist & may be appropriate for individual patients.
Ulcer with >2 cm of inflammation with extension to fascia	As above, plus coliforms possible	Oral therapy: (AM-CL-ER plus TMP-SMX-DS) or [(CIP or Levo or Moxi) plus linezolid] Dosages in footnote⁹		
Extensive local inflammation plus systemic toxicity. Treatment modalities of limited efficacy & expensive: (wound vac) (Ln 366:1704 2005), growth factor (becaplermin), and hyperbaric oxygen (CID 43:188, 193, 2006)	As above, plus anaerobic bacteria. Role of enterococci unclear.	Parenteral therapy: (Vanco plus β-lactam/β-lactamase inhibitor), or (vanco plus carbapenem) Other alternatives: 1. Dapto or linezolid for vanco 2. (CIP or Levo or Moxi or aztreonam) plus metronidazole for β-lactam/β-lactamase inhibitor 3. Ceftobiprole Dosages in footnote⁹		
Onychomycosis: See Table 11, page 96, fungal infections				
Puncture wound: Nail/Toothpick	P. aeruginosa	Cleanse. Tetanus booster. Observe.		See page 4. 1–2% evolve to osteomyelitis. After toothpick injury (PIDJ 23:80, 2004): S. aureus, Strep sp. and mixed flora.
GALLBLADDER				
Cholecystitis, cholangitis, biliary sepsis, or common duct obstruction (partial; 2° to tumor, stones, stricture)	Enterobacteriaceae 68%, enterococci 14%, bacteroides 10%, Clostridium sp. 7%, rarely candida	PIP-TZ or AM-SB or TC-CL or ERTA If life-threatening: IMP MER or Dori	OR OR IP Ceph 3 + metro Aztreonam + metro CIP + metro OR Moxi Dosages in footnote 3	In severely ill pts, antibiotic therapy complements adequate biliary drainage. 15–30% pts will require decompression: surgical, percutaneous or ERCP-placed stent. Whether antimicrobial therapy should always cover pseudomonas & anaerobes is uncertain. Ceftriaxone associated with biliary sludge of drug(by ultrasound) in 6%, symptomatic 0.9%. (AJM 322:1821, 1990); clinical relevance still unclear but has led to surgery (MMWR 42:39, 1993).

¹ **TMP-SMX-DS** 2 tabs po bid, **minocycline** 100 mg po bid, **Pen VK** 500 mg po qid, (O Ceph 2, 3: **cefprozil** 500 mg po q12h; **cefdinir** 300 mg q12h or 600 mg po q24h; **cefpodoxime** 200 mg po q12h). **CIP** 750 mg po bid. **Levo** 750 mg po q24h.

² **AM-CL-ER** 2000/125 mg po bid, **TMP-SMX-DS** 2 tabs po bid, **CIP** 750 mg po bid, **Levo** 750 mg po q24h, **linezolid** 600 mg po bid

³ **Danco** 1 gm IV q12h, (**parenteral β-lactams: AM-SB** 3 gm IV q6h, **PIP-TZ** 3.375 gm IV q6h or 4.5 gm IV q8h or 4 hr infusion of 3.375 gm; TC-CL 3.1 gm IV q6h); **carbapenems: ERTA** 1 gm IV q24h, **IMP** 0.5 gm IV q6h, **MER** 1.0 gm IV q8h); **aztreonam** 2 gm IV q8h, **linezolid** 600 mg per kg IV q24h, **daptomycin** 6 mg per kg IV q24h; **CIP** 400 mg IV q12h, **Levo** 750 mg IV q24h; **metro** 1 gm IV loading dose & then 0.5 gm IV q6h or 1gm IV q12h; **ceftobiprole** 500 mg (2-hr infusion) q8h.

NOTE: All dosage recommendations are for adults (unless otherwise indicated) and assume normal renal function.

Abbreviations on page 2.

TABLE 1 (12)

ANATOMIC SITE/DIAGNOSIS/ MODIFYING CIRCUMSTANCES	ETIOLOGIES (usual)	SUGGESTED REGIMENS*		ADJUNCT DIAGNOSTIC OR THERAPEUTIC MEASURES AND COMMENTS
		PRIMARY	ALTERNATIVE[1]	
GASTROINTESTINAL				
Gastroenteritis—Empiric Therapy (laboratory studies not performed or culture, microscopy, toxin results NOT AVAILABLE) (Ref.: *NEJM 350:38, 2004*)				
Premature infant with necrotizing enterocolitis	Associated with intestinal flora	Treatment and rationale as for diverticulitis/peritonitis, page 19. See Table 16, page 177 for pediatric dosages.		Pneumatosis intestinalis on x-ray confirms diagnosis. Bacteremia-peritonitis in 30–50%. If Staph. epidermidis isolated, add vanco (IV).
Mild diarrhea (≤3 unformed stools/day, minimal associated symptomatology)	Bacterial (see Severe, below), viral, parasitic. Viral usually causes mild to moderate disease. For traveler's diarrhea, see page 17.	Fluids only + lactose-free diet, avoid caffeine		**Rehydration: For po fluid replacement, see Cholera, page 17.** **Antimotility:** Loperamide (Imodium) 4 mg, then 2 mg after each loose stool to max. of 16 mg per day. Bismuth subsalicylate (Pepto-Bismol) 2 tablets (262 mg) po qid. Do not use if suspect hemolytic uremic syndrome.
Moderate diarrhea (≥4 unformed stools/day &/or systemic symptoms)		Antimotility agents (see Comments) + fluids		**Hemolytic uremic syndrome (HUS):** Risk in children infected with E. coli 0157:H7 8–10%. Early treatment with TMP-SMX or FQs ↑ risk of HUS (*NEJM 342:1930 & 1990, 2000*). Controversial meta-analysis: *JAMA 288:996 & 311:1, 2002*.
Severe diarrhea (≥6 unformed stools/day, &/or temp ≥101°F, tenesmus, blood, or fecal leukocytes)	Shigella, salmonella, C. jejuni, E. coli 0157:H7, toxin-positive C. difficile, Klebsiella oxytoca, E. histolytica. For typhoid fever, see page 54	FQ [CIP 500 mg po q12h or Levo 500 mg po q24h] times 3–5 days	TMP-SMX-DS po bid times 3–5 days. Campylobacter resistance to TMP-SMX common in tropics.	**Norovirus:** Etiology of over 90% of non-bacterial diarrhea (± nausea/vomiting). Lasts 12–60 hrs. Hydrate. No effective antiviral. **Other potential etiologies:** Cryptosporidia—no treatment in immunocompetent host (see Table 13A & JID 770:272, 1994). Cyclospora—usually chronic diarrhea, responds to TMP-SMX (see Table 12A & MM 123:409, 1995).
NOTE: Severe afebrile bloody diarrhea should ↑ suspicion of E. coli 0157:H7 infection— causes only 1–3% all cases diarrhea in US—but causes up to 38% cases of bloody diarrhea (CID 32:573, 2001)		If recent antibiotic therapy add: Metro 500 mg po tid times 10–14 days	(C. difficile toxin colitis possible) Vanco 125 mg po qid times 10–14 days	Klebsiella oxytoca identified as cause of antibiotic-associated hemorrhagic colitis (cytotoxin positive): NEJM 355:2418, 2006.
Gastroenteritis—Specific Therapy (results of culture, microscopy, toxin assay AVAILABLE) (Ref.: *NEJM 350:38, 2004*)				
If culture negative, probably **Norovirus** (Norwalk) or rarely (in adults) **Rotavirus**—see Norovirus, page 137	Aeromonas/Plesiomonas	CIP 500 mg po bid times 3 days.	TMP-SMX-DS po bid times 3 days	Although no absolute proof, increasing evidence as cause of diarrheal illness.
	Amebiasis (Entamoeba histolytica, Cyclospora, Cryptosporidia and Giardia), see Table 13A			
NOTE: In 60 hospital pts with unexplained WBCs ≥15,000, 35% had C. difficile toxin present (AJM 115:543, 2003; CID 34:1585, 2002)	**Campylobacter jejuni** CAUTION: See Comment on FQ resistance. Fever in 53–83%; H/O bloody stools 37% (CID 44:696 & 701, 2007).	Azithro 500 mg po q24h x 3 days or CIP 500 mg po bid (See Comment)	Erythro stearate 500 mg po qid x 5 days	**↑ worldwide resistance to FQs** varies by region from 10% (USA) to 84% (Thailand) (AAC 47:2358, 2003). Erythro resistance rarely reported (CID 37:131, 2003). **Post-Campylobacter Guillain–Barré:** assoc. 15% of cases (Ln 366:1653, 2005). Assoc. with small bowel lymphoproliferative disease; may respond to antimicrobials (NEJM 350:239, 2003). **Reactive arthritis** another potential sequelae. See Traveler's diarrhea, page 17.

[1] H/O = history of

Abbreviations on page 2.   NOTE: All dosage recommendations are for adults (unless otherwise indicated) and assume normal renal function.

TABLE 1 (13)

ANATOMIC SITE/DIAGNOSIS/ MODIFYING CIRCUMSTANCES	ETIOLOGIES (usual)	SUGGESTED REGIMENS* PRIMARY	ALTERNATIVE[1]	ADJUNCT DIAGNOSTIC OR THERAPEUTIC MEASURES AND COMMENTS
GASTROINTESTINAL/Gastroenteritis—Specific Therapy (continued)				
Differential diagnosis of toxin-producing diarrhea • C. difficile • Klebsiella oxytoca • S. aureus • Shiga toxin producing E. coli (STEC)	**C. difficile** toxin positive antibiotic-associated colitis (CID 45:222, 2007). po meds okay; WBC <20,000.	Metro 500 mg po tid or 250mg qid x 10-14 days	Vanco 125 mg po qid x 10-14 days / Teicoplanin[NUS] 400 mg po bid x 14 days	Probiotics role in prevention and/or treatment unclear (Med Lett 49:55, 2007; CID 45:5122, 2007). **D/C antibiotic if possible; avoid antimotility agents, hydration, enteric isolation.** Relapse in 10-20%. **Nitazoxanide** 500mg po bid for 7-10 days equivalent to **Metro** po in phase 3 study[NUS] (CID 43:421, 2006)
	po meds okay; Sicker; WBC >20,000.	Vanco 125 mg po qid x 10-14 days	Metro 500 mg po tid x 10 days	Vanco superior to metro in sicker pts (CID 40:1586, 1591 & 1598, 2005 & 45: 302, 2007). Relapse in 10-20% (not due to resistance (JAC 56:988, 2005)
	Post-treatment relapse	1st relapse Vanco 125 mg po qid x 10 days	2nd relapse Vanco as above + rif 300 mg po bid / 3rd relapse: See Comment	**3rd relapse: Vanco** taper (all doses 125mg po): week 1 - qid, week 2 - bid, week 3 – q24h; week 4 - qod; wks 5&6 - q 3 d. Last resort: stool transplant (CID 36:580, 2003) Other options: 1) After initial vanco, rifaximin[NUS] 400-800 mg daily divided bid po tid x 2 wks (CID 44:846, 2007; rifaximin-resistant C. diff. reported (Abstr C2-2059a, ICAAC, 2007)); 2) nitazoxanide[NUS] 500 mg bid x 10d (JAC 59:705, 2007).
	Post-op ileus; severe disease with toxic megacolon	Metro 500 mg IV q6h + vanco via nasogastric tube (or naso-small bowel tube) ± retrograde catheter in cecum. See comment for dosage.		Vanco instillation into bowel, add 500mg vanco in 1 liter of saline and perfuse at 1-3mL/min to maximum of 2gm in 24 hrs (CID 690:2002). **Note: IV vanco not effective.** (M.G. Report of benefit of IV tigecycline: Clin Inf Dis 35:1311, 2009) NSAIDs & lack of benefit (An J Infect Control 36:132).
	E. coli O157:H7— H/O bloody stools 63% shiga toxin producing E. Coli (STEC)	NO TREATMENT with antimicrobials and anti-motility drugs; may enhance toxin release and ↑ risk of hemolytic uremic syndrome (HUS) (NEJM 342:1930 & 1990, 2000). Hydration important (Ln 365:1073, 2005).		NOTE: 5-10% of pts develop HUS (approx. 10% with HUS die or have permanent renal failure); 50% HUS pts have some degree of renal impairment (CID 38:1298, 2004). Non O157:H7 STEC emerging as cause of bloody diarrhea and/or HUS; EIA for shiga toxin available (CID 43:1587, 2006). Suggested that stopping NSAIDs helps. Ref: NEJM 365:2418, 2006
	Klebsiella oxytoca- antibiotic-associated	Responds to stopping antibiotic		Recently recognized cause of food poisoning, manifest as febrile gastroenteritis. Percentage with complicating bacteremia/meningitis unknown. Not detected in standard stool culture (NEJM 336:100 & 130, 1997).
	Listeria monocytogenes	AMP 50 mg/kg IV per day	TMP-SMX 20 mg/kg per day IV div q6-8h	Treat if <1yr old or >50yr old. If immunocompromised, if vascular
	Salmonella, non-typhi— For typhoid (enteric) fever, see page 54. Fever 57%, H/O bloody stools in 34%	If pt asymptomatic or illness mild, antimicrobial therapy not indicated. If septic (see typhoid fever, page 54). CIP 500 mg po bid x 5-7 days. Resistance ↑ (Ln 353:1590, 1998)	Azithro (gm po once, then 500 mg q24h) x 6 days (AAC 43:1441, 1999)	resistance to TMP-SMX and chloro. Ceftriaxone, cefotaxime usually active (Page 22), or fluoroquinolone & FQ resistance in US, Asia (CID 40:315, 2005; Ln 363:1285, 2004). Primary treatment of enteritis is fluid and electrolyte replacement. No adverse effects from FQs in children (Ln 348:547, 1996). If immunocompromised, treat 14 days.
	Shigella Fever in 58%, H/O bloody stools 51%	FQs po: CIP 500mg bid or (Levo 500 mg q24h) x 3 days.	TMP-SMX-DS po bid x 3 days) or (azithro 500 mg x1, then 250 mg q24h x 4 days)	Peds doses: TMP-SMX 5/25mg/kg po x 3 days. For severe disease, ceftriaxone 50-75mg/kg per day x 2-5 days. CIP suspension 10mg/kg bid x 5 days. (Ln 352:522, 1998). CIP superior to ceftriaxone in children (LnID 3:537, 2003). Immunocompromised children & adults: Treat for 7-10 days.
	Staphylococcus aureus See Comment	See Comment for peds rx per dose		Azithro causes increase in QT interval in trial in children (PIDJ 22:374, 2003). Case reports of toxin-mediated pseudo-membranes in small bowel) (CID 39:747, 2004). Clinda to stop toxin production reasonable if organism susceptible.

[1] **H/O** = history of

NOTE: All dosage recommendations are for adults (unless otherwise indicated) and assume normal renal function.

Abbreviations on page 2.

17

TABLE 1 (14)

ANATOMIC SITE/DIAGNOSIS/ MODIFYING CIRCUMSTANCES	ETIOLOGIES (usual)	SUGGESTED REGIMENS*		ADJUNCT DIAGNOSTIC OR THERAPEUTIC MEASURES AND COMMENTS
		PRIMARY	ALTERNATIVE†	
GASTROINTESTINAL/Gastroenteritis—Specific Therapy *(continued)*				
(continued from above)	**Spirochetosis** (*Brachyspira pilosicoli*)	Benefit of treatment unclear. Susceptible to **metro, ceftriaxone**, and **Moxi** (AAC 47:2354, 2003).		Anaerobic intestinal spirochete that colonizes colon of domestic & wild animals plus humans. Case reports of diarrhea with large numbers of the organism present (AAC 39:340, 2001; Am J Clin Path 120:828).
	Vibrio cholerae Treatment decreases duration of disease, volume losses, & duration of excretion (NEJM 364:2452, 2500, 2006) Increasing number of failures (11/06).	**Primary rx is hydration** (see Comments) **Azithromycin** 1gm po once, 6% achieve	**Primary Rx is hydration CIP** 1 gm po once but high failure rate. Peds dosage in Comments	Primary rx is fluid. **IV** use (per liter) 4gm NaCl, 1gm KCl, 6.5 gm Na lactate, 8gm glucose. **PO** use (per liter potable water): 1 level teaspoon table salt + 4 heaping teaspoons sugar (JTMH 84:73, 1981). Add orange juice or 2 bananas for K+. Volume given = fluid loss. Mild dehydration, give 5% body weight; for moderate, 7% body weight. (Refs: CID 20:1485, 1995; TRSM 89:103, 1995). Peds azithro: 20mg/kg (to 1gm max.) x 1 (Ln 360:1722, 2002). CIP 20 mg/kg (Ln 360:1085, 2003).
	Vibrio parahaemolyticus	Antimicrobial rx does not shorten course. Hydration		Shellfish source common. Treat severe disease: **FQ**, **doxy**, **FQ Ceph 3**
	Vibrio vulnificus	Usual presentation is skin lesions & bacteremia, life-threatening; treat early, **ceftaz + doxy**—see page 49; **levo** (AAC 46:3580, 2002)		
	Yersinia enterocolitica Fever in 68%, bloody stools in 26%	No treatment unless severe. If severe, combine **doxy** 100mg IV bid + (**tobra** or **gent** 5mg/kg per day once q24h) **TMP-SMX + FQs** are alternatives.		Mesenteric adenitis pain can mimic acute appendicitis. Lab diagnosis difficult: requires "cold enrichment" and/or yersinia selective agar. Desferrioxamine therapy increases severity, discontinue if on it. In Fe overload states predispose to yersinia (CID 27:1362 & 1367, 1998).
Gastroenteritis—Specific Risk Groups-Empiric Therapy				
Anoreceptive intercourse Proctitis (distal 15 cm only) Colitis	Herpes viruses, gonococci, chlamydia, syphilis. *See Genital Tract, page 20* Shigella, salmonella, campylobacter, E. histolytica (see Table T3A)		**FQ** (e.g., **CIP** 500 mg po) q12h x 3 days. See Table T3A	
HIV-1 infected (AIDS): >10 days diarrhea Acid-fast organisms: Other:	Cryptosporidium parvum, Cyclospora cayetanensis Isospora belli, microsporidia (Enterocytozoon bieneusi, Septata intestinalis) G. lamblia		See Table T3A See Table T3A	
Neutropenic enterocolitis or "typhlitis" (CID 27:695 & 700, 1998)	Mucosal invasion by **Clostridium septicum.** Occasionally caused by C. sordellii or P. aeruginosa	As for perirectal abscess, diverticulitis, pg 19. Ensure empiric regimen includes drug active vs Clostridia species; e.g., **pen G, AMP or clinda**. Empiric regimen should have predictive activity vs P. aeruginosa		Tender right lower quadrant. Surgical resection controversial but may be necessary. **NOTE:** Resistance of clostridia to clindamycin reported.
Traveler's diarrhea, self-medication. Patient usually afebrile (CID 44:338 & 347, 2007)	**Acute:** 60% due to diarrheagenic E. coli; shigella, salmonella, or campylobacter. C. difficile, amebiasis (see Table 13) If **chronic:** cyclospora, crypto-sporidia, giardia, isospora	**For Latin America & S.E. Asia and elsewhere: Azithro** 1gm po x 1 dose OR other **FQ** (**Levo** 500mg x 1 dose or 500mg once daily x 3 days OR (**Levo, Moxi** or **CIP**) po daily x 3 days (dose in footnote¹) Add **imodium** 4 mg (2 caps) po x 1, then 2mg after each loose stool to max 16mg/day.	Geographic variability in likely etiology. Increasing resistance of campylobacter to FQs (esp. in SE Asia, now perhaps also resistance to levo & moxi). Single dose azithro + Imodium as effective as levo + Imodium (CID 45:294 & 301, 2007). Azithro: peds dose: 5–10mg/kg x1 dose. Rifaximin approved for age 12 or older. Adverse effects similar to placebo. No loperamide if fever or blood in stool. **CIP and rifaximin** equivalent therapy vs non-invasive pathogens (AJTMH 74:1060, 2006)	For peri-rectal abscess, diverticulitis, pg 19. **OR rifaximin** 200 mg po bid x 3 days.

¹ **FQ** dosage po for self-rx traveler's diarrhea—mild disease: **CIP** 750 mg x 1; severe disease: **CIP** 500mg bid x 3 days. **Oflox** 300 mg po bid x 3 days; severe 500mg bid x 3 days: **Levo** 500 mg. **Moxi** 400 mg probably would work but not FDA-approved indication.

Abbreviations on page 2. *NOTE: All dosage recommendations are for adults (unless otherwise indicated) and assume normal renal function.*

18

TABLE 1 (15)

ANATOMIC SITE/DIAGNOSIS/ MODIFYING CIRCUMSTANCES	ETIOLOGIES (usual)	SUGGESTED REGIMENS*		ADJUNCT DIAGNOSTIC OR THERAPEUTIC MEASURES AND COMMENTS
		PRIMARY	ALTERNATIVE†	
GASTROINTESTINAL/Gastroenteritis—Specific Risk Groups—Empiric Therapy *(continued)*				
Prevention of Traveler's diarrhea	Not routinely indicated. Current recommendation is to take **FQ + Imodium** with 1st loose stool.		Alternative during 1st 3wk & only if activities are essential: **Rifaximin 200 mg po bid** *(AnIM 142:805 & 861, 2005).*	
Gastrointestinal Infections by Anatomic Site: Esophagus to Rectum				
Esophagitis	Candida albicans, HSV, CMV	See Sanford Guide to HIV/AIDS Therapy and Table 11A, page 96		
Duodenal/Gastric ulcer; gastric cancer, MALT lymphomas (not 2° NSAIDs) *(Can J Gastro 19:399, 2005; Ann J Med 114:364, 140, 2006; Am J Gastro 102:1808, 2007)*	**Helicobacter pylori** See Comment Prevalence of pre-treatment resistance increasing	**Rx q12h po for 14 days: Bismuth** (see footnote[3]), **bismuth subsalicylate 2 tabs qid + tetracycline 500 mg qid + omeprazole 20 mg bid.** **Rx q12h po for 14 days:** (**Omeprazole 20 mg[1] or rabeprazole 20 mg[1] + amox 1 gm + clarithro 500 mg**) all po bid OR sequential therapy: (**Rabeprazole 20 mg + amox 1 gm) bid x 5 d, then (rabeprazole 20 mg + clarithro 500 mg + tinidazole 500 mg) bid for another 5 days.**		**Dx: Stool antigen**—Monoclonal EIA >90% sens. & specific. *(Amer J Gastro 101:921, 2006).* Other tests: Urea breath test, if endoscoped, rapid urease &/or histology &/or culture. **Antimicrobial resistance increasing** *(LnID 6:699, 2006).* Resistance to amox & metronidazole common, clarithro resistance, up to 23%, metro 20–30% *(Dig Liver Dis 35:541, 2003).* **Treatment success:** Correlates with active drugs & pt compliance. **Rx duration** varies between 7–14 days, we suggest that regimen times 14 days to ↑ compliance & hopefully efficacy *(7–9% ↑ cures with 14 days) (Aliment Pharmacol Ther 14:603, 2000).* **Test of cure:** Repeat stool antigen and/or urea breath test >8 wks post-treatment.
Small intestine: Whipple's disease *(NEJM 356:55, 2007)* See *Infective endocarditis, culture-negative, page 27*	Tropheryma whipplei	**initial 10–14 days** (**Pen G** 6–24 million units IV q24h + **streptomycin** 1 gm IM/IV q24h) OR **ceftriaxone** 2gm IV q24h Then, **for approx. 1 year** **TMP-SMX-DS** 1 tab po bid	**TMP-SMX-DS** 1 tab po bid **Doxy** 100 mg po bid) + **Pen VK** 500 mg qid	Refs for sequential therapy: AnIM 146:556, 2007. Therapy based on empiricism and retrospective analyses. TMP-SMX: CNS relapses during TMP-SMX rx reported. Interesting in vitro susceptibility study: combination of doxy & hydroxychloro-quine bactericidal *(AAC 48:747, 2004).* Cultivated from CSF in pts with intestinal disease and no neurologic findings *(JID 188:797 & 801, 2003).* Early experience with combination of doxy 100 mg bid plus hydroxychloroquine 200 mg tid in patients without neurologic disease *(NEJM 356:55, 2007).*
Inflammatory bowel disease: Ulcerative colitis, Crohn's disease Mild to moderate *Ref.: Ln 359:331, 2002*	Unknown	**Sulfasalazine** (1gm po qid) or **mesalamine (5ASA)** 1 gm po qid	CIP + metro had no benefit *(Gastro 123:33, 2002)* **Coated mesalamine** (Asacol) 800 mg tid or (and equally effective) **Corticosteroid enemas**	Check stool for E. histolytica. Try aminosalicylates 1st in mild/mod. disease. See review article for more aggressive therapy.
Severe Crohn's disease *Ref: CID 44:256, 2007*	Unknown	**Etanercept**	In randomized controlled trial. **Infliximab/adalimumab**	Screen for latent TBc before blocking TNF *(MMWR 53:683, 2004).* If possible, delay anti-TNF drugs until TBc prophylaxis complete. For other anti-TNF risks: NEJM 351:42, 2004.

* Can substitute other **proton pump inhibitors** for omeprazole or rabeprazole for esomeprazole 20 mg *(FDA-approved),* lansoprazole 30mg *(FDA-approved),* pantoprazole 40mg *(not FDA-approved for this indication)*

[3] **bismuth preparations:** (1) In U.S. **bismuth subsalicylate (Pepto-Bismol)** 262 mg tabs; adult dose for helicobacter is 2 tabs (524 mg) qid. (2) Outside U.S., colloidal bismuth subcitrate (De-Nol) 120mg chewable tablets; dose is 1 tablet qid. (3) Another treatment option: Ranitidine bismuth citrate 400 mg; give with metro 500 mg and clarithro 500 mg—all bid times 7 days. Worked despite metro/clarithro resistance *(Gastro 114:A323, 1998).*

NOTE: All dosage recommendations are for adults (unless otherwise indicated) and assume normal renal function.

Abbreviations on page 2.

TABLE 1 (16)

ANATOMIC SITE/DIAGNOSIS/ MODIFYING CIRCUMSTANCES	ETIOLOGIES (usual)	SUGGESTED REGIMENS*		ADJUNCT DIAGNOSTIC OR THERAPEUTIC MEASURES AND COMMENTS
		PRIMARY	ALTERNATIVE§	
GASTROINTESTINAL/Gastrointestinal Infections by Anatomic Site: Esophagus to Rectum *(continued)*				
Diverticulitis, perirectal abscess, peritonitis Also see Peritonitis, *page 42* CID 37:997, 2003	Enterobacteriaceae, occasionally P. aeruginosa, Bacteroides sp., enterococci	**Outpatient rx—mild diverticulitis, drained perirectal abscess:** [(**TMP-SMX-DS** bid) or (**CIP** 750 mg bid or **Levo** 750 mg q24h)] + **metro** 500 mg q6h. All po x 7–10 days.	(**AM-CL-ER** 1000/62.5 mg 2 tabs po bid x 7–10 days **OR** **Moxi** 400 mg po q24h x 7-10 days	Must "cover" both Gm-neg. aerobic & Gm-neg. anaerobic bacteria. **Drugs active only vs anaerobic Gm-neg. bacilli:** clinda, metro. **Drugs active only vs aerobic Gm-neg. bacilli:** APAG¹, P Ceph 2/3/4 (see Table 10C, page --), aztreonam, AP Pen, CIP, Levo. **Drugs active vs both aerobic/anaerobic Gm-neg. bacteria:** cefoxitin, cefotetan, TC-CL, PIP-TZ, AM-SB, ERTA, Dori, IMP, MER, Moxi, & tigecycline. Increasing resistance of Bacteroides species (AAC 51:1649, 2007):
		Mild-moderate disease—Inpatient—Parenteral Rx: (e.g., focal peri-appendiceal peritonitis, peri-diverticular abscess, endomyometritis) **PIP-TZ** 3.375 gm IV q6h or 4.5 gm IV q8h or **AM-SB** 3 gm IV q6h, or **TC-CL** 3.1 gm IV q6h or **ERTA** 1 gm IV q24h or **MOXI** 400 mg IV q24h	[(**CIP** 400 mg IV q12h) or (**Levo** 750 mg IV q24h)] + (**metro** 500 mg IV q6h or 1 gm IV q12h) **OR tigecycline** 100 mg IV 1ˢᵗ dose & then 50 mg IV q12h **OR Moxi** 400 mg IV q24h								Cefoxitin	Cefotetan	Clindamycin
---	---	---	---
% Resistant:	5-30	17–87	19-35

Resistance to metro, PIP-TZ rare. Few case reports of metro resistance *(CID 40:e67, 2005; J Clin Micro 42:4127, 2004).*
 Ertapenem less active vs P. aeruginosa/Acinetobacter sp. than IMP, MER or Dori.
 Concomitant surgical management important, esp. with moderate-severe disease. **Role of enterococci remains debatable.** Probably pathogenic in infections of biliary tract. Probably need drugs active vs enterococci in pts with valvular heart disease.

 Severe penicillin/cephalosporin allergy: (aztreonam 2 gm IV q6h) + (**metro** (500 mg IV q6h) or (1 gm IV q12h)) **OR** [(**CIP** 400 mg IV q12h) or (**Levo** 750 mg IV q24h) + **metro**].

(Continuation of PRIMARY / ALTERNATIVE columns for Severe life-threatening disease:)

Severe life-threatening disease, ICU patient: **IMP** 500 mg IV q6h or **MER** 1 gm IV q8h **or Dori** 500 mg q8h (1-hr infusion). | **AMP + metro + (CIP** 400 mg IV q12h or **Levo** 750 mg IV q24h) **OR (AMP** 2gm IV q6h + **metro** 500 mg IV q6h + aminoglycoside¹ (see Table 10D, page 93)]

---

¹ **APAG** = antipseudomonal aminoglycosidic aminoglycoside, e.g., amikacin, gentamicin, tobramycin

Abbreviations on page 2.   NOTE: All dosage recommendations are for adults (unless otherwise indicated) and assume normal renal function.

TABLE 1 (17)

ANATOMIC SITE/DIAGNOSIS/ MODIFYING CIRCUMSTANCES	ETIOLOGIES (usual)	SUGGESTED REGIMENS*		ADJUNCT DIAGNOSTIC OR THERAPEUTIC MEASURES AND COMMENTS
		PRIMARY	ALTERNATIVE†	
GENITAL TRACT: Mixture of empiric & specific treatment. Divided by sex of the patient. For sexual assault (rape), see Table 15A, page 167. **See Guidelines for Dx of Sexually Transmitted Diseases, MMWR 55 (RR-11), 2006 and focused commentary in CID 44(Suppl 3), 2007.**				
Both Women & Men: Chancroid	H. ducreyi	**Ceftriaxone** 250 mg IM single dose OR azithro 1 gm po single dose	**CIP** 500 mg bid po x 3 days OR **erythro base** 500 mg qid po x 7 days.	In HIV+ pts, failures reported with single dose azithro (CID 21:409, 1995). Evaluate after 7 days, ulcer should objectively improve.
Chlamydia, et al, non-gono-coccal or post-gonococcal urethritis, cervicitis **NOTE: Assume concomitant N. gonorrhoeae** Chlamydia conjunctivitis, see page 11	Chlamydia 50%, Myco-plasma hominis. Other known etiologies (10–15%): trichomonas, herpes simplex virus, Mycoplasma genitalium. Refs: JID 193:333, 336, 2006.	**(Doxy** 100 mg po bid x 7 days) or **azithro** 1 gm po as single dose). Evaluate & treat sex partner **In pregnancy: erythro base** 500 mg po qid x 7 days OR **amox** 500 mg po tid x 7 days.	**Erythro base** 500 mg qid po x 7 days) or **Offlox** 300 mg (q12h po x 7 days) or **Levo** 500 mg (q24h) x 7 days) **In pregnancy: erythro** 1 gm po x 1 **Doxy & Oflox contra-indicated**	**Diagnosis:** Nucleic acid amplification tests for C. trachomatis & N. gonorrhoeae on urine samples equivalent to cervix or urethra specimens (AnIM 142:914, 2005). **For recurrent or persistent disease:** either metro 2 gm po x 1 or either erythro base 500 mg po qid x 7 days or erythro ethylsuccinate 800 mg po x 7 days. **Evaluate & treat sex partners.**
Recurrent/persistent urethritis	Occult trichomonas, tetra-resistant U. urealyticum.	**Metro** 2 gm po x 1, **PLUS erythro base** 500 mg po qid x 7 days.	**Erythro ethylsuccinate** 800 mg po x 7 days	In men with NGU, 20% infected with trichomonas (JID 188:465, 2003). Another option: (metro or tinidazole 2gm po x 1 dose) plus azithro 1 gm po x 1 dose.
Gonorrhea [MMWR 55 (RR-11), 2006]. **FQs no longer recommended for treatment of gonococcal infections (MMWR 56:332, 2007).**				
Conjunctivitis (adult)	N. gonorrhoeae	**Ceftriaxone** 1 gm IM or IV times one dose		Consider saline lavage of eye times 1
Disseminated gonococcal infection (DGI, dermatitis-arthritis syndrome)	N. gonorrhoeae	**(Ceftriaxone** 1 gm IV q24h) or **(cefotaxime** 1 gm q8h IV) or **(ceftizox-ime** 1 gm q8h IV)—see Comment	**Spectinomycin** NUS 2 gm IM q12h—see Comment	Continue IV regimen for 24hr after symptoms ↓; reliable pts may be dis-charged 24hr after sx resolve to complete 7 days IV with **cefixime† 400 mg po bid.** R/O meningitis/ endocarditis. **Treat presumptively for concomitant C. trachomatis**
Endocarditis	N. gonorrhoeae	**Ceftriaxone** 1–2 gm IV q24h x 4wk.		Ref: JID 157:1281, 1988
Pharyngitis	N. gonorrhoeae	**Ceftriaxone** 125 mg IM x 1		If chlamydia not ruled out: **Azithro** 1 gm po x 1 or **doxy** 100 mg po bid x 7 days. Some suggest test of cure culture after 1wk. **Spectinomycin, cefixime, cefpodoxime & cefuroxime not effective**
Urethritis, cervicitis, proctitis (uncomplicated) For proctitis, see page 24. Diagnosis: nucleic acid amplification test (NAAT) on urine or urethral swab—see AnIM 142:914, 2005. **NO FQs: MMWR 56:332, 2007.**	N. gonorrhoeae (50% of pts with urethritis, cervicitis have infection not ruled out) and C. trachomatis **—treat for both unless NAAT indicates single pathogen)**	**Ceftriaxone** 125 mg IM x 1) or **(cefpodoxime** 400 mg po x 1 **PLUS — if chlamydia infection not ruled out: Azithro** 1 gm po x 1 or **(doxy** 100 mg po bid x 7 days)	**(cefixime† 400 mg po x 1) or (ceftriaxone** 125 mg IM x 1) Severe allergy/ceph allergy? Maybe azithro comment. Understanding risk of FQ-resistance, could try FQ therapy with close follow-up.	**Treat for both GC and C. trachomatis unless single pathogen by NAAT.** Screen for syphilis. Other alternatives for GC: Spectinomycin NUS 2 gm IM x 1 Other single cephalosporins: ceftizoxime 500 mg IM, cefoxitin 2 gm IM + probenecid 1 gm po. **Azithro** 1 gm po x1 effective for chlamydia but need 2 gm po for GC; not recommended for GC due to GI side-effects, expense & rapid emergence of resistance.

---

† Cefixime tablets not available (Aug 07); generic oral suspension, 100 mg/5 mL, is manufactured.

* Cefixime tablets not available (Aug 07); generic oral suspension, 100 mg/5 mL, is manufactured.

Abbreviations on page 2.   NOTE: All dosage recommendations are for adults (unless otherwise indicated) and assume normal renal function.

TABLE 1 (18)

ANATOMIC SITE/DIAGNOSIS/ MODIFYING CIRCUMSTANCES	ETIOLOGIES (usual)	SUGGESTED REGIMENS* PRIMARY	SUGGESTED REGIMENS* ALTERNATIVE¹	ADJUNCT DIAGNOSTIC OR THERAPEUTIC MEASURES AND COMMENTS
GENITAL TRACT/ Both Women & Men (continued)				
Granuloma inguinale (Donovanosis)	Klebsiella (formerly Calymmatobacterium) granulomatis	**Doxy** 100 mg po bid x 3-4wks OR **TMP-SMX-DS** q12h x 3wk	**Erythro** 500 mg po qid x 3wks OR **CIP** 750 mg po x 4wks OR **azithro** 1 gm po q wk x 3wks	Clinical response usually seen in 1wk. Rx until all lesions healed, may take 4wk. Treatment failures & recurrence seen with doxy & TMP-SMX-DS. Improve with FQ and chloro. Ref. CID 25:24, 1997 If improvement not evidence in first few days, some experts add gentamicin 1 mg/kg IV q8h.
Herpes simplex virus	See Table 14A, page 137			
Human papilloma virus (HPV)	See Table 14A, page 137			
Lymphogranuloma venereum	Chlamydia trachomatis, serovars, L1, L2, L3	**Doxy** 100 mg po bid x 21 days	**Erythro** 0.5 gm po qid x 21 days	Dx based on serology; biopsy contraindicated because sinus tracts develop. Nucleic acid amplification tests for C. trachomatis will be positive. In MSM, presents as fever, rectal ulcer, anal discharge. (CID 39:996, 2004).
Phthirus pubis (pubic lice, "crabs") & scabies	Phthirus pubis & Sarcoptes scabiei	See Table 13, page 125		
Syphilis (JAMA 290:1510, 2003): **Early, primary, secondary, or latent <1yr**	**Syphilis & HIV:** LnID 4:456, 2004; MMWR 53:RR-15, 2004 and 55: RR-11, 2006 T. pallidum NOTE: Test all pts with syphilis for HIV; test all HIV patients for latent syphilis.	**Benzathine pen G (Bicillin L-A)** 2.4 million units IM x 1 NOTE: **Azithro** 2 gm po x 1 dose but use is problematic due to **emerging azithro resistance** (See Comment)	(**Doxy** 100 mg po bid x 14 days) or **tetracycline** 500 mg po qid x 14 days) or (**ceftriaxon** 1 gm IM/IV q24h x 8–10 days). Follow-up mandatory.	If early or congenital syphilis, **quantitative VDRL at 0, 3, 6, 12 & 24 mo** after rx. If 1° or 2° syphilis, VDRL should ↓ 2 tubes at 6mo, 3 tubes 12mo, & 4 tubes 24mo. Early latent: 2 tubes ↓ at 12mo. With 1°, 50% will be RPR seronegative at 24mo, 24% neg. FTA/ABS at 2-3yrs (AnIM 114:1005, 1991). If titers fail to fall, examine CSF; if CSF (+), treat as neurosyphilis; if CSF is negative, retreat with benzathine Pen G 2.4 m.u. IM x 3wks. **Azithro-resistant syphilis** documented in California, Ireland, & elsewhere (CID 44:S130, 2007). NOTE: Use of **benzathine procaine penicillin** is inappropriate!!
More than 1 yr's duration (latent of indeterminate duration, cardiovascular, late benign gumma)		**Benzathine pen G (Bicillin L-A)** 2.4 million units IM q week x 3 = 7.2 million units total	**Doxy** 100mg po bid x 28 days or **tetracycline** 500mg po qid x 28 days	No published data on efficacy of alternatives. The value of routine lumbar puncture in asymptomatic late syphilis is being questioned in the U.S., i.e.: no LP, rx all patients as primary recommendation. **Indications for LP (CDC): neurologic symptoms, treatment failure, serum non-treponemal titer >1:32, other evidence of active syphilis (aortitis, gumma, iritis), non-penicillin rx, + HIV test.**
Neurosyphilis—Very difficult to treat. Includes ocular (retrobulbar neuritis) syphilis. **All need CSF exam.**	For penicillin desensitization method, see Table 7, pg 74 And MMWR 55 (RR-11):33-35, 2006.	**Pen G** 3–4 million units IV q4h x 10–14 days	(**Procaine pen G** 2.4 million units IM q24h + **probenecid** 0.5gm po qid both x 10–14 days—See Comment)	**Ceftriaxone** 2 gm (IV or IM) q24h x 14 day. 23% failure rate reported (AnIM 93:481, 1992). For penicillin allergy, either desensitize or obtain infectious diseases consultation. **Serologic criteria for response to rx: 4-fold titer ↓ in VDRL titer over 6-12mo.** (CID 28 (Suppl. 1):S21, 1999).
HIV infection (AIDS) CID 44:S130, 2007.		Treatment same as HIV uninfected with closer follow-up. LP on all HIV-infected pts with late syphilis and serum RPR ≥1:32. Recommend CSF exam of all HIV+ pts regardless of stage of syphilis. Treat early neurosyphilis 10-14 days regardless of CD4 count. MMWR 56:625, 2007.		HIV+ plus RPR ≥1:32 plus CD4 count ≤350/mcL increases risk of neurosyphilis nearly 19-fold—examine CSF (JID 189:369, 2004); also, CSF changes less likely regardless of CD4 count. Reviews of syphilis & HIV: LnID 4:456, 2004; MMWR 53:RR-15, 2004.

Abbreviations on page 2.   NOTE: All dosage recommendations are for adults (unless otherwise indicated) and assume normal renal function.

TABLE 1 (19)

ANATOMIC SITE/DIAGNOSIS/ MODIFYING CIRCUMSTANCES	ETIOLOGIES (usual)	SUGGESTED REGIMENS*		ADJUNCT DIAGNOSTIC OR THERAPEUTIC MEASURES AND COMMENTS
		PRIMARY	ALTERNATIVE†	
GENITAL TRACT/Both Women & Men (continued)				
Pregnancy and syphilis		Same as for non-pregnant; some recommend 2nd dose (2.4 million units) **benzathine pen G** 1 wk after initial dose esp. in 3rd trimester or with 2° syphilis	Skin test for penicillin allergy. Desensitize if necessary, as parenteral pen G is only therapy with documented efficacy!	Monthly quantitative VDRL or equivalent. If 4-fold ↑, re-treat. Doxy, tetracycline contraindicated. Erythro not recommended because of high risk of failure to cure fetus.
Congenital syphilis	T. pallidum	**Aqueous crystalline pen G** 50,000 units/kg per dose IV q12h x 7 days, then q8h for 10 day total.	**Procaine pen G** 50,000 units/kg IM q24h for 10 days	Another alternative: Ceftriaxone ≤30 days old, 75 mg/kg IV/IM q24h; >30 days old 100 mg/kg IV/IM q24h. Treat 10–14 days. If symptomatic, ophthalmologic exam indicated. If more than 1 day of rx missed, restart entire course. **Need serologic follow-up!**
Warts, anogenital	See Table 14, page 137			
Women:				
Amnionitis, septic abortion	Bacteroides, esp. Prevotella bivius; Group B, A. streptococci; Enterobacteriaceae; C. trachomatis	[(**Cefoxitin** or **TC-CL** or **Dori**WEDA4 or **IMP** or **MER** or **AM-SB** or **ERTA** or **PIP-TZ**) + **doxy**] OR [**Clinda** + (**aminoglycoside** or **ceftriaxone**)]	[(**Cefotetan** or **TC-CL** or **IMP** or **MER** or **AM-SB** or **ERTA** or **PIP-TZ**) + **doxy**] OR [**Clinda** + (**aminoglycoside** or **ceftriaxone**)] Dosage: see footnote¹	D&C of uterus. In septic abortion, Clostridium perfringens may cause fulminant intravascular hemolysis. In postpartum patients with enigmatic fever and/or pulmonary emboli, **consider septic pelvic vein thrombophlebitis** (see Vascular, septic pelvic vein thrombophlebitis, page 58) Alter discharge: doxy or continue clinda. **NOTE:** IV clinda effective for C. trachomatis, no data on po clinda (CID 19/720, 1994).
Cervicitis, mucopurulent Treatment based on results of nucleic acid amplification test	N. gonorrhoeae Chlamydia trachomatis	Treat for Gonorrhea, page 20. Treat for non-gonococcal urethritis, page 20		Criteria for dx: yellow or green pus on cervical swab; >10 WBC/oil field. Gram stain for GC, if negative rx for C. trachomatis. If in doubt, send swab or urine for culture, EIA or nucleic acid amplification test and rx for both.
Endomyometritis/septic pelvic phlebitis Early postpartum (1st 48 hrs)	Bacteroides, esp. Prevotella bivius, Group B, A streptococci; Enterobacteriaceae; C. trachomatis	[(**Cefoxitin** or **TC-CL** or **ERTA** or **IMP** or **MER** or **AM-SB** or **PIP-TZ**) + **doxy**] OR [**Clinda** + (**aminoglycoside** or **ceftriaxone**)] Dosage: see footnote¹		See Comments under Amnionitis, septic abortion, above
Late postpartum (48 hrs to 6 wks) (usually after vaginal delivery)	Chlamydia trachomatis, M. hominis	**Doxy** 100 mg IV or po q12h times 14 days		Tetracyclines not recommended in nursing mothers; discontinue nursing. M. hominis sensitive to tetra, clinda, not erythro (CCTID 17:5:200, 1993).
Fitzhugh–Curtis syndrome	C. trachomatis, N. gonorrhoeae	Treat as for pelvic inflammatory disease immediately below.		Perihepatitis (violin-string adhesions)

¹ **P Ceph 2** cefoxitin 2 gm IV q6–8h, cefotetan 2 gm IV q12h; cefuroxime 750 mg IV q8h); **TC-CL** 3.1 gm IV q4–6h; **AM-SB** 3 gm IV q6h; **PIP-TZ** 3.375 gm q6h or for nosocomial pneumonia 4.5 gm IV q6h or 4-hr infusion of 3.375 gm q8h; **doxy** 100 mg IV q12h; **clinda** 450–900 mg IV q8h; **APAG** (gentamicin, see Table 10D, page 100); **ceftriaxone** 2 gm IV q8h; **ceftriaxone** 1 gm IV q24h; **MER** 1 gm IV q8h; **azithro** 1 gm IV q24h; **ertapenem** 1 gm IV q24h (1-hr infusion); **IMP** 0.5 gm IV q6h; **doripenem** 500 mg IV q8h (1-hr infusion); **linezolid** 600 mg IV/po q12h; **vanco** 1 gm IV q12h.

TABLE 1 (20)

ANATOMIC SITE/DIAGNOSIS/ MODIFYING CIRCUMSTANCES	ETIOLOGIES (usual)	SUGGESTED REGIMENS*		ADJUNCT DIAGNOSTIC OR THERAPEUTIC MEASURES AND COMMENTS
		PRIMARY	ALTERNATIVE[1]	
GENITAL TRACT/Women (continued)				
Pelvic Inflammatory Disease (PID), salpingitis, tubo-ovarian abscess				
Outpatient rx: limit to pts with temp <38°C, WBC <11,000 per mm³, minimal evidence of peritonitis, active bowel sounds & able to tolerate oral nourishment	N. gonorrhoeae, chlamydia, bacteroides, Enterobacteriaceae, streptococci	**Outpatient rx:** [(ceftriaxone 250 mg IM or IV x 1) **+ metro** 500 mg po bid x 14 days] **+ (doxy** 100 mg po bid x 14 days)]. **OR (cefoxitin** 2 gm IM with **probenecid** 1 gm po both as single dose) plus **(doxy** 100 mg po bid times 14 days)]	**Inpatient regimens:** [(Cefotetan 2 gm IV q12h or **cefoxitin** 2 gm IV q6h) **+ doxy** 100 mg IV/po q12h] [**Clinda** 900 mg IV q8h) **+ gentamicin** 2 mg/kg loading dose, then 1.5 mg/kg q8h or 4.5 mg/kg once per day), then **doxy** 100 mg po bid x 14 days]	Another alternative parenteral regimen: **AM-SB** 3 gm IV q6h + **doxy** 100 mg IV/po q12h Remember: Evaluate and treat sex partner. FQs not recommended due to increasing resistance (MMWR 56:332, 2007 & www.cdc.gov/std/treatment)
CID 44:953 & 961, 2007; MMWR 55(RR-11), 2006 & www.cdc.gov/std/treatment				
Vaginitis—MMWR 51(RR-6), 2002 or CID 35 (Suppl 2):S135, 2002				
Candidiasis Pruritus, thick cheesy discharge, pH <4.5 See Table 11A, page 96	Candida albicans 80–90%. C. glabrata, C. tropicalis may be increasing—they are less susceptible to azoles	**Oral azoles** **Fluconazole** 150 mg po x 1: **Itraconazole** 200 mg po bid x 1 day	**Intravaginal azoles:** variety of strengths—from 1 dose to 7-14 days. Drugs available (all end in -azole): butocon, clotrim, micon, tiocon, tercon (doses: Table 11A, footnote page 98)	Nystatin vag. tabs times 14 days less effective. Other rx for azole-resistant strains: gentian violet, boric acid. If recurrent candidiasis (4 or more episodes per yr): 6 mos. suppression with: fluconazole 150 mg po q week or itraconazole 100 mg po q24h or clotrimazole vag. suppositories 500 mg q week.
Trichomoniasis Copious foamy discharge, pH >4.5 Treat sexual partners—see Comment	Trichomonas vaginalis	**Metro** 2 gm as single dose or 500 mg po bid x 7 days OR **Tinidazole** 2 gm po single dose **Pregnancy:** See Comment	**For rx failure:** Re-treat with metro 500 mg po bid x 7 days. If 2nd failure: metro 2 gm po q24h x 3–5 days. If still failure, suggest ID consultation and/or contact CDC: 770-488-4115 or www.cdc.gov/std.	Treat male sexual partners (2 gm metronidazole as single dose). Nearly 20% men with NGU are infected with trichomonas (JID 188:465, 2003). Another option if metro-resistant: **Tinidazole** 500 mg po bid x 14 days. Ref. CID 33:1341, 2001. **Pregnancy:** No data indicating metro teratogenic or mutagenic [MMWR 51(RR-6), 2002]
Bacterial vaginosis Malodorous vaginal discharge, pH >4.5. Data on recurrence & review: JID 193:1475, 2006	Etiology unclear: associated with Gardnerella vaginalis, mobiluncus, Mycoplasma hominis, Prevotella sp. & Atopobium vaginae et al.	**Metro** 0.5 gm po bid x 7 days or **metro vaginal gel** (1 applicator intravaginally) 1x/day x 5 days OR **Tinidazole** (2 gm po once daily x 2 days or 1 gm po once daily x 5 days)	**Clinda** 0.3 gm po bid x 7 days or 2% **clinda vaginal cream** (1 applicator) at bedtime x 7 days or **clinda ovules** 100 mg intravag-inally at bedtime x 3 days.	Reported 50% ↑ in cure rate if azstiran from sex or use condoms: CID 44:213 & 220, 2007. Treatment of male sex partner **not** indicated unless balanitis present. Metro extended release tabs 750 mg po q24h x 7 days available; no published data. **Pregnancy:** Treat same as non-pregnancy, except avoid clindamycin cream (↑ risk premature birth). Atopobium resistant to metro in vitro; suscept. To clinda (BMC Inf Dis 6:51, 2006); *importance unclear.*

[1] 1 applicator contains 5 gm of gel with 37.5 mg metronidazole

Abbreviations on page 2.   NOTE: All dosage recommendations are for adults (unless otherwise indicated) and assume normal renal function.

TABLE 1 (21)

ANATOMIC SITE/DIAGNOSIS/ MODIFYING CIRCUMSTANCES	ETIOLOGIES (usual)	SUGGESTED REGIMENS*		ADJUNCT DIAGNOSTIC OR THERAPEUTIC MEASURES AND COMMENTS
		PRIMARY	ALTERNATIVE†	
GENITAL TRACT (continued)				
Men:				
Balanitis	Candida 40%, Group B strep, gardnerella	Oral **azoles** as for vaginitis		Occurs in 1/4 of male sex partners of women infected with candida. Exclude circinate balanitis (Reiter's syndrome). Plasma cell balanitis (non-infectious) responds to hydrocortisone cream.
Epididymo-orchitis				
Age <35 years	N. gonorrhoeae, Chlamydia trachomatis	**Ceftriaxone** 250 mg IM x 1 + **doxy** 100 mg po bid x 10 days		Also: bedrest, scrotal elevation, and analgesics.
Age >35 years or homosexual men (insertive partners in anal intercourse)	Enterobacteriaceae (coliforms)	**FQ: CIP-ER** 500 mg 1x/day or **CIP** 400 mg IV bid or **Levo** 750 mg IV(po page 22) 1x/day) x10-14 days	**AM-SB 3 TC-CL, PIP-TZ:** see footnote	Midstream pyuria and scrotal pain and edema. Also, bedrest, scrotal elevation, and analgesics. NOTE: Do urine NAAT (nucleic acid amplification test) to ensure absence of N. gonorrhoeae with concomitant risk of FQ-resistant gonorrhoeae.
Non-gonococcal urethritis—See *Chlamydia et al, Non-gonococcal urethritis, Table 1(17), page 20*				
Prostatitis—Review: *AJM 106:327, 1999*				
Acute ≤35 years of age	N. gonorrhoeae, C. trachomatis	**ceftriaxone** 250 mg IM x 1 then **doxy** 100 mg bid x 10 days		FQs no longer recommended for gonococcal infections. In AIDS pts, prostate may be focus of Cryptococcus neoformans.
≥35 years of age	Enterobacteriaceae (coliforms)	**FQ** (dosage: see *Epididymo-orchitis, >35 yrs, above*) or **TMP-SMX** 1 DS tablet (160mg TMP) po bid x 10-14 days		Treat as acute urinary infection, 14 days (not single dose regimen). Some authorities recommend 3-4wk therapy (*IDCP 4:325, 1995*). If uncertain, do urine test for C. trachomatis and of N. gonorrhoeae.
Chronic bacterial	Enterobacteriaceae 80%, enterococci 15%, P. aeruginosa	**FQ: CIP** 500 mg po bid x 4wk, **Levo** 750 mg po bid x 4wk—see Comment	**TMP-SMX-DS** 1 tab po bid x 1–3mo	With treatment failures consider infected prostatic calculi. FDA approved dose of levo is 500 mg; editors prefer higher dose.
Chronic prostatitis/chronic pain syndrome (New NIH classification, *JAMA 282:236, 1999*)	The most common prostatitis syndrome. Etiology is unknown, molecular probe data suggest infectious etiology (*Clin Micro Rev 11: 604, 1998*)	**α-adrenergic blocking agents are controversial** (*AnIM 133:367, 2000*).		Pt has evidence of prostatis but negative cultures and no cells in prostatic secretions. Rev: *JAC 46:157, 2000*. In randomized double-blind study, CIP and an alpha-blocker of no benefit (*AnIM 141:581 & 639, 2004*).
HAND (*Bites: See Skin*)				
Paronychia				
Nail biting, manicuring	Staph. aureus (maybe MRSA)	Incision & drainage; do culture	**TMP-SMX-DS** 2 tabs po bid while waiting for culture result.	See Table 6 for alternatives
Contact with oral mucosa—dentists, anesthesiologists, wrestlers	Herpes simplex (Whitlow)	**Acyclovir** 400 mg tid x 10 days	**Famciclovir** or **valacyclovir** should work, see Comment	Gram stain and routine culture negative. Famciclovir/valacyclovir doses used for primary genital herpes should work; see Table 14, page 13?
Dishwasher (prolonged water immersion)	Candida sp.	**Clotrimazole** (topical)		Avoid immersion of hands in water as much as possible.

TABLE 1 (22)

ANATOMIC SITE/DIAGNOSIS/ MODIFYING CIRCUMSTANCES	ETIOLOGIES (usual)	SUGGESTED REGIMENS*		ADJUNCT DIAGNOSTIC OR THERAPEUTIC MEASURES AND COMMENTS
		PRIMARY	ALTERNATIVE[1]	
HEART				
Infective endocarditis—Native valve—empirical rx awaiting cultures—No IV illicit drugs Valvular or congenital heart disease including mitral valve prolapse but no modifying circumstances See Table 15C, page 171 for prophylaxis	NOTE: Diagnostic criteria include evidence of continuous bacteremia (multiple positive blood cultures), definite embolic event, and echocardiographic (transthoracic or transesophageal) evidence of valvular vegetations. Refs.: Table 15A, pg 167 Viridans strep 30-40%, "other" strep 15-25%, enterococci 5-18%, staphylococci 20-35%	[[Pen G 20 million units IV q24h, continuous drip or q4h) or (AMP 12 gm IV q24h, continuous drip or q4h)] + (nafcillin or oxacillin 2 gm IV q4h) + gentamicin 1 mg/kg IV q8h] or IV q8h (see Comment)	[(Vanco 15 mg/kg IV q12h (not to exceed 2 gm q24h unless serum levels monitored) + gentamicin 1 mg/kg[1] IM or IV q8h) OR dapto 6 mg/kg IV q24h]	If patient not acutely ill and not in heart failure, we prefer to wait for blood culture results. If initial 3 blood cultures neg, after 24-48 hrs, obtain 2-3 more blood cultures before empiric therapy started. Nafcillin/oxacillin + gentamicin may not be adequate coverage of enterococci, hence addition of penicillin G pending cultures. When blood cultures +, modify regimen from empiric to specific based on organism, in vitro susceptibility, clinical experience. **Gentamicin** used for synergy; peak levels need not exceed 4 mcg per mL.
Infective endocarditis—Native valve ± evidence rt-sided endocarditis—empiric therapy	S. aureus All others rare	Vanco 1 gm IV q12h	Dapto 6 mg/kg IV q24h Approved for right-sided endocarditis.	Quinupristin-dalfopristin cidal vs S. aureus if both constituents active. In controlled clinical trial, dapto equivalent to vanco plus 4 days of gentamicin for right-sided endocarditis. (NEJM 355:653, 2006).
Infective endocarditis—Native valve—culture positive (NEJM 345:1318, 2001; CID 36:615, 2003; JAC 54:971, 2004[2])	Viridans strep, S. bovis	[(Pen G 12-18 million units/day IV divided q4h x 4wk) OR (ceftriaxone IV 1g/kg q8h IV x2wks)] OR (Pen G 12-18 million units/day IV divided - q4h (ceftriaxone 2 gm IV q24h x 4wk)	(Ceftriaxone 2 gm IV q24h + gentamicin 1 mg per kg IV q24h x 2wks) - if allergy, Vanco 15 mg/kg IV q12h to 2 gm/day max unless serum levels measured x 4 weeks	Also effective: (ceftriaxone 2 gm q24h) + (netilmicin[N4] 4 mg/kg q24h) x2 wks (CID 21:1406, 1996). Target peak 3mcg/mL, trough <1 mcg/mL. If very obese pt, recommend consultation for dosage adjustment. Infuse vanco over 2.1 hr to avoid "red man" syndrome. **S. bovis suggests occult bowel pathology (New name: S. gallolyticus).** Since relapse rate may be greater in pts II for >3 mos, prior to start of rx, the penicillin-gentamicin synergism theoretically may be advantageous in **acidic IV fluids, rapid renal clearance and rising MICs (AAC 48:4463, 2004)**
Viridans strep, S. bovis, with penicillin G **MIC ≤0.1mcg/mL** Note: New name for S. bovis, biotype I is S. gallolyticus.				**Note:** Dropped option of continuous infusion of Pen G due to instability
Viridans strep, S. bovis, gallolyticus) with penicillin G **MIC >0.1 to <0.5mcg/mL**	Viridans strep, S. bovis, nutritionally variant streptococci (e.g. S. Abiotrophia) tolerant strep[3]	(Pen G 18 million units/day IV (divided q4h) x 4 wks PLUS gentamicin 1 mg/kg IV q8h x 2 wks NOTE: Low dose of gentamicin	Vanco 15 mg/kg IV q12h to max 2 gm/day unless serum levels documented x 4 wks	**Note:** IgE-mediated pen G in pt with allergy, that is not IgE-mediated (e.g., anaphylaxis). Alternatively, can use Vanco. (See Comment above on pen G and vanco.) **NOTE: If necessary to remove infected valve & valve culture neg., 2 weeks antibiotic treatment post-op sufficient (CID 41:1785, 2005).**
For viridans strep or S. bovis with **pen G MIC >0.5** and enterococci susceptible to AMP/pen G, vancomycin. NOTE: Int. Dis consultation suggested	For **Susceptible enterococci**—viridans strep, S. bovis, **nutritionally variant streptococci**. New names are: > Abiotrophia sp. & Granulicatella sp.[3]	(Pen G 18-30 million units per day IV, divided q4h x 4-6 wks) PLUS (gentamicin 1 mg/kg IV q8h x 4-6 wks) OR (ceftriaxone 2 gm/day IV, divided q4h + gent as above x 4-6 wks)	Vanco 15 mg/kg IV q12h to max of 2 gm/day unless serum levels measured PLUS gentamicin 1.5 - 1.5 mg/kg q8h x 4-6 wks NOTE: Low dose of gent	4 wks of rx if symptoms <3 mos.; 6 wks of rx if symptoms >3 mos. Vanco for pen-allergic pts; do not use cephalosporins. Do not give gent once-q24h for enterococcal endocarditis. Target gent levels: peak 3 mcg/mL, trough <1 mg/mL. Vanco target serum levels: peak 30-50 mcg/mL, trough <15 mcg/mL. **NOTE:** Because of ↑ frequency of resistance (see below), all enterococci causing endocarditis should be tested in vitro for susceptibility to penicillin, gentamicin and vancomycin plus β lactamase production.

[1] Assumes estimated creatinine clearance ≥80 mL per min, see Table 17.

[2] Ref. for Guidelines of British Soc. for Antimicrob. Chemother. Includes drugs not available in U.S.: flucloxacillin IV, teicoplanin IV. JAC 54:971, 2004.

[3] Tolerant streptococci = MBC 32-fold greater than MIC

Abbreviations on page 2.   NOTE: All dosage recommendations are for adults (unless otherwise indicated) and assume normal renal function.

TABLE 1 (23)

ANATOMIC SITE/DIAGNOSIS/ MODIFYING CIRCUMSTANCES	ETIOLOGIES (usual)	SUGGESTED REGIMENS*		ADJUNCT DIAGNOSTIC OR THERAPEUTIC MEASURES AND COMMENTS
		PRIMARY	ALTERNATIVE†	
HEART/Infective endocarditis—Native valve—culture positive (continued)				
Enterococci: MIC streptomycin >2000 mcg/mL, MIC gentamicin >500-2000 mcg/mL, no resistance to penicillin	Enterococci, high-level aminoglycoside resistance	Pen G or AMP IV as above **x 8-12 wks** (approx. 50% cure)	If prolonged rx or AMP fails, consider surgical removal of infected valve. See Comment	10-25% E. faecalis, and 45-50% E. faecium resistant to high-level gents. May be sensitive to streptomycin, check MIC. Case report of success with combination of AMP, IMP, and vanco (Scand J Inf Dis 29:628, 1997). Cure rate of 67% with IV AMP 2 gm q4h plus ceftriaxone 2 gm q12h x 6 wks (AnIM 146:574, 2007).
Enterococci, penicillin resistance β-lactamase production test is **positive & no gentamicin** resistance	Enterococci, penicillin resistance	AM-SB 3 gm IV q6h **PLUS gentamicin** 1-1.5 mg/kg q8h IV **x 4-6 wks.** **Low dose of gent**	AM-SB 3 gm IV q6h PLUS **vanco** 15 mg/kg IV q12h (check levels if >2 gm) **x 4-6 wks**	β-lactamase **not** detected by MIC tests with standard inocula. Detection requires testing with the chromogenic cephalosporin nitrocefin. Once-q24h **gentamicin rx not** efficacious in animal model of E. faecalis endocarditis (JAC 49:457, 2002)—hence give gent q8h.
Enterococci: β-lactamase test neg., pen G/ AMP resistance	Enterococci, intrinsic pen G/AMP resistance	**Vanco** 15 mg/kg IV q12h (check levels if >2 gm) **PLUS gent** 1-1.5 mg/kg IV q8h **x 4-6 wks**		Desired vanco serum levels: peak 20-50 mcg/mL, trough 5-12 mcg/mL. Gentamicin used for synergy; peak levels need not exceed 4 mcg/mL.
Enterococci: Pen/AMP resistant + high-level gent/strep resistant + vanco resistant; usually VRE Consultation suggested	Enterococci, vanco-resistant, usually E. faecium	No reliable effective rx. Can try quinupristin-dalfo-pristin (Synercid) or linezolid—see Comment, footnote¹ and Table 5	**Teicoplanin** active against a subset of vanco-resistant enterococci, but bacteriostatic. **Dapto** is an option.	Synercid activity limited to E. faecium and is usually bacteriostatic, therefore expect high relapse rate. Dose: 7.5 mg per kg IV (via central line) q8h. **Linezolid** active most enterococci, but bacteriostatic. Dose: 600 mg IV or po q12h. Linezolid failed in rx with E. faecalis endocarditis (CID 37:e29, 2003). **Dapto:** clinical experience in CID 41:1134, 2005.
Staphylococcal endocarditis **Aortic and/or mitral valve infection—MSSA**	Staph. aureus, methicillin-sensitive	**Nafcillin (oxacillin)** 2 gm IV q4h **x 4-6 wks PLUS gentamicin** 1 mg/kg IV q8h **x 3-5 days**	[**Cefazolin** 2 gm IV q8h x 4-6wk) PLUS gentamicin 1 mg/kg q8h x 3-5 days]. **Low dose of gent!** OR **Vanco** 15 mg/kg IV q12h (check levels if >2 gm per day] **x 4-6 wks**	If IgE-mediated penicillin allergy, 10% cross-reactivity to cephalosporins (AnIM 141:16, 2004). Cefazolin failures reported (CID 37:1194, 2003). With pen-allergic patient and positive skin test, desensitize or use vanco. For Staph. aureus endocarditis, pro-con review favor q8h dosing times no more than 3-5 days. At present, favor q8h dosing. vanco ± RIF (if sensitive) ↑ recognition of IV catheter-associated S. aureus endocarditis. May need TEE to detect vegetation (CID 115:106 & 115, 1999). If TEE neg, may only need 2 wks of therapy.
Aortic and or mitral valve—MRSA	Staph. aureus, methicillin-resistant	**Vanco** 1 gm IV q12h x 4-6 wks	**Dapto** for right-sided endocarditis	Daptomycin. Approved for Staphylococcus aureus bacteremia and in **right-sided** endocarditis based on randomized study (NEJM 355:653 & 727, 2006). **Note:** 1/3 of microbiological failures in dapto treated pts. Resistance developed during
Tricuspid valve infection (usually IVDUs): **MSSA**	Staph. aureus, methicillin-sensitive	**Nafcillin (oxacillin)** 2 gm IV q4h **PLUS gentamicin** 1 mg/kg IV q8h x 2 wks **NOTE: low dose of gent**	If **penicillin allergy:** use **vanco** gent 1 mg/kg IV q12h x 2 wks OR **Dapto** 6 mg/kg IV q24h (avoid if concomitant left-sided endocarditis)	Success with **4-week oral** regimen: CIP 750 mg bid + RIF 300 mg bid. Less than 10% pts had MRSA (LnI 2:1071, 1989; AJM 101:68, 1996). High failure rate with 2 wks of vanco + gentamicin (CID 33:120, 2001). Can try longer duration rx of **vanco ± RIF (if sensitive)**

---

¹ Three interesting recent reports: (1) Successful rx of vanco-resistant E. faecium endocarditis with Synercid without change in MIC (CID 25:163, 1997); (2) resistance to Synercid emerged during therapy of E. faecium bacteremia (CID 24:90, 1997); and (3) super-infection with E. faecalis occurred during Synercid rx of E. faecium (CID 24:91, 1997).

Abbreviations on page 2.   NOTE: All dosage recommendations are for adults (unless otherwise indicated) and assume normal renal function.

TABLE 1 (24)

ANATOMIC SITE/DIAGNOSIS/ MODIFYING CIRCUMSTANCES	ETIOLOGIES (usual)	SUGGESTED REGIMENS* PRIMARY	ALTERNATIVE†	ADJUNCT DIAGNOSTIC OR THERAPEUTIC MEASURES AND COMMENTS
HEART/Infective endocarditis—Native valve—culture positive (continued)				
Methicillin resistant (MRSA)	Staph. aureus, methicillin-resistant	**Vanco** 15 mg/kg IV q12h x 4-6 wks	**Dapto** 6 mg/kg IV q24h x 4-6wk (equiv to **vanco** for rt-sided endocarditis, both Daptv & dapto did poorly if lt-sided endocarditis (NEJM 355: 653, 2006). (See Comments & table 6, pg 73)	For MRSA, no difference in duration of bacteremia or fever between pts rx with vanco vs dapto (see JAC 58:273, 2006). Quinupristin-dalfopristin another option. See Table 6, page 23. **Linezolid:** Limited experience (see JAC 58:273, 2006) in patients with few treatment options; 64% cure rate; clear failure in 21%; thrombocytopenia in 31%.
Slow-growing fastidious Gm-neg. bacilli	HACEK group (see Comments). Change to HABCEK if add Bartonella	**Ceftriaxone** 2 gm IV q24h x 4 wks [Bartonella resistant — see below]	**Ceftriaxone** 2 gm IV q24h x 6 wks + **gentamicin** 1 mg/kg IV/IM q8h x 4 wks	HACEK (acronym for **H**aemophilus parainfluenzae, **H.** aphrophilus, **A**ctinobacillus, **C**ardiobacterium, **E**ikenella, **K**ingella). H. aphrophilus resistant to vanco, clinda and methicillin. Penicillinase-positive HACEK organisms should be susceptible to AM-SB + gentamicin.
Bartonella species Circ 111:3167, 2005	B. henselae, B. quintana	**Ceftriaxone** 2 gm IV q24h x 6 wks + **gentamicin** 1 mg/kg q8h x 14 days] + **doxy** 100 mg IV/po bid x 6 wks		**Doc:** Immunofluorescent antibody titer ≥1:800, blood cultures only occ. positive; or PCR of tissue from surgery. **Surgery:** Over ½ pts require valve surgery; relation to cure unclear. B. quintana transmitted by body lice among homeless; asymptomatic colonization of RBCs described (Ln 360:226, 2002).
Infective endocarditis—"culture negative" Fever, valvular disease, and ECHO vegetations ± emboli and neg. cultures. Rev. Medicine 84:162, 2005		Etiology in 348 cases studied by serology, culture, histopath, & molecular detection: C. burnetti 48%, Bartonella sp. 28%, and rarely (Abiotrophia elegans (nutritionally variant strep), Mycoplasma hominis, Legionella pneumophila, Tropheryma whipplei—together 1%), & rest without etiology identified (most on antibiotic). Ref: NEJM 356:715, 2007.		
Infective endocarditis—empiric therapy (cultures pending) S. aureus now most common etiology (NEJM 297:1354, 2007).				
Early (<2mo post-op)	S. epidermidis, S. aureus, Rarely, Enterobacteriaceae, diphtheroids, fungi.	**Vanco** 15 mg/kg IV q12h + **RIF** 300 mg po q8h + **gentamicin** 1 mg/kg IV q8h		**Vanco:** Surgical consultation advised especially if etiology is S. aureus, evidence of heart failure, presence of diabetes and/or renal failure, or concern for valve ring abscess (JAMA 297:1354, 2007; CID 44:364, 2007).
Late (>2mo post-op)	S. epidermidis, viridans strep, enterococci, S. aureus	**Vanco** 15 mg/kg IV q12h + **RIF** 300 mg po q8h x 6 wks + **gentamicin** 1 mg/kg IV q8h		
Infective endocarditis—Prosthetic valve—positive blood cultures	Staph. epidermidis	Methicillin sensitive: (**Nafcillin** 2 gm IV q12h + **RIF** 300 mg po q8h x 14 days. Methicillin resistant: (**Vanco** 1 gm IV q12h + **RIF** 300 mg po q8h x 6 wks + **gentamicin** 1 mg/kg IV q8h times 14 days. See effective endocarditis, native valve, culture positive, page 25		If S. epidermidis is susceptible to nafcillin/oxacillin, then substitute nafcillin (or oxacillin) for vanco
Surgical consultation advised; retrospective data analysis showed ↓ mortality if pts with S. aureus endocarditis if valve replaced during antibiotic rx (CID 26:1302 & 1310, 1998); also retrospective study showed ↑ risk of death 2° neuro events in assoc. with Coumadin rx (AMM 159:473, 1999)	Staph. aureus			
	Viridans strep, enterococci			
	Enterobacteriaceae or P. aeruginosa	Aminoglycoside (**tobra** if P. aeruginosa) + **Ceph 3 AP** or **P Ceph 4**		Early surgery for APAG, but no clinical data. In theory, could substitute CIP or FQ for APAG.
	Candida, aspergillus	**Ampho B** ± an azole, e.g. fluconazole (Table 11, page 96)		High mortality. Valve replacement plus antifungal therapy standard therapy but some success with antifungal therapy alone (CID 22:262, 1996).
Infective endocarditis—Q fever NEJM 356:715, 2007.	Coxiella burnetti	**Doxy** 100 mg po bid + **hydroxychloroquine** 600 mg/day x 1.5-3 yrs (if infection of native valve) x 5 yrs (if infection of prosthetic valve) Pregnancy: Need long term TMP-SMX (see CID 45:548, 2007)		**Dx:** Complement-fix or ELISA IgG antibody to phase I antigen diagnostic of acute Q fever. A titer of >1:200 to phase I antigen diagnostic of chronic infection (JCM 43:4038, 2005; 44:2283, 2006). Want doxy serum conc. >5 mcg/mL (JID 188:1322, 2003).

† Case report of dapto success: Heart & Lung 34:69, 2005.

* Abbreviations on page 2.

¹ All dosage recommendations are for adults (unless otherwise indicated) and assume normal renal function.

28

TABLE 1 (25)

ANATOMIC SITE/DIAGNOSIS/ MODIFYING CIRCUMSTANCES	ETIOLOGIES (usual)	SUGGESTED REGIMENS*		ADJUNCT DIAGNOSTIC OR THERAPEUTIC MEASURES AND COMMENTS
		PRIMARY	ALTERNATIVE†	
HEART *(continued)*				
Pacemaker/defibrillator infections	S. aureus, S. epidermidis, rarely others	Device removal + **vanco** 1 gm IV q12h + **RIF** 300 mg po bid	Device removal + **dapto** 6 mg per kg IV q24h**[NFL]** + **RIF** (no data)	**Duration of rx after device removal:** For "pocket" or subcutaneous infection, 10–14 days; if lead-assoc. endocarditis, 4–6 wks depending on organism. Refs.: *Circulation 108:2015, 2003; NEJM 350:1422, 2004*
Pericarditis, purulent— empiric therapy *Rev. Medicine 82:385, 2003*	Staph. aureus, Strep. pneumoniae, Group A strep, Enterobacteriaceae	**Vanco + CIP** (Dosage, see footnote¹)	**Vanco + CFP** (see footnote¹)	Drainage required if signs of tamponade. Forced to use empiric vanco due to high prevalence of MRSA.
Rheumatic fever with carditis *Ln 366:155, 2005*	Post-infectious sequelae of Group A strep infection (usually pharyngitis)	ASA, and usually prednisone 2 mg/kg po q24h for symptomatic treatment of fever, arthritis, arthralgia. May not influence carditis.		Clinical features: Carditis, polyarthritis, chorea, subcutaneous nodules, erythema marginatum. For Jones criteria: *Circulation 87:302, 1993. Prophylaxis: see page 54*
Ventricular assist device-related infection *Ref. LnID 6:426, 2006*	S. aureus, S. epidermidis, aerobic gm-neg bacilli, Candida sp	After culture of blood, wounds, drive line, device pocket and maybe pump. **Vanco** 1 gm IV q12h + **Clp** 400 mg IV q12h or **levo** 750 mg IV q24h) + **fluconazole** 800 mg IV q24h.		Can substitute **daptomycin** 6 mg/kg/d for **vanco**, **cefepime** 2 gm IV q12h for FQ, and (**vori, caspo, micafungin or anidulafungin**) for **fluconazole**
JOINT—Also see Lyme Disease, page 52				
Reactive arthritis (See Comment for definition)		Only treatment is non-steroidal anti-inflammatory drugs		Definition: Urethritis, conjunctivitis, arthritis, and sometimes uveitis and rash. Arthritis: asymmetrical oligoarthritis of ankles, knees, feet, sacroiliitis. Rash: palms and soles—keratoderma blennorrhagica; circinate balanitis of glans penis. HLA-B27 positive predisposes to Reiter's.
Reiter's syndrome	Occurs wks after infection with C. trachomatis, Campylobacter jejuni, Yersinia enterocolitica.			
Poststreptococcal reactive arthritis (See Rheumatic fever, above)	Immunologic reaction after strep pharyngitis: (1) arthritis onset in <10 days, (2) lasts months, (3) unresponsive to ASA	Treat strep pharyngitis and then NSAIDs (prednisone needed in some pts)		A reactive arthritis after a β-hemolytic strep infection in absence of sufficient Jones criteria for acute rheumatic fever. Ref.: *Mayo Clin Proc 75:144, 2000.*
Septic arthritis: Treatment requires both adequate drainage of purulent joint fluid and appropriate antimicrobial therapy. collection of blood and joint fluid for culture; review Gram stain of joint fluid. For full differential, see *Ln 351:197, 1998.*			**There is no need to inject antimicrobials into joints.** Empiric therapy after	
Infants <3mo (neonate)	Staph. aureus, Enterobacteriaceae, Gp B strep, N. gonorrhoeae	If MRSA no concern: **Nafcillin or oxacillin** +	If MRSA concern: **Vanco + P Ceph 3**	Blood cultures frequently positive. Adjacent bone involved in 2/3 pts. Group B strep and gonococci most common community-acquired etiologies.
		+ P Ceph 3 (Dosage, see Table 16, page 177)		
Children (3mo–14yr)	Staph. aureus 27%, S. pyogenes & Group A strep 14%, H. influenzae 3%, Gm-neg. bacilli 6%, other (GC, N. meningitidis) 14%, unknown 36%	**Vanco** + **P Ceph 3** (CFP 750 mg po bid or 400 mg IV q8h; See Table 16 for dosing) Steroids—see Comment		Marked ↓ in H. influenzae since use of conjugate vaccine. **NOTE:** Septic arthritis due to salmonella has no association with sickle cell disease, unlike salmonella osteomyelitis. Duration of treatment varies with specific microbial etiology. Short-course steroid: Benefit reported *(PIDJ 22:883, 2003)*

¹ **APAG** (see Table 10D, page 100), **IMP** 0.5 gm IV q6h, **MER** 1 gm IV q8h, **nafcillin** or **oxacillin** 2 gm IV q4h, **TC-CL** 3.1 gm IV q6h or 4.5 gm q8h, **AM-SB** 3 gm IV q6h, **PIP-TZ** 3.375 gm IV q6h or **P Ceph 1** (cephalothin 2 gm IV q4h or cefazolin 2 gm IV q8h), **CIP** 750 mg po bid or 400 mg IV q12h; **RIF** 600 mg po q24h, **aztreonam** 2 gm IV q8h; **CFP** 2 gm IV q12h

Abbreviations on page 2. NOTE: All dosage recommendations are for adults (unless otherwise indicated) and assume normal/renal function.

TABLE 1 (26)

ANATOMIC SITE/DIAGNOSIS/ MODIFYING CIRCUMSTANCES	ETIOLOGIES (usual)	SUGGESTED REGIMENS* PRIMARY	ALTERNATIVE†	ADJUNCT DIAGNOSTIC OR THERAPEUTIC MEASURES AND COMMENTS
JOINT/Septic arthritis (continued)				
Adults (review Gram stain): See page 52 for *Lyme Disease* and page — for gonococcal arthritis				
Acute monoarticular				
At risk for sexually-transmitted disease	**N. gonorrhoeae** (see page 20), S. aureus, streptococci, rarely aerobic Gm-neg. bacilli	**Gram stain negative:** **Ceftriaxone** 1 gm IV q24h or **cefotaxime** 1gm IV q8h or **ceftizoxime** 1 gm IV q8h	If Gram stain shows cocci in clusters use: **vanco** 1 gm IV q12h	For treatment comments, see *Disseminated GC, page 20*
Not at risk for sexually-transmitted disease	S. aureus, streptococci, Gm-neg bacilli	**All empiric choices guided by Gram stain** **Vanco − P Ceph 3** *For treatment duration, see Table 3, page 64* *For dosage, see footnote page 33* *See Table 2, Table 11, & Table 12*	[**Vanco − (CIP or Levo)**]	Differential includes gout and chondrocalcinosis (pseudogout). **Look for crystals in joint fluid.** **NOTE:** See Table 6 for MRSA treatment.
Chronic monoarticular	Brucella, nocardia, mycobacteria, fungi			If GC, usually associated petechiae and/or pustular skin lesions and tenosynovitis. Consider Lyme disease if exposure areas known to harbor infected ticks. *See page 52.*
Polyarticular, usually acute	**Gonococci** B. burgdorferi, acute rheumatic fever; viruses, e.g., hepatitis B, rubella vaccine, parvo B19	Gram stain usually negative for GC. If sexually active, culture urethra, cervix, anal canal, throat, blood, joint fluid, and then: **ceftriaxone** 1 gm IV q24h		Expanded differential incl gout, pseudogout, reactive arthritis (HLA-B27 pos.). Treat based on culture results x 14 days (assumes no foreign body present).
Septic arthritis, post intra-articular injection	MSSE/MRSE 40%, MSSA/MRSA 20%, P. aeruginosa, Propionibacteria	**NO empiric therapy.** Arthroscopy for culture/sensitivity, crystals, washout		
Infected prosthetic joint *CID 36:1157, 2003; JAC 53:127, 2004; NEJM 351:1645, 2004.* *See surgical options in Comments*	See below	**No empiric therapy.** Need culture & sens. results. Surgical options in comment.		**Surg. options: 1. 2-stage:** Remove infected prosthesis & leave spacer, anti-microbics, then new prosthesis. Highest cure rate (CID 42:216, 2006). **2. 1-stage:** Remove infected prosthesis, debride, new prosthesis, then antibiotics. **3. Extensive debridement & leave prosthesis in place during** antibiotic therapy; 53% failure rate, esp. if ≥8 of symptoms (CID 42:471, 2006). Other: Remove prosthesis & treat ± bone fusion of joint. Last option: debridement of chronic antimicrobial suppression. **RIF** combo highly successful vs staph—slow-growing, & biofilm-producing bacteria. Never use **RIF** alone due to rapid development of resistance (JAMA 279:1537, 1575, 1998). **RIF + Fusidic acid** another option (Cl.Micro.&Inf. 2(53):89, 2006). Limited linezolid experience is favorable (JAC 55:387, 2005). Watch for toxicity if over 2 wks of therapy, Table 10C, page 87. **Depto** experience IDCP 14:144, 2006. AAC 39:2423, 1995
	S. epidermidis - CoNS - S, A, B, or G, viridans strep	Debridement & prosthesis retention: **Pen G** or **ceftriax**) iv x 4 wks. Cured 17/19 pts (CID 36:847, 2003)	(**Dapto** IV + RIF PO) x6wk	
	MSSE/MSSA	(**Vanco** IV + RIF po) OR		
	MRSE/MRSA	(**Vanco** IV + RIF po) x 6 wks	(CIP or Levo—if susceptible—po) + (RIF po) OR (Dapto + RIF) x6wk	
Drug dosages in footnote[1]	P. aeruginosa	**Ceftaz** IV + (**CIP** or **Levo** po)	(**CIP** or **Levo**)	
For dental prophylaxis, see Table 15B				
Rheumatoid arthritis	TNF inhibitors (adalimumab, etanercept, infliximab) ↑ risk of TBc, fungal infection and malignancy (MMWR 53:683, 2004)			TNF inhibitors (adalimumab, etanercept, infliximab). Treat latent TBc first
Septic bursitis; Olecranon bursitis; prepatellar bursitis	Staph. aureus >80%, M. tuberculosis (rare), M. marinum (rare)	(**Nafcillin** or **oxacillin** 2 gm IV q4h or **dicloxacillin** 500 mg po qid) if MSSA *Other doses, see footnote page 33*	(**Vanco** 1 gm IV q12h or **linezolid** 600 mg po bid) if MRSA	**Initially aspirate q24h and treat for a minimum of 2-3 weeks.** Surgical excision of bursa should not be necessary if treated for at least 3 weeks. Ref.: *Semin Arth & Rheum 24:391, 1995.*

---

[1] **Aqueous Pen G** 2 million units IV q4h; **cefazolin** 1 gm IV q8h; **cefotaxime** 1 gm IV q8h; **ceftriaxone** 1 gm IV q24h; **nafcillin** or **oxacillin** 2 gm IV q4h; **vancomycin** 1 gm IV q12h; Daptomycin 6mg/kg IV q24h, **RIF** 300 mg IV/po bid; **CIP** 750 mg IV/po bid, **Levo** 750 mg IV/po qd). **Levo** 750 mg IV/po bid; **ceftazidime** 2 gm IV q8h

Abbreviations on page 2. NOTE: All dosage recommendations are for adults (unless otherwise indicated) and assume normal renal function.

TABLE 1 (27)

ANATOMIC SITE/DIAGNOSIS/ MODIFYING CIRCUMSTANCES	ETIOLOGIES (usual)	SUGGESTED REGIMENS* PRIMARY	SUGGESTED REGIMENS* ALTERNATIVE[†]	ADJUNCT DIAGNOSTIC OR THERAPEUTIC MEASURES AND COMMENTS
KIDNEY, BLADDER AND PROSTATE [For review, see AJM 113(Suppl 1A):1S, 2002 & NEJM 349:259, 2003]				
Acute uncomplicated urinary tract infection (cystitis-urethritis) in females [NOTE: Routine urine culture not necessary]	Enterobacteriaceae (E. coli) Staph. saprophyticus, enterococci	**Local E. coli resistant to TMP-SMX <20% & no allergy:** TMP-SMX-DS bid x 3 days. If sulfa allergy: **nitrofurantoin** 100 mg po bid x 5 days or **fosfomycin** 3 gm po x one dose	**Local E. coli resistant ≥20% or TMP-SMX allergy:** then 3 days of CIP 250 mg bid, **CIP-ER** 500 mg q24h, **Levo** 250 mg q24h OR **Moxi** 400 mg q24h OR **Nitrofurantoin** 100 mg bid OR single 3 gm dose of fosfomycin	self-rx works (AnIM 135:9, 2001)). Try to spare FQs (CID 39:75, 2004) 7-day rx recommended in pregnancy; [discontinue or do not use sulfonamides (TMP-SMX) near term (2 weeks before EDC) because of potential ↑ in kernicterus]. If failure on 3-day course, culture and rx 2 weeks. **Fosfomycin** 3 gm po times 1 less effective vs E. coli than multi-dose TMP-SMX or FQ (Med Lett 39:66, 1997). Fosfo active vs E. faecalis; poor activity vs other coliforms **Moxifloxacin & gemifloxacin:** Neither approved for UTIs. Moxi equivalent to comparator drugs in investigational clinical trials (on file with Bayer). **Phenazopyridine (Pyridium)** non-prescription OTC agent to relieve dysuria: 200 mg po tid times 2 days. Hemolysis if G6PD deficient
NOTE: Resistance of E. coli to TMP-SMX approx. 15–20% (CID 36:183, 2003) & correlates with microbiological clinical failure (CID 34:1061 & 1165, 2002). **Recent reports of E. coli resistant FQs as well.** 5-day nitrofurantoin ref: AnIM 167:2207, 2007				
Risk factors for STD Dipstick: positive leukocyte esterase or hemoglobin, neg. Gram stain	C. trachomatis	**Doxy** 100 mg po bid x 7 days	**Azithro** 1 gm po single dose	Pelvic exam for vaginitis & herpes simplex, urine LCR/PCR for GC and C. trachomatis
Recurrent (3 or more episodes/ year) in young women	Any of the above bacteria	Eradicate infection, then TMP-SMX po q24h long term	**TMP-SMX** 1 single-strength tab po q24h long term	A cost-effective alternative to continuous prophylaxis is self-administered single dose rx (TMP-SMX-DS, 2 tabs, 320/1600 mg) at symptom onset. Another alternative: 1 DS tablet TMP-SMX post-coitus.
Child: ≤5 yrs old & grade 3–4 reflux	Coliforms	TMP-SMX (2 mg TMP/10 mg SMX) per kg po q24h) or **nitrofurantoin** 2 mg per kg po q24h)		**CIP** approved as alternative drug ages 1–17 yrs.
Recurrent UTI in postmenopausal women	E. coli & other Enterobacteriaceae, enterococcus, S. saprophyticus	Treat as for uncomplicated UTI. Evaluate for potentially correctable urologic structural abnormalities. See Comment.		Definition: ≥3 culture + symptomatic UTIs in 1 year or 2 UTIs in 6 months. Urologic factors: (1) cystocele, (2) incontinence, (3) ↑ residual urine volume (250 mL).
See CID 30:152, 2000			**Nitrofurantoin** may be less effective than vaginal cream in decreasing frequency, but Editors worry about pulmonary fibrosis with long-term Nfr x (CID 36:1862, 2003)	
Acute uncomplicated pyelonephritis (usually women 18–40 yrs) with definite costovertebral tenderness) >102°F; definite costovertebral tenderness. Report of hemolyticuremic syndrome as result of toxin-producing E. coli UTI (NEJM 335:635, 1996). **If male, look for obstructive uropathy or other complicating pathology.**	Enterobacteriaceae (most likely E. coli), enterococcus (Gm stain of uncentrifuged urine may allow identification of Gm-neg. bacilli vs Gm+ cocci)	An **FQ** po times 7 days: **CIP** 500 mg bid or **CIP-ER** 1000 mg q24h, **Levo** 750 mg q24h, **Ofloxacin** 400 mg bid, **Moxi**[NEW] 400 mg q24h possibly ok—see comment	**AM-CL, DS Ceph.** or **TMP-SMX-DS** po. Treat for 14 days. Dosage as footnote as FQs (JAMA 293:949, 2005)	NOTE: Culture of urine and blood indicated prior to therapy. In randomized double-blind trial, bacteriologic and **clinical success higher for 7 days of CIP than for 14 days of TMP-SMX:** failures correlated with TMP-SMX in vitro resistance (JAMA 283:1583, 2000). **CIP** worked with 7 days of therapy for nosocomial pneumonia 4.5 gm IV q8h, **gentamicin** (see Table 10C, page 93) **Moxi** urine concentrations high (Internat J Antimicrob Agents 24:168, 2004). **Levo:** Alternative approved dose is 750 mg IV po x 5 days.
Moderately ill (outpatient) NOTE: May need one IV dose due to nausea				

[1] **AM-CL** 875/125 mg po q12h or 500/125 mg po tid or 2000/125 mg po bid, **aztreonam** 2 gm IV q8h, **FQ (IV) CIP** 400 mg IV q12h, **Levo** (250 mg or 500 mg IV q24h for mild uncomplicated disease, 750 mg IV q24h for hospital UTI), **CIP-ER** po dose 1000 mg q24h, **cefotan** 2 gm IV q8h, **P Ceph 3 cefotaxime** 1 gm IV q12h for uncomplicated infections, up to 2 gm IV q4h for life-threatening infections; **ceftriaxone** 1–2 gm IV q24h (use 2 gm/day under age 65)), **AP Pen (PIP** 3 gm IV q6h), **PIP-TZ** 3.375 gm IV q6h or for nosocomial pneumonia 4.5 gm IV q8h, **gentamicin** (see Table 10C, page 100), **TMP-SMX** 2.0 mg per kg (TMP) IV q6h, **P Ceph 3 AP (ceftazidime** 2 gm IV q8h), **P Ceph 4 (CFP** 2 gm IV q12h), **Dori** 500 mg IV q8h (1-hr infusion), **IMP** 0.5 gm IV q6h, **MER** 1 gm IV q8h, **Naticillin** or **oxacillin** 2 gm IV q4h, **Ceph 4** see active as FQs above. **Metronidazole** 500 mg po q8h or 15 mg per kg IV q12h (max. 4 gm per day). **Vanco** 1 gm IV q12h, **linezolid** 600 mg IV/po q12h

NOTE: All dosage recommendations are for adults (unless otherwise indicated) and assume normal renal function.

Abbreviations on page 2.

TABLE 1 (28)

ANATOMIC SITE/DIAGNOSIS/ MODIFYING CIRCUMSTANCES	ETIOLOGIES (usual)	SUGGESTED REGIMENS*		ADJUNCT DIAGNOSTIC OR THERAPEUTIC MEASURES AND COMMENTS
		PRIMARY	ALTERNATIVE†	
KIDNEY, BLADDER AND PROSTATE	**Acute uncomplicated pyelonephritis** (continued)			
Hospitalized	E. coli most common, enterococcus 2° in frequency	**FQ** (IV) or (**AMP** + **genta-micin**) or **Ceph 3** or **AP Pen.** Treat for 14 days. *Dosages in footnote 1 page 33* Do not use cephalosporins for suspect or proven enterococcal infection	**TC-CL** or **AM-SB** or **PIP-TZ** or **ERTA** or **Dori**. 500 mg q8h. Treat for 14 days.	Treat IV until pt afebrile 24–48 hrs, then complete 2-wk course with oral drugs (as Moderately ill, above). If no clinical improvement in 3 days, we recommend imaging. On CT, if single focal mass-like lesion, avg. response requires 6 days; if lesions diffuse, avg. response 13 days. (AJM 93:289, 1992) If pt hypotensive, prompt imaging (Echo or CT) is recommended to ensure absence of obstructive uropathy. NOTE: Cephalosporins & ertapenem not active vs enterococci.
Complicated UTI/catheters (Obstruction, reflux, azotemia, transplant, **Foley catheter-related, R/O obstruction**)	Enterobacteriaceae, P. aeruginosa, enterococci, rarely S. aureus (CID 42:46, 2006)	(**AMP** + **gent**) or **PIP-TZ** or **TC-CL** or **Dori** or **IMP** or **MER** for up to 2-3 wks	IV **FQ CIP Gati Levo** for up to 2-3 wks Switch to **FQ** or **TMP-SMX** when possible	Not all listed drugs predictably active vs enterococci or P. aeruginosa. **CIP** approved in children (1-17 yrs) as alternative. Not 1st choice secondary to ↑ increased incidence joint adverse effects. Peds dose: 6-10 mg/kg (400 mg max) IV q8h or 10-20 mg/kg (750 mg max) **po** q12h. **Levo:** FDA approved dose of 750 mg IV/po x 5 days
Asymptomatic bacteriuria. IDSA Guidelines CID 40:643, 2005			For dosages, see footnote 1 page 33	
Preschool children		Base regimen on C&S, not empirical		Diagnosis requires 10⁵ CFU per mL urine of same bacterial species in 2 specimens obtained 3-7 days apart.
Pregnancy	Aerobic Gm-neg bacilli & Staph. hemolyticus	Screen 1st trimester. If positive, rx 3-7 days with **amox**. **nitrofurantoin**. O **Ceph**, **TMP-SMX**, or **TMP** alone		Screen monthly for recurrence. Some authorities treat continuously until delivery (stop TMP-SMX 2 wks before EDC). ↑ resistance of E. coli to TMP-SMX
Before and after invasive uro-logic intervention, e.g., Foley catheter	Aerobic Gm-neg bacilli	Obtain urine culture and then rx 3 days with TMP-SMX DS, bid		In one study, single dose 2.1 TMP-SMX DS 80% effective (AJM 114:713, 1991). Clinical benefit of antimicrobial-coated Foley catheters is uncertain (AnIM 144:116, 2006).
Neurogenic bladder – see "spinal cord injury" below		No therapy in asymptomatic patient; intermittent catheterization if possible		Ref: AJM 113(1A):67S, 2002 – Bacteriuria in spinal cord injured patient
Asymptomatic, advanced age, male or female Ref: CID 40:643, 2005		No therapy indicated unless in conjunction with surgery to correct obstructive uropathy; measure residual urine vol. in females; prostate exam/PSA in males.		
Malacoplakia	E. coli	**Bethanechol chloride** + (**CIP** or **TMP-SMX**)		Chronic pyelo with abnormal inflammatory response. See CID 29:444, 1999
Perinephric abscess				
Associated with staphylococcal bacteremia	Staph. aureus	If **MSSA**, **Nafcillin/ oxacillin** or **cefazolin** (Dosage, see footnote page 29)	If **MRSA: Vanco** 1 gm IV q12h OR **dapto** 6 mg/kg IV q24h	Drainage, surgical or image-guided aspiration.
Associated with pyelonephritis	Enterobacteriaceae	See pyelonephritis, complicated UTI above		Drainage, surgical or image-guided aspiration
Prostatitis		See prostatitis, page 24		
Spinal cord injury pts with UTI	E. coli, Klebsiella sp., enterococci	**CIP** 250 mg po bid x 14 days		If fever, suspect assoc. pyelonephritis. Microbiologic cure greater after 14 vs 3 days of CIP (CID 39:658 & 665, 2004). For asymptomatic bacteriuria see AJM 113(1A):67S, 2002.
LIVER *(for spontaneous bacterial peritonitis, see page 42)*				
Cholangitis		See Gallbladder, page 14		
Cirrhosis & variceal bleeding	Esophageal flora	(**Norfloxacin** 400 mg po bid or **CIP** 400 mg IV q12h) daily for max. of 7 days	**Ceftriaxone** 1 gm IV once daily for max. of 7 days	Short term prophylactic antibiotics in cirrhotics with G-I hemorr, with or without ascites, decreases rate of bacterial infection & ↑s survival (Hepatology 46:922, 2007).

Abbreviations on page 2.   NOTE: All dosage recommendations are for adults (unless otherwise indicated) and assume normal renal function.

TABLE 1 (29)

ANATOMIC SITE/DIAGNOSIS/ MODIFYING CIRCUMSTANCES	ETIOLOGIES (usual)	SUGGESTED REGIMENS* PRIMARY	ALTERNATIVE†	ADJUNCT DIAGNOSTIC OR THERAPEUTIC MEASURES AND COMMENTS
LIVER (continued)				
Hepatic abscess Pyogenic abscess ref.: CID 39:1654, 2004	Enterobacteriaceae (esp. Klebsiella sp.), bacteroides, enterococci, Entamoeba histolytica, Yersinia entero-colitica (rare) For echinococcus, see Table 13, page 125. For cat-scratch disease (CSD), see pages 41 & 51.	Metro + (ceftriaxone or cefotax OR TC-CL or PIP-TZ or AM-SB or CIP or levo. (Dosage, see footnote page 33) AMP + aminoglycoside + metro traditional & effective. If AMP-resistant Gm-neg. bacilli ↑ and aminoglycoside toxicity an issue	Metro (for amoeba) + either IMP, MER or Dori (Dosage, see footnote page 33)	**Serological tests for amebiasis should be done on all patients;** if neg. surgical drainage or percutaneous aspiration. In pyogenic abscess, ½ have identifiable GI source or underlying biliary tract disease. If amoeba serology positive, treat with **metro** alone without surgery. Empiric **metro** included for both E. histolytica & bacteroides. **Hemochromatosis** associated with Yersinia enterocolitica liver abscess (CID 18:938, 1994). Regimens listed are effective for yersinia. Klebsiella pneumoniae genotype K1 associated ocular & CNS Klebsiella infections (CID 45:284, 2007).
Leptospirosis	Leptospirosis, see page 53			
Peliosis hepatitis in AIDS pts	Bartonella henselae and B. quintana	See page 51		
Post-transplant infected "biloma" (CID 39:517, 2004)	Enterococci (incl. VRE), candi-da, Gm-neg. bacilli (P. aeru-ginosa 8%), anaerobes 5%	Linezolid 600 mg IV bid + CIP 400 mg IV q12h	Dapto 6 mg/kg per day + Levo 750 mg IV q24h + fluconazole 400 mg IV q24h	Suspect if fever & abdominal pain post-transplant. Exclude hepatic artery throm-bosis. Presence of candida and/or VRE have bad prognosticators.
Viral hepatitis	Hepatitis A, B, C, D, E, G	See Table 14, page 136		

NOTE: bid = twice a day, tid = 3 times a day, qid = 4 times a day.

LUNG/Bronchi

Bronchiolitis/wheezy bronchitis (expiratory wheezing)				
Infants/children (≤ age 5) See RSV, Table 14B page 150 Ref.: Ln 368:312, 2006	**Respiratory syncytial virus** (RSV) 50%, parainfluenza 25%, human metapneumovirus	Antibiotics not useful, mainstay of therapy is oxygen. Riba-virin for severe disease: 6 gm vial (20 mg/mL) in sterile H2O by SPAG-2 generator over 18-20 hrs daily times 3-5 days.		RSV most important. Rapid diagnosis with antigen detection methods. For prevention a humanized mouse monoclonal antibody, **palivizumab**. See Table 14, page 150. RSV immune globulin IV no longer available. Review Red Book of Peds 2006, 27th Ed.
Bronchitis				
Infants/children (≤ age 5)	< Age 2: Adenovirus, age 2-5: Respiratory syncytial virus/parainfluenza 3 virus, human metapneumovirus	Antibiotics not indicated	Antibiotics not indicated Antitussive ± inhaled bronchodilators	RSV most important in < 1 yr of age
Adolescents and adults with acute tracheobronchitis (Acute bronchitis) Ref.: NEJM 355:2125, 2006	Usually viral: M. pneumoniae 5%, C. pneumoniae 5%. See Persistent cough, below			M. pneumoniae & C. pneumoniae ref. LnID 1:334, 2001. Rare pt with the C. pneumo infection may require 6 wks of clarithro to clear organism (J Med Micro 52:265, 2003)
Persistent cough (>14 d.), afebrile during community outbreak: Pertussis (whooping cough) 10-20% adults with cough >14 d. have pertussis (MMWR 54 (RR-14), 2005) Review: Chest 130:547, 2006	Bordetella pertussis & occ. Bordetella parapertussis. Also consider asthma, gastroesophageal reflux, post-nasal drip	**Peds doses:** Azithro/clarithro po OR erythro estolate OR erythro base OR TMP-SMX (doses in footnote[*] page 33)	**Adult doses:** Azithro 500 mg/day	250 mg q24h days 2-5 OR erythro estolate 500 mg po qid times 14 days OR TMP-SMX-DS 1 tab po bid times 14 days OR clarithro 500 mg po bid or 1 gm ER q24h times 7 days)	**3 stages of illness:** catarrhal (1-2 wks), paroxysmal coughing (2-4 wks), and convalescence (1-2 wks). Treatment may abort or eliminate pertussis in catarrhal stage, but does not shorten paroxysmal stage. **Diagnosis:** PCR on nasopharyngeal secretions or 1 pertussis-toxin antibody. **Azithro** works best (PIDJ 22:847, 2003). Hypertrophic pyloric stenosis reported in infants under 6 wks of age given erythro (MMWR 48:1117, 1999).

Abbreviations on page 2.   NOTE: All dosage recommendations are for adults (unless otherwise indicated) and assume normal renal function.

TABLE 1 (30)

ANATOMIC SITE/DIAGNOSIS/ MODIFYING CIRCUMSTANCES	ETIOLOGIES (usual)	SUGGESTED REGIMENS*		ADJUNCT DIAGNOSTIC OR THERAPEUTIC MEASURES AND COMMENTS
		PRIMARY	ALTERNATIVE[1]	
LUNG/Bronchi/Bronchitis/Persistent cough (continued)				
Prophylaxis of household contacts		Drugs and doses as per treatment immediately above		Recommended by Am. Acad. Ped. Red Book 2006 for all household or close contacts; community-wide prophylaxis not recommended.
Acute bacterial exacerbation of chronic bronchitis (ABECB), adults (almost always smokers with COPD). Pertinent refs.: Chest 118: 193, 2000; NEJM 347:465, 2002: CID 39:980 & 987, 2004; AnIM 165:891, 2005; Thorax 61:535, 2006	Viruses 20–50%. C. pneumoniae 5%, M. pneumoniae <1%; role of S. pneumo, H. influenzae, M. catarrhalis controversial. Tobacco use, air pollution contribute. Non-pathogenic H. haemophilus may be mistaken for H. influenza (JID 195:81, 2007).	Severe ABECB: ↑ dyspnea, ↑ sputum viscosity/purulence, &/or low O₂ sat.; (2) inhaled anticholinergic bronchdilator; (3) oral corticosteroid; (4) non-invasive positive pressure ventilation. **For mild or moderate disease, no antimicrobial treatment** or (Doxy, amox, TMP-SMX, or O Ceph). **For severe disease,** AM-CL, azithro/clarithro, or O Ceph or Moxi). Placebo-controlled studies: Pul Pharm & Therap 14:449, 2001; In 358:2020, 2001.	**Role of antimicrobial therapy debated even for severe disease. For mild or moderate disease, no antimicrobial treatment** or (Doxy, amox, TMP-SMX, or O Ceph). **For severe disease,** AM-CL, azithro/clarithro, or O Ceph or Moxi).	↑ sputum volume. For severe ABECB: (1) consider chest x-ray, esp. if febrile &/or tobacco use; **Drugs & doses in footnote[1]. Duration** varies with drug, range 3–10 d. Limit Gemi to 5 d to decrease risk of rash
Fever, cough, myalgia during influenza season	Influenza A & B	Oseltamivir 75 mg po bid x 5 d (see Table 14A)		**Complications: Influenza pneumonia, secondary bacterial pneumonia** (S. pneumo, S. aureus, S. pyogenes, H. influenzae). S. aureus TSS. Ref: LnID 6:296, 2006.
Bronchiectasis. Ref: NEJM 346:1383, 2002	H. influ, P. aeruginosa, and rarely S. pneumo.	Gemi, levo, or moxi x 7-10 d		Many potential etiologies: obstruction, ↓ immune globulins, cystic fibrosis, dyskinetic cilia, tobacco, prior severe or recurrent necrotizing bronchitis; e.g. pertussis.
Acute exacerbation				
Prevention	Not applicable	One option: **Erythro** 500 mg po bid or **azithro** 250 mg q24h x 8 wks (JAMA 290:1749, 2003; Eur Resp J 13:361, 1999)		
Specific organisms	Aspergillus (see Table 11) MAI (Table 12) and P. aeruginosa (Table 5)			
Pneumonia				
Neonatal: Birth to 1 month	Viruses: CMV, rubella, H. simplex. Bacteria: Group B strep, listeria, coliforms, S. aureus, P. aeruginosa. Other: Chlamydia trachomatis, syphilis	**AMP + gentamicin ± cefotaxime** Add **vanco** if MRSA a concern. For chlamydia therapy, **erythro** 12.5 mg per kg po or IV qid times 14 days.		Blood cultures indicated. Consider C. trachomatis if afebrile pneumonia, staccato cough. IgM > 1:8: therapy with erythro or sulfisoxazole. If MRSA documented, **vanco.** **TMP-SMX, linezolid** alternatives. **Linezolid** dosage birth to age 11 yrs is **10 mg per kg q8h.** Ref: PIDJ 22(Suppl.):S158, 2003.

[1] **TMP-SMX adult:** 1 double-strength tab (160 mg TMP) po bid; **peds** (>6 mo of age) 8 mg/kg/d TMP component, div bid x 14 d. **doxy** 100 mg po bid, **amox** 500 mg po tid, **AM-CL** 875/125 mg po bid or 500/125 mg po tid or 2000/125 mg po bid, adult dose cfb of 500 mg CD (extended release) po q12h; **cefdiforen** 200 mg q8h or 400 mg po q24h; **cefixime** 400 mg po q24h, **cefpodoxime proxetil** 200 mg po q12h; **cefprozil** 500 mg po q12h; **loracarbef** 400 mg po q12h; **cefbuten** 400 mg po q24h; **cefuroxime axetil** 250 or 500 mg po q12h; **cefdinir** 300 mg q12h or 600 mg q24h; **azithro** 500 mg po initial dose then 250 mg q24h times 4 or 500 mg po q24h times 3 days; **clarithro** 500 mg po q12h or **clarithro ER** 1000 mg po q24h times 7 days; **clarithromycin** 500 mg po bid; **erythro base** 8 mg/kg/d po div q6h x 14 d; **Oflox** 400 mg po bid; **CIP** 750 mg po q12h, **Levo** 500 mg po q24h times 5 days, **Moxi** 400 mg po q24h. **Peds oral doses: Azithro** 10 mg/kg/d on day1, then 5 mg/kg q24h x 4 days; **clarithro** 7.5 mg/kg po q12h times 5-7 days; **erythro estolate** 40 mg/kg/d divided q8-12h times 14 days, **erythro base** 40 mg/kg/d divided q6h times 14 days.

NOTE: CIP and cefbuten have relatively poor in vitro activity vs S. pneumo.

NOTE: All dosage recommendations are for adults (unless otherwise indicated) and assume normal renal function.

Abbreviations on page 2.

TABLE 1 (31)

ANATOMIC SITE/DIAGNOSIS/ MODIFYING CIRCUMSTANCES	ETIOLOGIES (usual)	SUGGESTED REGIMENS*		ADJUNCT DIAGNOSTIC OR THERAPEUTIC MEASURES AND COMMENTS
		PRIMARY	ALTERNATIVE†	
LUNG/Bronchi/Pneumonia (continued)				
CONSIDER TUBERCULOSIS IN ALL PATIENTS; ISOLATE ALL SUSPECT PATIENTS				
Age 1–3 months (Adapted from NEJM 346:429, 2002)				
Pneumonia syndrome. Usually afebrile	C: trachomatis, RSV, parainfluenza virus 3, human metapneumovirus, S. pneumoniae, Bordetella (rare), S. aureus (rare)	**erythro** 12.5 mg/kg q6h x 14 days or po **azithro** 10 mg/kg x dose, then 5 mg/kg x 4 days.	**Inpatient: If afebrile erythro** 10 mg/kg IV q6h or po **azithro** 2.5 mg/kg IV q12h (see Comment). **If febrile, add cefotaxime** 200 mg/kg per day div q8h	Pneumonitis syndrome: cough, tachypnea, dyspnea, diffuse infiltrates, afebrile. Usually requires hospital care. Reports of hypertrophic pyloric stenosis after erythro under age 6 wks; not sure about azithro; bid azithro dosing theoretically might ↓ risk of hypertrophic pyloric stenosis. If lobar pneumonia, give AMP 200–300 mg per kg per day for S. pneumoniae. No empiric coverage for S. aureus, as it is rare etiology.
			For RSV, see Bronchiolitis, page 32	
Age 4 months–5 years For RSV, see bronchiolitis, page 32, & Table 14 Refs: NEJM 346:429, 2002; LnID 364:1141, 2004	RSV, human metapneumovirus, other resp. viruses, S. pneumo, H. flu, mycoplasma, S. aureus (rare), M. tb.	**Outpatient: Amox** 100 mg/kg/day div q8h. **Inpatient (not ICU):** No antibiotic if viral or IV **AMP** 200 mg/kg per day div q6h	**Inpatient (ICU): Cefotaxime** 200 mg per kg per day IV div q8h or **ceftriaxone** 50–75 mg per kg per day IV once per day	Common 'other' viruses: rhinovirus, influenza, parainfluenza, adenovirus (PIDJ 19:293, 2000). Often of mild to moderate severity. S. pneumo, non-type B H. flu in 4–20%. Treat for 10–14 days. NOTE: High frequency of resistance of DRSP to cefuroxime. See Table 5, page 71, for treatment of drug-resistant S. pneumo.
Age 5 years–15 years, Non-hospitalized, immunocompetent NEJM 346:429, 2002; PIDJ 21:592, 2002	Mycoplasma, Chlamydophilia pneumoniae, S. pneumoniae, S. pneumoniae, Mycobacterium tuberculosis Respiratory viruses: mixed, e.g. influenza Bacterial/viral infection in 23% (Peds 113:701, 2004) Legionella (especially in pts with malignancy) Ln Inf Dis 6:529, 2006	[**Amox** (100mg/kg per day) + (**Clarithro** 500mg po bid or **erythro** 500 mg po qid (if ≥8 yrs old) or **azithro** 10 mg/kg po x1, then 0.5 gm po x1, then 0.25 gm/day. Peds dose 10mg/kg, then 5mg/kg per day, max. 250 mg]	[**Amox** (100mg/kg per day) + (**Doxy** 100 mg bid (if ≥8 yrs old) or **erythro** 500 mg qid. (Peds dose: 10 mg/kg q6h)]	If otherwise healthy and not concomitant with (or post-) influenza, S. pneumo & S. aureus uncommon in this subset; suspect S. pneumo if sudden onset and large amount of purulent sputum. **Macrolide-resistant S. pneumo** an issue. Higher prevalence of macrolide-resistant S. pneumo in pts <5 yrs old (JAMA 286:1857, 2001). Mycoplasma PCR/viral culture usually not done for outpatients. **Mycoplasma requires 2–3 wks of therapy.** C. pneumoniae up to 6 wks. (LnID 1:334, 2001; J Med Micro 52:265, 2003). Macrolide-resistant M. pneumo reported (AAC 50:709, 2006). Linezolid approved for peds use for pen-susceptible & multi-drug resistant S. pneumo (including bacteremia) & methicillin-sensitive S. aureus.
Children, hospitalized, immunocompetent– 2–18 yrs	S. pneumoniae, viruses, mycoplasma, consider S. aureus if abscesses or necrotizing, esp. during influenza season	**See Comment regarding macrolide resistance** **Ceftriaxone** 50 mg per kg per day IV (to max. 2 gm per day) + **azithro** 10 mg per kg per day IV div q12h.		**Alternatives are a problem in children:** If proven S. pneumo resistant to azithro & ceftriaxone (or severe ceftriaxone allergy): IV vanco, linezolid, or off-label respiratory-FQ. No doxy under age 8. Linezolid reported efficacious in children (PIDJ 22:677, 2003). Cefuroxime failures vs drug-resistant S. pneumo (CID 29:462, 1999).

Ceftriaxone... **vanco** 40mg/kg/day divided q6h.

NOTE: All dosage recommendations are for adults (unless otherwise indicated) and assume normal renal function.

TABLE 1 (32)

ANATOMIC SITE/DIAGNOSIS/ MODIFYING CIRCUMSTANCES	ETIOLOGIES (usual)	SUGGESTED REGIMENS*		ADJUNCT DIAGNOSTIC OR THERAPEUTIC MEASURES AND COMMENTS
		PRIMARY	ALTERNATIVE†	
LUNG/Bronchi/Pneumonia (continued)				
Adults (over age 18)—IDSA/ATS Guideline for CAP in adults: CID 44 (Suppl 2): S27, 2007.				**Azithro/clarithro:** Pro: appropriate spectrum of activity more in vitro resistance than clinical failure (Chest 131:1205, 2007). If pen G resist S. pneumo, up to 50%+ resistance to azithro/clarithro. Influence of prior macrolide use on macrolide resistance S. pneumo (CID 40:1288, 2005).
Prognosis prediction: CURB-65 (AnIM 118:384, 2005):	**Community-acquired, not hospitalized**			
C: confusion = 1 pt	Varies with clinical setting.	**No co-morbidity:**	**No co-morbidity:**	
U: BUN >19 mg/dl = 1 pt	**No co-morbidity:** Atypicals—M. pneumoniae, et al.,"S. pneumo, viral	Azithro 0.5 gm po times 1 then 0.25 gm po times 4	**Respiratory FQ** (see footnote¹)	
R: RR >30 /min = 1 pt		**OR** clarithro 500 mg po bid	OR	
B: BP <90/60 = 1 pt	**Co-morbidity present:** (DM, COPD, liver, renal, CHF)	OR clarithro-ER 1 gm po q24h	**(azithro or clarithro) + (high dose amox, high dose AM-CL, or cefdinir, cefpodoxime, or cefprozil)**	**Amoxicillin:** Pro: Active 90–95% S. pneumo at 3-4 gm per day Con: No activity vs atypicals or β-lactamase + H. influenzae. Need 3-4 gm per day
Age ≥65 = 1 pt			OR	
If score = 1, ok for outpatient therapy; if >1, hospitalize. The higher the score, the higher the mortality.	Alcoholism: S. pneumo, anaerobes, coliforms Bronchiectasis incl. Cystic fibrosis, page 39 COPD: H. influenzae, M. catarrhalis, S. pneumo IVDU: Hematogenous S. aureus Post-CVA aspiration: Oral flora incl. S. pneumo, anaerobes Post-influenza: S. pneumo and S. aureus	If prior antibiotic within 3 months: **azithro or clarithro + (amox 1 gm or AM-CL)** or **Respiratory FQ**	**telithromycin—see comment, page 36** Doses in footnote³	**AM-CL:** Pro: Spectrum of activity includes β-lactamases + H. influenzae, M. catarrhalis, MSSA, & Bacteroides sp. Con: No activity atypicals
		Duration of rx:		**Cephalosporins**—Cefditoren, cefpodoxime, cefprozil, cefuroxime & others—see footnote³
		S. pneumo—Not bacteremic: until afebrile 3 days		Pro: Active 75–85% S. pneumo & H. influenzae. Cefuroxime least active & higher mortality rate when S. pneumo resistant (CID 37:230, 2003)
		—Bacteremic: 10-14 days reasonable		Con: Inactive vs atypical pathogens
		C. pneumoniae—Unclear. Some reports suggest 21 days. Some bronchitis pts required 5–6 wks of clarithro (J Med Micro 52:265, 2003)		**Doxycycline:** Pro: Active vs S. pneumo & H. influenzae, atypicals, & bioterrorism agents (anthrax, plague, tularemia)
		Legionella—10-21 days		Con: Resistance of S. pneumo 18–20% (CID 35:633, 2002). Sparse clinical data (AnIM 159: 266, 1999; CID 37:870, 2003).
		Necrotizing pneumonia 2° to coliforms, S. aureus, S. aureus: ≥2 weeks		**FQs—Respiratory FQs:** Moxi, levo & gemi Pro: In vitro & clinically effective vs pen-resistant & pen-sensitive S. pneumo. Gemi only available po
		Cautions: 1. If local macrolide resistance to S. pneumoniae >25%, use alternative empiric therapy.		**NOTE: dose of Levi is 750 mg q24h.** Q24h dosing.
		2. Esp. during influenza season, look for S. aureus.		Con: Geographic pockets of resistance with clinical failure (NEJM 346:747, 2002). Important drug-drug interactions (see Table 22A, page 198). Reversible rash in young females given Gemi for >7 days.
Community-acquired—NOT in the ICU	Etiology by co-morbidity & risk factors as above Culture sputum & blood (Legionella urinary antigen indicated). In general, the sicker the pt, the more valuable culture data. Look for S. aureus.	**Ceftriaxone** 1 gm IV q24h + **azithro** 500 mg IV	**Levo** 750 mg IV q24h or **Moxi** 400 mg IV q24h	**Ceftriaxone/cefotaxime:**
Treat for minimum of 5 days, afebrile for 48-72 hrs, with stable BP, adequate oral intake, and room air O₂ saturation >90%. (COID 20:177, 2007).		OR	**Gati** 400 mg IV q24h (gati no longer marketed in US due to hypo- and hyperglycemic reactions)	Pro: Drugs of choice for pen-sens. S. pneumo, active H. influenzae, M. catarrhalis, & MSSA
		Ertapenem 1 gm q24h plus **azithro** 500 mg IV	No rigid time window for first dose; if in ER, first dose in ER. OK for admitting diagnosis of "uncertain." (Chest 130:16, 2006).	Con: Not active atypicals or pneumonia due to bioterrorism pathogens. Add macrolide vs atypicals and perhaps their anti-inflammatory activity.

---

¹ Atypical pathogens: Chlamydophila pneumoniae, C. psittaci, Legionella sp., M. pneumoniae, C. burnetii (Q fever) (Ref: LnID 3:709, 2003)

² Respiratory FQs with enhanced activity vs S. pneumo with HLR to penicillin in US due to hypo- and hyperglycemic reactions), **Gemi** 320 mg po q24h, **Levo** 750 mg IV/po q24h. **Moxi** 400 mg IV/po q24h. Ketoralide: **telithro** 800 mg po q24h (physicians warned about rare instances of hepatotoxicity).

³ **O Ceph dosage: Cefdinir** 300 mg po q12h; **cefditoren pivoxil** 200 mg, 2 tabs po bid; **cefpodoxime proxetil** 200 mg po q12h; **high dose amox** 1 gm po tid; **high dose cefprozil** 500 mg po q12h. **AM-CL—use AM-CL-ER** 1000/62.5 mg, 2 tabs po bid; **telithromycin** 800 mg po q24h times 7-10 days.

Abbreviations on page 2.   *NOTE: All dosage recommendations are for adults (unless otherwise indicated) and assume normal renal function.*

TABLE 1 (33)

ANATOMIC SITE/DIAGNOSIS/ MODIFYING CIRCUMSTANCES	ETIOLOGIES (usual)	SUGGESTED REGIMENS* PRIMARY	ALTERNATIVE†	ADJUNCT DIAGNOSTIC OR THERAPEUTIC MEASURES AND COMMENTS
LUNG/Bronchi/Pneumonia/Adults (over age 18) *(continued)*				
Community-acquired, hospitalized—IN ICU Empiric therapy NOTE: Not all ICU admissions meet DSSATS CAP Guideline criteria for severe CAP. Do not believe that all ICU pneumonia patients need 2 drugs with activity vs. gram-negative bacilli. 4 example clinical settings are outlined.	Severe COPD pt with pneumonia: *S. pneumoniae*, *H. influenzae*, *Moraxella* sp., *Legionella* sp. Rarely *S. aureus*. Culture sputum, blood and maybe pleural fluid. Look for respiratory viruses. Urine antigen for *Legionella* and *S. pneumoniae*. Sputum PCR for *Legionella*.	Levo 750 mg IV q24h or Moxi 400 mg IV q24h	(Ceftriaxone 1 gm IV q24h + azithro 500 mg IV q24h) + ERTA 1 gm IV q24h + azithro 500 mg IV q24h (see Comment)	**Telithromycin:** *Pro:* Virtually no resistant *S. pneumo*. Active vs atypical pathogens (*Antim* 24:4-15, 2006; *NEJM* 355:2260, 2006). *Con:* Concern of severe hepatotoxicity (*Ann* 144:415, 2006). Only advisable po. Transient reversible blurry vision due to paralysis of lens accommodation; avoid in myasthenia gravis pts **(Black Box Warning)**. **Various studies** indicate improved outcome when azithro added to a β-lactam (*CID* 36:389 & 1239, 2003; *AnM* 164:1837, 2001 & 159:2562, 1999). Similar results in prospective study of critically ill pts with pneumococcal bacteremia (*CID* 36:170-440, 2004).
			Addition of a macrolide to beta-lactam lowers mortality for patients with bacteremic pneumococcal pneumonia (*CID* 36:389, 2003). Benefit NOT found with use of FQ or tetracycline in "atypicals" (*Chest* 131:466, 2007). Combination therapy benefited patients with concomitant "shock." (*CCM* 35:1493 & 1617, 2007).	**Ertapenem** could substitute for ceftriaxone; need azithro for atypical pathogens. Do not use if suspect *P. aeruginosa*. **Legionella:** Not all *Legionella* species detected by urine antigen; if suspicious culture or PCR on airway secretions. In patients with normal sinus rhythm and not receiving beta-blockers, relative bradycardia suggests *Legionella*, psittacosis, Q-fever, or typhoid fever (*Clin Micro Infect* 6:633, 2000).
Community-acquired, hospitalized—IN ICU Empiric therapy	**if concomitant with or post-influenza** *S. aureus* and *S. pneumoniae* possible.	Vanco 1 gm IV q12h + (Levo 750 mg IV q24h or moxi 400 mg IV q24h)	Linezolid 600 mg IV bid + (levo or moxi)	At risk for gm-neg rod pneumonia due to: alcoholism with necrotizing pneumonia, underlying chronic bronchiectasis (e.g. cystic fibrosis), chronic tracheostomy and/or mechanical ventilation, febrile neutropenia and pulmonary infiltrates, septic shock, underlying malignancy, or organ failure.
Community-acquired, hospitalized—IN ICU Empiric therapy NOTE: Not all ICU admissions meet DSSATS CAP Guideline criteria for severe CAP. Do not believe that all ICU pneumonia patients need 2 days with activity vs. gram-negative bacilli. Hence. 4 example clinical settings are outlined.	Suspect aerobic gm-neg bacilli incl *P. aeruginosa* and/or life-threatening infection (see comment). Hypoxic and/or hypotensive "Cover" *S. pneumo* & *Legionella*	Anti-pseudomonal beta-lactam + (respiratory FQ or aminoglycoside). Add azithro if no FQ Drugs and doses in footnote†	If severe IgE-mediated beta-lactam allergy: (aztreonam + FQ) or (aztreonam + aminoglycoside + azithro)	Microbiologic documentation of pneumonia due to an aerobic gn-neg rod in the community and admitted to the ICU is an uncommon event (*AnM* 162:1849, 2002, *CCID* 16:135, 2003; *AJRCCM* 160:397, 1999).
Community-acquired, hospitalized—IN ICU Empiric therapy	Risk of Pen G-resistant *S. pneumoniae* 2° antibiotic use in last 3 months.	High dose IV amp (or Pen G) + azithro + respiratory FQ	Beta-lactam allergy: vanco + azithro	Empiric therapy vs MRSA decreases risk of mortality (*CCM* 34:2069, 2006). If Pen G MIC>4 mcg/mL, vanco. Very rare event.

NOTE: q24h = once q24h; bid = twice q24h; tid = 3 times a day, qid = 4 times a day.
† Antipseudomonal beta-lactams: **Aztreonam** 2 gm IV q8h; **piperacillin** 3 gm IV q4h; **piperacillin/tazobactam** 3.375 gm IV q6h or 4.5 gm IV q8h or 4-hr infusion of 3.375 gm q8h[high dose for Pseudomonas]; **cefepime** 2 gm IV q12h; **ceftazidime** 2 gm IV q8h; **doripenem** 500 mg IV q8h as 1 or 4 hr infusion; **imipenem/cilastatin** 500 mg IV q6h; **meropenem** 1 gm IV q8h; **gentamicin or tobramycin** (see Table 10D, pg 93). Respiratory FQs: **levofloxacin** 750 mg IV q24h or **moxifloxacin** 400 mg IV q24h; **high-dose ampicillin** 400 mg IV q24h; **azithromycin** 500 mg IV q24h; **vanco** 1 gm IV q12h.

Abbreviations on page 2.   **NOTE:** *All dosage recommendations are for adults (unless otherwise indicated) and assume normal renal function.*

TABLE 1 (34)

ANATOMIC SITE/DIAGNOSIS/ MODIFYING CIRCUMSTANCES	ETIOLOGIES (usual)	SUGGESTED REGIMENS*		ADJUNCT DIAGNOSTIC OR THERAPEUTIC MEASURES AND COMMENTS
		PRIMARY	ALTERNATIVE†	
LUNG/Pneumonia/Adult *(continued)*				
IDSA/ATS Guideline for CAP in adults: CID 44(Suppl 2): S27-S72, 2007.				
Hospital-acquired—usually **with mechanical ventilation** (empiric therapy) Diagnosis confirmed by quantitative cultures (see Comment)	Highly variable depending on clinical setting: S. pneumo, S. aureus, P. aeruginosa, stenotropho-monas, acinetobacter, anaerobes all possible	**IMP** 0.5 gm IV q6h or **Dori** 500 mg IV q8h (1 or 2 hr infusion) **or MER** 1 gm IV q8h) plus, if suspect legionella or bioterrorism, **respiratory FQ (Levo or Moxi)**	**[Cefepime or high-dose PIP-TZ]** + **tobra**. Add **resp. FQ** if suspect legionella or bioterrorism. NOTE: Regimen not active vs **MRSA**—see specific rx below	Dx of ventilator-associated pneumonia: Fever & lung infiltrates often **not** pneumonia (Chest 106:221, 1994). Quantitative cultures helpful: bronchoalveolar lavage (>10⁴ per mL, pos.) or protect. spec. brush (>10³ per mL pos.) Ref.: AJRCCM 165:867, 2002; AnIM 132:621, 2000. **Microbial etiology:** No empiric regimen covers all possibilities. Regimens listed above majority of **S. pneumo, legionella, & most coliforms**. Regimens not active vs MRSA, Stenotrophomonas & others; see below. Specific therapy see culture results known.
Vent-Assoc: Pneumonia Guidelines: AJRCCM 171:388, 2005; Reviews: Chest 130:597, 2006; JAMA 297:1583, 2007.			See Comment regarding diagnosis Dosages: See footnotes pages 22, 33, & 35	**Ventilator-associated pneumonia—Prevention:** If possible, keep head of bed elevated 30° or more. Remove N-G, endotracheal tubes as soon as possible. If available, continuous subglottic suctioning Chlorhexidine oral care may help. Refs. Chest 130:251, 2006; CCM 32:1396, 2004; AJRCCM 173:1297, 1348, 2006.
Hospital- or community-acquired, neutropenic pt (<500 neutrophils per mm³)	Any of organisms listed under community- & hospital-acquired + fungi (aspergillus) See Table 11	Duration of therapy, see footnote³ See Hospital-acquired, immediately above. Vanco not included in initial therapy unless high suspicion of infected IV access or drug-resistant S. pneumo. Ampho not used improving, then po therapy → see Alternative column See Comment		See consensus document on management of febrile neutropenic pt: CID 34:730, 2002.
Adults—Selected specific therapy after culture results (sputum, blood, pleural fluid, etc.) available. Also see Table 2, page 61				
Burkholderia (Pseudo-)mallei, B. pseudomallei (etiology of melioidosis) Ref.: J Cl 361:1715, 2003	Gram-negative	**Initial parenteral rx: Ceftazidime** 2 gm IV per kg IV q6h **or IMP** 20 mg per kg IV q8h. minimum 10 days &	**Post-parenteral po rx:** 1000/62.5, 2 tabs po bid times 20 wks (children); **Chloro** 10 mg per kg q6h times 8 wks; **Doxy** 2 mg per kg bid times 20 wks; **TMP-SMX** 5 mg per kg (TMP component) bid times 20 wks	For oral regimen, use **AM-CL-ER** Children **<8 yrs old & pregnancy:** High % of comensal H. hemolyticus Even with compliance, relapse rate is 10%. Max. daily ceftazidime dose: 6 gm. Tigecycline. No clinical data but active in vitro (AAC 50:1555, 2006).
Adults—Selected specific therapy after culture results (sputum, blood, pleural fluid, etc.) available. Also see Table 10C, pages 67				
Haemophilus influenzae β-lactamase negative β-lactamase positive		**AMP** IV, **amox** po, **TMP-SMX**, **azithro/clarithro**, **doxy**. **AM-CL**, **O Ceph 2/3**, **O Ceph 3**, **FQ**, **azithro/clarithro**, **telithro**⁴ Dosage: Table 10C	**AMP** IV or **Levo** IV or **Moxi** IV. See Table 10C, pages 67 & 67 for dosages. Treat for 7–14 days (CID 37:1734, 2004)	25–35% strains β-lactamase positive. ↑ resistance to both TMP-SMX and doxy. See Table 10C, page 65 for doses. High % of comensal H. hemolyticus misidentified as H. influenzae (JID 195:81, 2007).
Klebsiella species & other coliforms	**Hospitalized/ immunocompromised**	**Dori, IMP** or **MER**, if resistant, **polymyxin E (colistin)** or **B** Usually several weeks of therapy. **Azithro** IV or **Levo** IV or **Moxi** IV. See Table 10C, pages 67		ESBL inactivates all cephalosporins, β-lactam/β-lactamase inhibitor drug activity not predictable, co-resistance to all FQs & others common. Ref.: AJRCCM 171:388, 2005.
—ESBL pos. &	β-lactamase positive			
Legionella species Relative bradycardia common feature				**Legionella** website: www.legionella.org Two studies show superiority of **Levo** over macrolides (CID 40:794 & 800, 2005). **Gemi** should work if po therapy possible.

---

† If Acinetobacter sp. susceptibility to IMP & MER may be discordant (CID 41:758, 2005).

² **PIP-TZ** dose 4.5 gm IV q6h or 3.375 gm IV q6h: higher dose, 3.375 gm q4h, with **tobra** for P. aeruginosa pneumonia.

³ Dogma on duration of therapy not possible with so many variables: i.e, certainty of diagnosis, infecting organism, severity of infection and number/severity of co-morbidities. Agree with efforts to de-escalate & shorten course. Treat at least 7-8 days. Need clinical evidence of response: fever resolution, improved oxygenation, falling WBC. Refs. AJRCCM 171:388, 2005; CID 43:S75, 2006; COID 19:185, 2006.

⁴ **Telithro** = telithromycin 800 mg po q24h. Rare severe hepatotoxic reactions reported (AnIM 144:415, 2006; NEJM 355:2260, 2006).

⁵ **ESBL** = Extended spectrum beta-lactamase

Abbreviations on page 2. NOTE: All dosage recommendations are for adults (unless otherwise indicated) and assume normal renal function.

TABLE 1 (35)

ANATOMIC SITE/DIAGNOSIS/MODIFYING CIRCUMSTANCES	ETIOLOGIES (usual)	SUGGESTED REGIMENS*		ADJUNCT DIAGNOSTIC OR THERAPEUTIC MEASURES AND COMMENTS
		PRIMARY	ALTERNATIVE†	
LUNG/Pneumonia/Adults—Selected specific therapy after culture results *(continued)*				
Moraxella catarrhalis	93% β-lactamase positive	AM-CL, O Ceph 2/3, P Ceph 2/3, macrolide, 1 telithro	FQ, TMP-SMX. Doxy another option.	*(see footnote 4 on page 37)*
Pseudomonas aeruginosa	Often ventilator-associated	PIP-TZ 3.375 gm IV q4h or 4-hr infusion of 3.375 gm q8h) + tobra 5 mg/kg IV once q24h (see Table 10D, page 93) Could substitute cefepime or carbapenem (Dori, IMP, MER) for PIP-TZ (if pt. strain is susceptible).	AM-CL, O Ceph 2/3, P Ceph 2/3, macrolide 1 telithro	**NOTE:** High-dose PIP-TZ for P. aeruginosa, other options: cefepime 2 gm IV q 12h. CIP 400 mg IV q12h + PIP-TZ. IMP 500mg IV q6h + CIP 400mg IV q12h; if multi-drug resistant, polymyxin—parenteral & perhaps by inhalation, 80 mg bid *(CID 41:754, 2005). Ref for 4-hr infusion of PIP-TZ: CID 44:357, 2007.*
Staphylococcus aureus Duration of treatment: 3 wks if just pneumonia, 4-6 wks if concomitant endocarditis and/or osteomyelitis.	Nafcillin/oxacillin susceptible	Nafcillin/oxacillin 2 gm IV q4h	Vanco 1 gm IV q12h or linezolid 600 mg IV q12h	Retrospective analysis of 2 prospective randomized double-blind studies of hospital-acquired **MRSA** showed enhanced survival with linezolid, p 0.03 *(Chest 124:1632, 2003);* efficacy perhaps related to superb linezolid lung concentrations. Concern of possible misinterpretation of post hoc subgroup analysis *(Chest 126:314, 2004).*
	MRSA	Vanco 1 gm IV q12h	Linezolid 600 mg IV q12h; if >10–14days check CBC q week.	
Stenotrophomonas maltophilia		TMP-SMX	TC-CL ± aztreonam	In vitro synergy refs.: *AAC 39:2220, 1995; CMR 11:57, 1998*
Streptococcus pneumoniae **Note:** Case fatality rate lower with combination therapy that includes azithro (AJM 107:345, 1999; CID 42:304, 2006)	Penicillin-susceptible	AMP 2 gm IV q6h, amox 1 gm po tid, macrolide¹, pen G IV², doxy, O Ceph 2, P Ceph 2/3, telithro 800 mg po q24h. See Table 10C, page 85 for other dosages		Refs.: *JAMA 283:2281, 2000; CID 42:614, 2006; JID 19:782, 2007.*
	Penicillin-resistant, high level	FQs with enhanced activity— Gemi, Levo, Moxi —see Table 5, page 72 for more data. If all options not acceptable (e.g., allergy), linezolid active until afebrile, 3-5 days (min. of 5 days).	Telithro 800 mg po q24h. Dosages Table 10C. Treat until afebrile, 3-5 days (min. of 5 days)	
Yersinia pestis (Plague)	Aerosol Y. pestis (See Table 1B(2)	Gentamicin 5 mg/kg IV q24h	Doxy 200 mg IV times 1, then 100 mg IV q12h	
LUNG—Other				
Anthrax Inhalation (applies to oropharyngeal & gastrointestinal forms): Treatment (Cutaneous: See page 46) Refs.: *MMWR 50:909, 2001;* www.bt.cdc.gov	Bacillus anthracis **To report possible bioterrorism event: 770-488-7100** Plague, tularemia see Table 1B, page 59 Chest x-ray; mediastinal widening & pleural effusion	**Adults (including pregnancy): CIP** 400 mg IV q12h) or **Levo** 500 mg IV q24h) or **doxy** 100 mg IV q12h) **plus clinda-mycin** 900 mg IV q8h &/or RIF 300 mg IV q12h Switch to po when able & lower CIP to 500 mg po bid, doxy to 100 mg po q8h, & RIF 300 mg po bid. Treat times 60 days. Other alternatives: *Table 1B, page 59*	**Children: CIP** 10 mg/kg IV q12h or 15 mg/kg po q12h) or **Doxy:** >8 y/o & >45 kg: 100 mg IV q12h; >8 y/o & ≤45 kg: 2.2 mg/kg IV q12h; ≤8 y/o: 2.2 mg/kg IV q12h) **plus clindamycin** 7.5 mg/kg IV q6h **and/or RIF** 20 mg/kg IV q24h (max. 600 mg/day) Treat times 60 days. See Table 16, page 177 for oral dosage.	1. Clinda may block toxin production 2. Rifampin penetrates CSF & intracellular sites. 3. Isolate shown penicillin-susceptible a. **Adults: Pen G** 4 million units IV q4h b. **Children: Pen G** <12 y/o: 50,000 units per kg IV q6h; >12 y/o: 4 million units IV q4h c. Constitutive & inducible β-lactamases—do not use pen or amp alone. 4. Do not use cephalosporins or TMP-SMX. 5. Erythro, azithro activity borderline; clarithro active. 6. No person-to-person spread. 7. Antitoxins in development 8. Moxi should work, but no clinical data 9. Case report of survival with use of anthrax immunoglobulin *(CID 44:968, 2007).*

---

¹ **Macrolide** = azithromycin, clarithromycin, dirithromycin, and erythromycin. Dirithromycin serum levels inadequate for bacteremic S. pneumo.

² **IV Pen G dosage:** Blood cultures neg., 1 million units IV q4h; blood cultures pos. & no meningitis, 2 million units IV q4h. Another option is continuous infusion (CI): 3 million units loading dose & then CI of 10-12 million units over 12 hrs *(Chest 112:1657, 1997).* If concomitant meningitis, 4 million units IV q4h.

Abbreviations on page 2. *NOTE: All dosage recommendations are for adults (unless otherwise indicated) and assume normal renal function.*

See Table 10C, page 85 for dosages

TABLE 1 (36)

ANATOMIC SITE/DIAGNOSIS/ MODIFYING CIRCUMSTANCES	ETIOLOGIES (usual)	SUGGESTED REGIMENS* PRIMARY	ALTERNATIVE[†]	ADJUNCT DIAGNOSTIC OR THERAPEUTIC MEASURES AND COMMENTS
LUNG—Other (continued)				
Prophylaxis for anthrax exposure	Info: www.bt.cdc.gov	**Adults (including pregnancy): CIP** 500 mg po bid or **Levo** 500 mg po q24h.) × 60 days. **Children: CIP** 20-30 mg/kg per day div q12h × 60 days.	**Adults (including pregnancy): Doxy** 100 mg po bid x 60 d. **Children** (see Comment): **Doxy** >8 y/o & >45kg: 100 mg po bid; >8 y/o & ≤45 & ≤8 y/o: 2.2mg/kg po bid. All for 60 days.	1. Once organism shows suscept. to penicillin, switch to amoxicillin 80 mg per kg per day div. q8h (max. 500 mg q8h); pregnant pt.to amoxicillin 500 mg po tid. 2. Do not use cephalosporins or TMP-SMX. 3. Other FQs (Gati, Moxi) should work but no clinical experience.
Aspiration pneumonia ± lung abscess Refs. *CID* 40:915 & 923, 2005	Transthoracic culture in 90 pts—% of total isolates: anaerobes 34%, Gm-pos. aerobes 26%, S. milleri 16%, Klebsiella pneumoniae 25%, nocardia 3%	**PIP-TZ** 3.375 gm IV q6h or 4-hr infusion of 3.375 gm q8h (*CID* 44:357. 2005) [or for nocardia, see Table 11, page 96]	**Ceftriaxone** 1 gm IV q24h **plus metro** 500 mg IV q6h or 1 gm IV q12h	Suggested regimens based on retrospective evaluation of 90 pts with cultures obtained by transthoracic aspiration (*CID* 40:915 & 923, 2005). Surprising frequency of Klebsiella pneumoniae. Note admin high IV/po q24h another option (*CID* 41:764, 2005). Note admin from clinda due to prevalence of Gm-neg bacilli.
Chronic pneumonia with fever, night sweats and weight loss	M. tuberculosis, coccidioidomycosis, histoplasmosis	See Table 11, Table 12. For risk associated with TNF inhibitors, see *CID* 41(Suppl 3):S187, 2005.		HIV+, foreign-born, alcoholism, contact with TB, travel into developing countries
Cystic fibrosis Acute exacerbation of pulmonary symptoms Refs. *Ln* 361:681, 2003; *AJRCCM* 168:918, 2003; *J PedS&ChildHealth* 42:601, 2006.	S. aureus or H. influenzae early in disease; P. aeruginosa later in disease	**For P. aeruginosa:** (Peds doses) **Tobra** 3.3 mg/kg q8h or 12 mg/kg IV q24h. Combine tobra with (**PIP** or **ticarcillin** 100 mg/kg q6h) **or ceftaz** 50 mg/kg q8h to max of 6 gm per day. If resistant to above, **CIP/Levo** used if P. aeruginosa susceptible. See footnote[*]	**For S. aureus: (1) MSSA—oxacillin/nafcillin** 2 gm IV q4h (Peds dose, *Table 16*). **(2) MRSA—vanco** 1 gm q12h & check serum levels. See Comment	May be hard to get pieracillin without tazobactam. Older children and adults need high dose PIP-TZ for P. aeruginosa (3.375 gm IV q4h). Extended infusion better. 4-hr infusion of 3.375 gm q8h. For pharmacokinetics of aminoglycosides in CF, *J PedS&ChildHealth 42:601, 2006.* For chronic suppression of P. aeruginosa, **inhaled phenol-free tobra** 300 mg bid x 28 d., then no rx 28 d., then repeat cycle (*AJRCCM 167:841, 2003*). *Inhaled aztreonam lysine in Phase III trials.*
Empyema Neonatal	Burkholderia (Pseudomonas) cepacia	**TMP-SMX** 5 mg per kg IV/po (TMP) IV q6h	**Chloro** 15-20 mg per kg IV/po q6h	B. cepacia has become a major pathogen. Patients develop progressive respiratory failure, 62% mortality at 1yr. **Fail to respond to aminoglycosides**, piperacillin, & ceftazidime. Patients with B. cepacia should be isolated from other CF patients.
		For other alternatives, see Table 2		
Empyema Neonatal	See Pneumonia, neonatal, page 33			Drainage indicated
Infants/children (1 month–5 yrs)	Staph. aureus, Strep. pneumoniae, H. influenzae	See Pneumonia, age 1 month–5 years, page 34		Drainage indicated

Empyema Refs. Pleural effusion review: *NEJM* 346:1971, 2002; *CID* 45:1480, 2007

[†] Other options. (Tobra + aztreonam 50 mg per kg IV q8h); (IMP 15-25 mg per kg IV q6h + tobra); **CIP commonly used in children**, e.g., CIP IV/po + ceftaz IV (*LnID* 3:537, 2003).

Abbreviations on page 2.

[*] Other options: (Tobra + aztreonam 50 mg per kg IV q8h + tobra). NOTE: All dosage recommendations are for adults (unless otherwise indicated) and assume normal renal function.

TABLE 1 (37)

ANATOMIC SITE/DIAGNOSIS/ MODIFYING CIRCUMSTANCES	ETIOLOGIES (usual)	SUGGESTED REGIMENS* PRIMARY	ALTERNATIVE†	ADJUNCT DIAGNOSTIC OR THERAPEUTIC MEASURES AND COMMENTS
LUNG—Other/Empyema (continued)				
Child >5 yrs to Adult, acute—Diagnostic thoracentesis, chest tube (± T-PA). For dosage, see Table 10 or footnote page 22. Microbiologic diagnosis *CID 42:1135, 2006.*	Staph. aureus: **Check for MRSA**. H. Influenzae	**Nafcillin or oxacillin** if MSSA	**Vanco**	In large multicenter double-blind trial, intrapleural streptokinase did not improve mortality, reduce the need for surgery or the length of hospitalization (*NEJM 352:865, 2005*). Success using S. pneumoniae urine antigen test on pleural fluid (*Chest 131:1442, 2007*).
Acute, with bacteremia—Strep. pneumoniae, Group A Strep. For dosage, see footnote page 22	Staph. aureus: **Check for MRSA**	**Cefotaxime or ceftriaxone** (Dosage, see footnote page 22)	**Ceftriaxone**	Usually complication of S. aureus pneumonia &/or bacteremia.
		Clinda 450–900 mg IV q8h if MSSA	**Vanco** if MRSA	
Subacute/chronic	Anaerobic strep, Strep. milleri, Bacteroides sp., Enterobacteriaceae, M. tuberculosis	**TMP-SMX** or **AM-SB**	**Cefoxitin** or **IMP** or **TC-CL** or **PIP-TZ** or **AM-SB** (Dosage, see footnote 1 page 22)	Pneumophic Grn-neg. bacilli. ↑ resistance to TMP-SMX. R/O tuberculosis or tumor. Drainage. Pleural biopsy with culture for mycobacteria and histology if TBc suspected.
Human immunodeficiency virus infection (HIV+): See SANFORD GUIDE TO HIV/AIDS THERAPY				
CD4 T-lymphocytes <200 per mm³ or clinical AIDS Acute cough, progressive dyspnea, & diffuse infiltrate. Prednisone first if suspect pneumocystis (see Comment)	Pneumocystis carnii most likely; also M. tbc, fungi, Kaposi's sarcoma, & lymphoma. NOTE: AIDS pts may develop pneumonia due to DRSP or other pathogens—see next box below	Rx listed here is for **severe** pneumocystis; see Table 13, page 125 for pts on regimens for **mild** disease. **Prednisone 1** (see Comment) **TMP-SMX** [IV: 15 mg per kg per day div q8h (TMP component) or po 2 DS (TMP component) q8h], total of 21 days	**Primaquine** 30 mg (qo) q8h + **(pentamidine** 4 mg per kg per day IV) times 21 days. See Comment	Diagnostic procedure of choice is sputum induction, if negative, bronchoscopy. Pts with PCP & <70 CD4 cells per mm³ should be on anti-PCP prophylaxis for life. **Prednisone** 40 mg bid po times 5 days then 40 mg q24h po times 5 days then 20 mg q24h po times 11 days **is indicated with PCP (pO₂ <70 mmHg), should be given at initiation of anti-PCP rx; don't wait until pt's condition deteriorates** (Table 13, page 125). If PCP studies negative, consider bacterial pneumonia, TBc, cocci, histo, crypto, Kaposi's sarcoma or lymphoma. **Pentamidine not active vs bacterial pathogens.**
CD4 T-lymphocytes normal	Strep. pneumoniae, H. influenzae, S. aureus, M. tuberculosis, Legionella rare, M. tbc	**Ceftriaxone** 1 gm IV q24h: **Clinda** (over age 65) 1 gm IV q24h) + **azithro.** Could use **Levo, Moxi** as alternative (see Comment)	**FQs: Levo** 750 mg q24h (first day 750 mg) or **Moxi** q24h	**Pneumocystis resistant to TMP-SMX, albeit rare, does exist.** If Gram stain of sputum shows Grm-neg. bacilli, options include **P Ceph 3 AP**, **FQs**. **Levo** 750 mg po/IV q24h. Gati not available in US due to hypo- & hyperglycemic reactions.
As above: Children	Same as adult (HIV + lymphoid interstitial pneumonia (LIP)	As for HIV + adults with pneumonia. If diagnosis is LIP, rx with steroids.		In children with AIDS, LIP responsible for 1/3 of pulmonary complications, usually <1 yr of age. PCP, which is seen at <1 yr of age. Clinically: clubbing, hepatosplenomegaly, salivary glands enlarged (take up gallium), lymphocytosis.
Viral (interstitial) pneumonia suspected (See Table 14, page 135)	Consider Adenovirus, coronavirus (SARS), hantavirus, influenza, metapneumovirus, parainfluenza virus, respiratory syncytial virus	**For influenza A or B:** see **tamiflu**† 75 mg po bid x 5 d or **zanamivir** 10 mg inhaled bid x 5 d. Start within 48 hrs of symptom onset.	**For influenza A: rimantadine** and **amantadine** not recommended because current circulating strains are resistant.	No known efficacious drugs for adenovirus (SARS), hantavirus, metapneumovirus, parainfluenza or RSV. Need travel (SARS) & exposure (Hanta) history. RSV and human metapneumovirus as serious as influenza in the elderly (*NEJM 352:1749 & 1810, 2005; CID 44:1152 & 1159, 2007*).
LYMPH NODES (approaches below apply to lymphadenitis without an obvious primary source)				
Lymphadenitis, acute Generalized	Etiologies: EBV, early HIV infection, syphilis, toxoplasma, tularemia, Lyme disease. Complete history and physical examination (*CID 39:138, 2004*).			History & physical examination directs evaluation. If nodes fluctuant, aspirate and base rx on Gram & acid-fast stains. **Kikuchi-Fujimoto** disease causes fever and benign self-
Regional				
Cervical—see cat-scratch disease (CSD), below				
Cervical disease (CSD), below	CSD (B. henselae), Grp A strep, Staph. aureus, anaerobes, M. TBc (scrofula), M. avium, M. scrofulaceum, M. malmoense, toxo, tularemia			Review of mycobacterial etiology: *CID 20:954, 1995.* **Kikuchi-Fujimoto** disease, systemic lupus erythematosus, and **Kikuchi-Fujimoto** disease (limited adenopathy). Treat specific agent(s).

Abbreviations on page 2.   NOTE: All dosage recommendations are for adults (unless otherwise indicated) and assume normal renal function.

TABLE 1 (38)

ANATOMIC SITE/DIAGNOSIS/ MODIFYING CIRCUMSTANCES	ETIOLOGIES (usual)	SUGGESTED REGIMENS*		ADJUNCT DIAGNOSTIC OR THERAPEUTIC MEASURES AND COMMENTS
		PRIMARY	ALTERNATIVE†	
LYMPH NODES/ Lymphadenitis, acute/Regional *(continued)*				
Inguinal				
Sexually transmitted	HSV, chancroid, syphilis, LGV			
Not sexually transmitted	GAS, S.A, tularemia, T. pestis, sporotrichosis			
Axillary	GAS, SA, CSD, tularemia, T. pestis, sporotrichosis			
Extremity, with associated nodular lymphangitis	Sporotrichosis, leishmania, Nocardia brasiliensis, Mycobacterium marinum, Mycobacterium chelonae, tularemia	Treatment varies with specific etiology		A distinctive form of lymphangitis characterized by subcutaneous swellings along inflamed lymphatic channels. Primary site of skin invasion usually present; regional adenopathy rare.
Cat-scratch disease— immunocompetent patient Axillary/epitrochlear nodes 46%, neck 26%, inguinal 17%	Bartonella henselae	**Azithro dosage—Adults** (>45.5 kg): 500 mg po x 1, then 250 mg/day x4 days. **Children** (<45.5 kg): liquid azithro 10 mg/kg x 1, then 5 mg/kg per day x 4 days. Rx is controversial	No therapy, resolves in 2–6 mos. Needle aspiration relieves pain in suppurative nodes. Avoid I&D.	**Clinical:** Approx. 10% nodes suppurate. Atypical presentation in < 5% pts, i.e., lung nodules, liver/spleen lesions. Parinaud's oculoglandular syndrome, CNS manifestations in 2% of pts (encephalitis, peripheral neuropathy, retinitis), FUO **Dx:** Cat exposure. Positive IFA serology. Rarely need biopsy. **Rx:** Only 1 prospective randomized blinded study, used azithro with ↑ rapidity of resolution of enlarged lymph nodes (PIDJ 17:447, 1998). **Note:** In elderly, endocarditis less frequent; lymphadenitis less frequent (CID 47:969, 2005)
MOUTH				
Odontogenic infection, including Ludwig's angina Can result in parapharyngeal space infection *(see page 44)*	Oral microflora: infection polymicrobial	**Clinda** 300–450 mg po q6h or 600 mg IV q6-8h	**(AM-CL,** 875/125 mg po bid or 500/125 mg tid or 2000/125 mg bid) or **cefotetan** 2 gm IV q12h	Surgical drainage & removal of necrotic tissue essential. β-lactamase producing organisms are ↑ in frequency Other parenteral alternatives: AM-SB, PIP-TZ, or TC-CL. For Noma (cancrum oris) see Ln 368:147, 2006.
Buccal cellulitis Children <5 yrs	H. influenzae	**Cefuroxime** or **ceftriaxone**	**AM-CL** or **TMP-SMX**	With Hib immunization, invasive H. influenzae infections have ↓ by 95%. Now occurring in infants prior to immunization.
		Dosage: See Table 16, page 177		
Herpetic stomatitis	Herpes simplex virus 1 & 2	See Table 14		
Aphthous stomatitis, recurrent	Etiology unknown	Topical steroids (Kenalog in Orabase) may ↓ pain and swelling; if AIDS, see SANFORD GUIDE TO HIV/AIDS THERAPY.		
MUSCLE				
"Gas gangrene" Contaminated traumatic wound Can be spontaneous without trauma (CID 28:159, 1999)	Cl. perfringens, other histotoxic Clostridium sp.	**(Clinda** 900 mg IV q8h) + **pen G** 24 million units/day div. q4-6h IV	**Ceftriaxone** 2 gm IV q12h or **erythro** 1 gm q6h IV (not by bolus)	Surgical debridement primary therapy. Hyperbaric oxygen adjunctive: efficacy debated, consider if debridement not complete or possible (NEJM 334:1642, 1996). Clinda decreases toxin production.
Pyomyositis Review: AJM 117:420, 2004	Staph. aureus, Group A strep, (rarely) Gm-neg. bacilli, variety of anaerobic organisms	**(Nafcillin** or **oxacillin** 2 gm IV q4h) or **IP Ceph 1** (**cefazolin** 2 gm IV q8h)] if **MSSA**	**Vanco** 1 gm IV q12h if **MRSA**	Common in tropics: rare, but occurs, in temperate zones (IDCP 7:265, 1998). Follows exercise or muscle injury, see Necrotizing fasciitis. Now seen in HIV/AIDS. Add **metro** if anaerobes suspected or proven (IDCP 8:252, 1999).
PANCREAS: Reviews—Ln 361:1447, 2003; JAMA 291:2865, 2004; NEJM 354:2142, 2006.				
Acute alcoholic (without necrosis) (idiopathic) pancreatitis	Not bacterial	None CT-diagnosed		[1]–9% become infected but prospective studies show no advantage of prophylactic antimicrobials (Ln 346:652, 1995). Observe for pancreatic abscesses or necrosis which require therapy.
Pancreatic abscess, infected pseudocyst, post-necrotizing pancreatitis	Enterobacteriaceae, enterococci, S. aureus, S. epidermidis, various anaerobes, candida	Need culture of abscess/infected pseudocyst for direct therapy		Can often get specimen by fine-needle aspiration.
Antimicrobial prophylaxis, necrotizing pancreatitis	As above	Controversial: Cochrane Database 2: CD002941, 2004 supports prophylaxis. Subsequent, double-blind, randomized, controlled study, showed no benefit (Gastroenterology 126:997, 2004). Consensus conference voted against prophylaxis (CCM 32:2524, 2004)		

Abbreviations on page 2. NOTE: All dosage recommendations are for adults (unless otherwise indicated) and assume normal renal function.

TABLE 1 (39)

ANATOMIC SITE/DIAGNOSIS/ MODIFYING CIRCUMSTANCES	ETIOLOGIES (usual)	SUGGESTED REGIMENS* PRIMARY	SUGGESTED REGIMENS* ALTERNATIVE†	ADJUNCT DIAGNOSTIC OR THERAPEUTIC MEASURES AND COMMENTS
PAROTID GLAND "Hot" tender parotid swelling	S. aureus, S. pyogenes, oral flora, & aerobic Gm-neg. bacilli (rare), mumps, rarely enteroviruses/influenza. **Nafcillin or oxacillin 2 gm IV q4h if MSSA, vanco if MRSA.**			Predisposing factors: stone(s) in Stensen's duct, dehydration. Therapy depends on ID of specific etiologic organism.
"Cold" non-tender parotid swelling	Granulomatous disease (e.g., mycobacteria, fungi, sarcoidosis, Sjögren's syndrome), drugs (iodides, et al.), diabetes, cirrhosis, tumors			History/lab results may narrow differential; may need biopsy for diagnosis
PERITONEUM/PERITONITIS: Reference—CID 31:997, 2003 Primary (spontaneous bacterial peritonitis, SBP) Refs: CID 27:669, 1998 ESBL ref: CID 28:683, 1999 Microbiology: CID 33:1513, 2001	Enterobacteriaceae 63%, S. pneumo 15%, enterococci 6–10%, anaerobes <1%. Extended β-lactamase (ESBL) positive Klebsiella species.	**Cefotaxime 2 gm IV q8h** (if life-threatening, q4h) OR **[ceftriaxone 2 gm IV q24h]**	**TC-CL or PIP-TZ or AM-SB** OR **[cefotaxime 2 gm IV q24h]**. **If resistant E. coli/Klebsiella species (ESBL+), then: [Dori, ERTA, IMP or MER]** or **[FQ: CIP, Levo, Moxi]**. Check in vitro susceptibility. *(Dosage in footnote¹).*	One-year risk of SBP in pts with ascites and cirrhosis as high as 29% (*Gastro* 104:1133, 1993). Dx: >250 PMN/mm³ of ascitic fluid, % pos. cultures ↑ if 10 mL of ascitic fluid added to blood culture bottles. **Duration of rx unclear:** Suggest 2wks if blood culture +. One report suggests repeat paracentesis after 48hrs of cefotaxime. If PMNs <250/mm³ & ascitic fluid sterile, success with 5 days of treatment (*AJM* 97:169, 1994). IV albumin (1.5gm/kg at dx & 1gm/kg on day 3) may ↓ frequency of renal impairment (p.0.002) & ↓ hospital mortality (p.0.01) [*NEJM* 341:403, 1999].
Prevention of SBP Cirrhosis & ascites For prevention after UGI bleeding, see Liver, page 31		**TMP-SMX-DS** 1 tab po 5 days/wk or **CIP** 750 mg po q.wk		**TMP-SMX** ↓ peritonitis or spontaneous bacteremia from 27% to 3% (*AnIM* 122:595, 1995). Ref. for CIP: *Hepatology* 22:1171, 1995
Secondary (bowel perforation, ruptured appendix, ruptured diverticula) Refs: *NEJM* 338:1521, 1998 & *CID* 37:997, 2003	Enterobacteriaceae, Bacteroides sp., enterococci, P. aeruginosa (3–15%)	**SUGGESTED REGIMENS—Inpatient/parenteral rx: Mild-moderate disease** (e.g., focal periappendiceal abscess, endomyometritis) **PIP-TZ** 3.375 gm IV q6h or 4.5 gm IV q8h or 4-hr infusion of 3.375 gm q8h **OR AM-SB** 3 gm IV q6h **OR TC-CL** 3.1 gm IV q6h **OR ERTA** 1 gm IV q24h **OR MOXI** 400 mg IV q24h **Severe life-threatening disease—ICU patient: IMP** 500 mg IV q6h or **MER** 1 gm IV q8h or **Dori** 500 mg IV q8h (1-hr infusion)	**[(CIP** 400 mg IV q12h or **Levo** 750 mg IV q24h) + (**metro** 500 mg q6h or 1 gm q12h)] OR [**aztreonam** 2 gm q12h + **metro**] OR **tigecycline** 100 mg IV times 1 dose, then 50 mg q12h **Severe life-threatening disease—ICU patient: [AMP + metro + (CIP** 400 mg IV q12h or **Levo** 750 mg IV q24h)] OR [**AMP** 2 gm q6h + **metro** 500 mg IV q6h + **APAG** (see Table 10D, page 93)]	Must "cover" both Gm-neg. aerobic & Gm-neg. anaerobic bacteria. **Drugs active only vs aerobic Gm-neg. bacilli:** APAG, P Ceph 2/3/4, aztreonam, AP Pen, CIP, Levo. **Drugs active vs both aerobic/anaerobic Gm-neg. bacteria:** cefoxitin, cefotetan, TC-CL, PIP-TZ, AM-SB, Dori, IMP, MER. Increasing resistance (R) of Bacteroides sp. (*AAC* 51:1649, 2007): % R — Cefoxitin 5–30 — Cefotetan 17–87 — Clindamycin 19–35 Essentially no resistance: **metro, PIP-TZ.** Case reports of metro resistance: *CID* 40:e67, 2005; *JCM* 42:4127, 2004. **Ertapenem** not active vs P. aeruginosa/Acinetobacter species. **In absence of ongoing fecal contamination, aerobic/anaerobic coverage of peritoneal exudate/abscess of help in guiding specific therapy.** Less need for aminoglycosides. With severe pen allergy can "cover" Gm-neg. aerobes with CIP or aztreonam. **Remember IMP/MER are β-lactams.**

Concomitant surgical management important

¹ Parenteral IV therapy for peritonitis: **TC-CL** 3.1 gm q6h. **PIP-TZ** 3.375 gm q6h or 4.5 gm q8h or 4-hr infusion of 3.375 gm q8h. **AM-SB** 3 gm q6h. **Dori** 500 mg IV q8h (1-hr infusion). **IMP** 0.5 gm q6h. **MER** 1 gm q8h. **FQ** [**CIP** 400 mg q12h; **Ofloxe** 400 mg q12h; **Levo** 750 mg q24h; **Moxi** 400 mg q24h]. **Moxi** 400 mg IV q24h. **cefotetan** 2 gm q12h; **cefoxitin** 2 gm q6h. **P Ceph 3** [**cefotaxime** 2 gm q4–8h; **ceftriaxone** 1–2 gm q24h; **ceftizoxime** 1–2 gm q6–8h]. **APAG** (see Table 10D, page 93). **AMP** 1 gm q6h. **cefepime** 2 gm q12h. **P Ceph 4** [**CFP** 2 gm q12h], cefpirome. **metro** 1 gm loading then 0.5 gm q6h or 1 gm q8h or 1 gm q8h q12h. **AP Pen** [**ticarcillin** 4 gm q6h; **PIP** 4 gm q6h, **aztreonam** 2 gm q8h]

Abbreviations on page 2.   NOTE: *All dosage recommendations are for adults (unless otherwise indicated) and assume normal renal function.*

TABLE 1 (40)

ANATOMIC SITE/DIAGNOSIS/ MODIFYING CIRCUMSTANCES	ETIOLOGIES (usual)	SUGGESTED REGIMENS*		ADJUNCT DIAGNOSTIC OR THERAPEUTIC MEASURES AND COMMENTS
		PRIMARY	**ALTERNATIVE†**	
PERITONEUM/PERITONITIS *(continued)*				
Associated with chronic ambulatory/peritoneal dialysis (defined as > 100 WBC per mL, >50% PMNs)	Staph. aureus (most common), Staph. epidermidis, P. aeruginosa, other Gm-neg. bacilli 11%, sterile 20%, M. fortuitum (rare)	If of moderate severity, can rx by adding drug to dialysis fluid—see Table 17 for dosage. Reasonable empiric options: **vancomycin** or **cefazolin** + **ceftazidime**. If severely ill, rx with same drugs IV (adjust dose for renal failure, Table 17) & via addition to dialysis fluid. Excellent ref: *Perit Dialysis Int 13:14, 1993*		For culture: concentrate several hundred mL of removed dialysis fluid by centrifugation. Gram stain concentrate and then inject into aerobic/anaerobic blood culture bottles and incubate. Gram stain positive in only ≤ 10%. If culture shows Staph. bacilli cultured, consider bowel perforation and catheter removal.
PHARYNX				
Pharyngitis/tonsillitis— Reviews: *NEJM 344:205, 2001; AnIM 139:113, 2002*. For relationship to acute rheumatic fever, see footnote[1] Rheumatic fever ref.: *Ln 366:155, 2005*	Group A,C,G strep, "viral", infectious mononucleosis (Group A, C, G strep) (*NEJM 339:156, 1993*). C. diphtheriae, A. haemolyticum, Mycoplasma pneumoniae In adults, only 10% pharyngitis due to Group A strep	**Pen V** po x 10 days or (if compliance unlikely) **benzathine pen G** IM x1 dose **See footnote[2] for adult and pediatric dosages** Acetaminophen effective for pain relief. Children—Linezolid should work. Adults—FQ	**O Ceph** 2 x 4–6 days *(CID 38:1526 & 1535, 2004)* or **clinda** or **azithro** x5 days or **clarithro** x 10 days or **dirithro** x 10 days Up to 35% of isolates resistant to erythro, azithro, clarithro, clinda *(AAC 48:473, 2004)* FQs no longer recommended due to high prevalence of resistance: *MMWR 55:332, 2007*	**Dx:** Rapid strep test or culture: *(JAMA 291:1587, 2004, & 292:167, 2004)*. Rapid strep test valid in adults: *An IM 166:640, 2006.* **Pen allergy & macrolide resistance:** No penicillin or cephalosporin-resistant S. pyogenes, but macrolide-resistant. **S. pyogenes** (7%, 2000–2003). Culture & susceptibility testing if clinical failure with macrolide *(CID 41:599, 2005)*. **S. pyogenes Groups C & G cause pharyngitis but not a risk for post-strep rheumatic fever.** To prevent rheumatic fever, eradicate Group A strep. Requires 10 days of pen V po. 4–6 days of po Ceph 2; 5 days of po azithro. 10 days of clarithro. In controlled trial, better eradication rate with 10 days clarithro (91%) than 5 days azithro (82%)*(CID 32:1798,2001).*
Gonococci	Gonococci	**Ceftriaxone** 125 mg IM x 1 dose+ (**azithro** or **doxy)** (see Comment)		Because of risk of concomitant genital C. trachomatis, add either (**azithro** 1 gm po times 1) or (**doxy** 100 mg po x2/d times 7 days).
Asymptomatic post-rx carrier Multiple repeated culture-positive episodes *(CID 25:574, 1997)*	Group A strep Group A strep	**No rx required** Clinda or AM-CL po		Routine post-rx throat culture not advised. Small % of pts have recurrent culture-pos. Group A strep with symptomatic tonsillo-pharyngitis. Hard to tell if true Group A strep infection or active viral infection in carrier 4 times to max. of 300 mg bid.(*J Ped 106:481 & 876, 1995)*
Whitish plaques, HIV+, (thrush) **Vesicular, ulcerative**	Candida albicans (see Table 11, page 96) Coxsackie A9, B1-5, ECHO (multiple types); Enterovirus 71; Herpes simplex 1, 2	Dosages in footnote[3] Antibacterial agents not indicated. For HSV-1,2: **acyclovir**		

---

*[1] Primary rationale for therapy is eradication of Group A strep (GAS) and prevention of acute rheumatic fever (ARF). Benzathine penicillin G has been shown in clinical trials to ↓ rate of ARF from 2.8 to 0.2%. This was associated with clearance of GAS on pharyngeal cultures (*CID 19:1110, 1994*). Subsequent studies have been based on cultures, not actual prevention of ARF. Treatment decreases duration of symptoms.*

*[2] Treatment of Group A strep: **All po unless otherwise indicated. PEDIATRIC DOSAGE: AM-CL** 45 mg per kg per day div. q12h times 10 days; **cefpodoxime proxetil** 10 mg per kg per day div. bid times10 days; **cefdinir** 7 mg per kg q12h times 10 days; **cefprozil** 15 mg per kg per day div. bid times 10 days; **cefpodoxime proxetil** 10 mg per kg per day bid times 5 days; **clinda** 20–30 mg per kg per day div. q8h times 10 days; **cefditoren** 200 mg tid times 10 days; **cefuroxime axetil** 250 mg bid times days; **cefpodoxime proxetil** 100 mg bid times 4 days; **cefdinir** 300 mg q12h times 5–10 days or 600 mg q24h times 10 days; **cefditoren** 200 mg bid; **cefprozil** 500 mg q24h times 10 days. **NOTE:** Only 1 and then 250 mg q24h times 4 days for 500 mg q24h times 10 days; **azithro** 500 mg day 1 and then 250 mg q24h times 4 days or 500 mg q24h times 3 days; **dirithromycin** 500 mg q24h times10 days.*

Abbreviations on page 2.   *NOTE: All dosage recommendations are for adults (unless otherwise indicated) and assume normal renal function.*

TABLE 1 (41)

ANATOMIC SITE/DIAGNOSIS/ MODIFYING CIRCUMSTANCES	ETIOLOGIES (usual)	SUGGESTED REGIMENS*		ADJUNCT DIAGNOSTIC OR THERAPEUTIC MEASURES AND COMMENTS
		PRIMARY	ALTERNATIVE†	
PHARYNX/ Pharyngitis/Tonsillitis or Vincent's angina	*(continued)* C. diphtheriae	**Antitoxin + erythro** 20–25 mg/kg IV q12h times 7–14 days (*JAC 35;717, 1995*) or **(benzyl pen G** 50,000 units/kg per day x 5 days, then po **pen VK** 50 mg/kg per day x 5 days)		Diphtheria occurs in immunized individuals. Antibiotics may ↓ toxin production, ↓ spread of organisms. Penicillin superior to erythro in randomized trial (*CID 27;845, 1998*).
	Vincent's angina (anaerobes/spirochetes)	**Pen G** 4 million units IV q4h	**Clinda** 600 mg IV q8h	May be complicated by F. necrophorum bacteremia, see jugular vein phlebitis, *Lemierre's, page 44*
Epiglottitis Children	H. influenzae (rare), S. pyogenes, S. pneumoniae, S. aureus	**Peds dosage: Cefotaxime** 50 mg per kg IV q8h or **ceftriaxone** 50 mg per kg IV q24h	**Peds dosage: AM-SB** 100–200 mg/kg per day div q6h or **clinda** 6–12 mg/kg TMP component /kg per day div q6h[25]	Have tracheostomy set "at bedside." Chloro is effective, but potentially less toxic alternative agents available. Review (adults): *JAMA 272;1358, 1994.*
Adults	Group A strep, H. influenzae (rare)	**Adult dosage:** *See footnote¹*		
Parapharyngeal space infection Poor dental hygiene, dental extractions, foreign bodies (e.g. toothpicks, fish bones)	Spaces include: sublingual, submandibular, submaxillary (Ludwig's angina, see footnote¹), lateral pharyngeal, retropharyngeal, pretracheal Polymicrobic: Strep sp., anaerobes, Eikenella corrodens	**(Clinda** 600–900 mg IV q8h) or **(pen G** 24 million units IV by cont. infusion or div. q4–6h IV) + **metro** 1 gm IV load and then 0.5 gm IV q6h)	**Cefoxitin** 2 gm IV q8h or **clinda** 600–900 mg IV q8h or **TC-CL** or **PIP-TZ** or **AM-SB** (Dosage, see footnote¹)	Close observation of airway. 1/3 require intubation, MRI or CT to identify abscess; if present, surgical drainage. **Metro** may be given 1 gm IV q12h.
Jugular vein septic phlebitis (Lemierre's disease) (*PIDJ 22;921, 2003; CID 31;524, 2000*)	Fusobacterium necrophorum in vast majority	**Pen G** 24 million units IV by cont. infusion or div. q4–6h	**Clinda** 600–900 mg IV q8h	Usual therapy includes external drainage of lateral pharyngeal space. Emboli, pulmonary and systemic common. Erosion into carotid artery can occur.
Laryngitis (hoarseness)/tracheitis	Viral (90%)	Not indicated		
Sinusitis, acute; current terminology: acute rhinosinusitis Obstruction of sinus ostia, viral infection, allergens Refs.: *Otolaryn-Head & Neck Surgery 130;S1, 2004; AnIM 134;495 & 498, 2001.* For rhinovirus infections (common cold), see Table 14, page 146. Pediatric Guidelines: *Peds 108;798, 2001*	Strep. pneumoniae 31%, H. influenzae 21%, M. catarrhalis 2%, Strep pyog 2%, anaerobes 6%, viruses 15%, S. aureus 4%. By CT scans, sinus mucosa inflamed in 87% of viral URIs; only 2% develop bacterial rhinosinusitis	Reserve antibiotic therapy for pts given decongestants/ analgesics for 7 days who have (1) maxillary/facial pain & (2) purulent nasal discharge; if severe illness (pain, fever), treat sooner—usually maxillary/facial pain & (2) purulent nasal discharge; if severe illness (pain, fever), treat sooner—usually requires hospitalization. For mild/mod. disease: Ask if antibiotics in prior month. Treatment deferred if NO recent antibiotic use vs recent antibiotic use. See below.		**Rx goals:** (1) Resolve infection, (2) prevent complications, e.g. subdural empyema, epidural abscess, brain abscess, meningitis and cavernous sinus thrombosis (*LnID 7;62, 2007*), (3) avoid chronic sinus disease, (4) avoid unnecessary antibiotic rx. High rate of spontaneous resolution. For pts with β-lactam/cephalosporin allergy, if severe IgE-mediated allergy, e.g. hives, anaphylaxis, treatment options: clarithro, azithro, TMP-SMX, doxy or FQs. Avoid FQs if under age 18. Dosages *in footnote²*, page 43. If allergy not skin rash, po cephalosporin OK. *(continued on next page)*

¹ **Ceftriaxone** 2 gm IV q24h; **cefotaxime** 2 gm IV q4–8h; **AM-SB** 3 gm IV q6h; **PIP-TZ** 3.375 gm IV q6h or 4-hr infusion of 3.375 gm q8h; **TC-CL** 3.1 gm IV q6h; **TMP-SMX** 8–10 mg per kg per day (based on TMP component) div q6h, q8h, or q12h.

Abbreviations on page 2.   *NOTE: All dosage recommendations are for adults (unless otherwise indicated) and assume normal renal function.*

TABLE 1 (42)

ANATOMIC SITE/DIAGNOSIS/ MODIFYING CIRCUMSTANCES	ETIOLOGIES (usual)	SUGGESTED REGIMENS*		ADJUNCT DIAGNOSTIC OR THERAPEUTIC MEASURES AND COMMENTS
		PRIMARY	ALTERNATIVE†	
PHARYNX/Sinusitis, acute; current terminology: acute rhinosinusitis (continued)				
acute rhinosinusitis		Antibiotic Use—NO: Amox-HD or AM-CL-ER or cefdinir or cefpodoxime or cefprozil	Antibiotic Use—YES: AM-CL-ER (adults) or resp. FQ (adults). For pen. allergy, see Comments. Use AM-CL susp. in peds.	Usual rx x 10 days. Results of 3 & 10 d. of TMP-SMX the same (JAMA 273:1015, 1995). Telithro, azithro, FQs often given for 5 days (see NOTE below). Watch for pts with fever & facial erythema; ↑ risk of S. aureus infection, requires IV nafcillin/oxacillin (antistaphylococcal penicillin), penicillinase-resistant for MSSA or vanco for MRSA)
		In general, treat 10 days (see Comment). Adult and pediatric doses, footnote1 and footnote2 on page 1 (Otitis)		Pts aged 1–18 y with clinical diagnosis of sinusitis randomized to placebo, amox, or AM-CL for 14 d. No difference in multiple measures of efficacy (Peds 107:619, 2001). Similar study in adults: AIM 163:1793, 2003. Hence, without bacteriologic endpoints, data are hard to interpret. NOTE: Levo 750 mg q24h x 5 d vs levo 500 mg q24h x 10 d: equivalent microbiologic and clinical efficacy (Otolaryngol Head Neck Surg 134:10, 2006)
Clinical failure after 3 days	As above, consider diagnostic tap/aspirate	Mild/Mod. Disease: AM-CL-ER (cefpo-doxime, cefprozil, or cefdinir)	Severe Disease: GatiNUS, Gemi, Levo, Moxi	
		Treat 10 days. Adult doses in footnote 2 & Comment See Table 1†, pages 94 & 96. Ref: NEJM 337:254, 1997		
Diabetes mellitus with acute keto-acidosis; neutropenia; deferox-amine rx	Rhizopus sp. ("mucor"), aspergillus			
Hospitalized + nasotracheal or nasogastric intubation	Gm-neg. bacilli 47% (pseu-domonas, acinetobacter, E. coli common), Gm+ (S. aureus) 35%, yeasts 18%. Polymicrobial in 80%	Remove nasotracheal tube and if fever persists, recommend sinus aspiration for C/S prior to empiric therapy Dori 500 mg IV q8h (1-hr infusion) or IMP 0.5 gm IV q6h or MER 1 gm IV q8h. Add vanco for MRSA	(Ceftaz 2 gm IV q8h + vanco) or (CFP 2 gm IV q12h + vanco)	After 7 d. of nasotracheal or gastric intubation: damage to ostiomeatal complex during acute bacterial disease, allergy ± polyps, occult sinusitis), but on transnasal puncture only 38% have x-ray "sinusitis" (AJRCCM 150:776, 1994). For pts requiring mechanical ventilation with nasotracheal tube for ≥1 wk, bacterial sinusitis occurs in <10% (CID 27:851, 1998). May need fluconazole if yeast on Gram stain of sinus aspirate. Review: CID 27:463, 1998
Sinusitis, chronic Adults	Prevotella, anaerobic strep, & fusobacterium—common anaerobes. Strep sp. haemophilus, P. aeruginosa, S. aureus, & moraxella-aerobes. (CID 35:428, 2002)	Antibiotics usually not effective		Otolaryngology consultation. If acute exacerbation, treat as acute Pathogenesis unclear and may be polyfactorial: damage to ostiomeatal complex during acute bacterial disease, allergy ± polyps, occult sinusitis, and/or odontogenic disease (periodontitis in maxillary teeth).
SKIN				
Acne vulgaris (JAMA 292:726, 2004; Ln 364:2188, 2004; Cochrane Database Syst Rev 2000, 2:CD002086)				
Comedonal acne, "blackheads," "whiteheads," earliest form, no inflammation	Excessive sebum production & gland obstruction. No Propionibacterium acnes	Once-q24h: Topical tretinoin (cream 0.025 or 0.05%) or gel 0.01 or 0.025%)	All once-q24h: Topical adapalene 0.1% gel OR azelaic acid 20% cream or tazarotene 0.1% cream	Goal is prevention. ↓ number of new comedones and create an environment unfavorable to P. acnes. Adapalene causes less irritation than tretinoin. Azelaic acid less potent but less irritating than retinoids. Expect 40–70% ↓ comedones in 12 weeks.

TABLE 1 (43)

ANATOMIC SITE/DIAGNOSIS/ MODIFYING CIRCUMSTANCES	ETIOLOGIES (usual)	SUGGESTED REGIMENS* PRIMARY	ALTERNATIVE†	ADJUNCT DIAGNOSTIC OR THERAPEUTIC MEASURES AND COMMENTS
SKIN/Acne vulgaris (*continued*)				
Mild inflammatory acne: small papules or pustules	Proliferation of P. acnes + abnormal desquamation of follicular cells	Topical **erythro** 3% + **benzoyl peroxide** 5%, bid	Can substitute **clinda** 1% gel for erythro	In random. controlled trial, topical benzoyl peroxide + erythro of equal efficacy to oral minocycline & tetracycline and not affected by antibiotic resistance of propionibacteria (*Ln 364:2188, 2004*).
Inflammatory acne: comedones, papules & pustules		Topical **erythro** 3% + **benzoyl peroxide** 5%, bid; & oral antibiotic. See Comment for mild acne	Oral drugs: (**doxy** 100 mg bid) or (**minocycline** 50 mg bid). **TMP-S, tetracycline, erythro, TMP-SMX, clinda**	Systemic **isotretinoin** reserved for pts with severe widespread nodular cystic lesions that fail oral antibiotic rx: 4–5 mo. course of 0.1–1 mg per kg per day.
common: deep nodules (cysts)	Progression of above events		Expensive extended release once-daily minocycline (Solodyn) 1 mg/kg/d (*Med Lett 48:95, 2006*).	Aggressive/violent behavior reported. Doxy can cause photosensitivity. Tetracyclines stain developing teeth. Minocycline side-effects: urticaria, vertigo, pigment deposition in skin or oral mucosa.
Acne rosacea	Skin mite: Demadex folliculorum	**Azelaic acid** gel bid, topical or **Metro** topical cream bid	Any of a variety of low dose oral tetracycline regimens (*Med Lett 49:5, 2007*).	
Anthrax, cutaneous, inhalation To report bioterrorism event: 770-488-7100. For info: www.bt.cdc.gov Refs: *JAMA 281:1735, 1999, & MMWR 50:909, 2001*	B. anthracis See Table, page 38, and Table 18, page 59	**Adults (including pregnancy):** CIP 500mg po bid or **Levo** 500mg IV/po q24h) × 60 days **Children:** CIP 20–30 mg/kg/day div q12h po (to max. 1 gm per day) × 60 days	**Adults (including pregnancy): Doxy** 100 mg po bid × 60 days **Children: Doxy** >8 y/o & >45kg: 100 mg po bid; >8 y/o & ≤45kg: 2.2 mg/kg po bid; ≤8 y/o: 2.2mg/kg po bid All for 60 days.	1. If penicillin susceptible, then:
Adults: Amox 500 mg po q8h times 60 days.
Children: Amox 80 mg per kg po q8h (max. 500 mg q8h)
2. Usual treatment of cutaneous anthrax is 7–10 days; 60 days in setting of bioterrorism with presumed aerosol exposure
3. Other FQs (Levo, Moxi) should work based on in vitro susceptibility data
Bacillary angiomatosis: For other in immunocompromised (HIV-1, bone marrow transplant) patients Also see SANFORD GUIDE TO HIV/AIDS THERAPY	Bartonella infections, see Cat-scratch disease lymphadenitis, page 41, and Bartonella, page 51 Bartonella henselae and quintana	**Clarithro** 500mg po bid or **azithro** 250mg po q24h or CIP 500–750mg po bid (see Comment)	**Erythro** 500 mg po qid or **doxy** 100 mg po bid	In immunocompromised pts with severe disease, doxy 100 mg po/IV bid + RIF 300 mg po bid reported effective (*IDC No. Amer 12:37, 1998; Adv PID 11:1, 1996*).
Bite: Remember tetanus prophylaxis—see Table 20. See Table 20E for rabies prophylaxis				
Bat, raccoon, skunk	Strep & staph from skin; rabies		**Doxy** 100 mg po bid	In Americas, **antirabies rx indicated**: rabies immune globulin + vaccine. (See Table 20E, page 196)
Cat: 80% get infected, culture & treat empirically.	**Pasteurella multocida**, Staph. aureus	**AM-CL** 875/125 mg po bid or 500/125 mg po tid	**Cefuroxime axetil** 0.5 gm po q12h or **doxy** 100 mg po bid. **Do not use cephalexin.** Sens. to FQs in vitro.	**P. multocida** resistant to **dicloxacillin, cephalexin, clinda; many strains resistant to erythro** (most sensitive to azithro but no clinical data). P. multocida: if infection develops within 24 hrs. Observe for osteomyelitis. If culture + only P. multocida, can switch to pen G IV or pen VK po. See Dog Bite.
Catfish sting	Toxins	See Comments		Pts with mod/severe pain: erythema, lymphangitis, sepsis treat immediately with local antibiotics as for dog bite below
Dog: Only 5% get infected; treat only if bite severe or bad co-morbidity (e.g. diabetes).	**P. multocida** S. aureus, Bacteroides sp., Fusobac-terium sp., EF-4, Capnocyto-phaga	**AM-CL** 875/125 mg po bid or 500/125 mg po tid (adults)	**Clinda** 300 mg po qid + FQ (adults) or **clinda** + **TMP-SMX** (children)	May become secondarily infected; AM-CL is reasonable empiric rx. May become secondarily infected with erythema strep cellulitis. Consider antirabies prophylaxis: rabies immune globulin + vaccine (Table 20C). Capnocytophaga in splenectomized pts may cause local eschar, sepsis with DIC. P. multocida resistant to diclox, cephalexin, clinda and erythro, sensitive to ceftriaxone, cefuroxime, cefprodoxime and FQs.

Abbreviations on page 2.   *NOTE: All dosage recommendations are for adults (unless otherwise indicated) and assume normal renal function.*

TABLE 1 (44)

ANATOMIC SITE/DIAGNOSIS/ MODIFYING CIRCUMSTANCES	ETIOLOGIES (usual)	SUGGESTED REGIMENS* PRIMARY	SUGGESTED REGIMENS* ALTERNATIVE†	ADJUNCT DIAGNOSTIC OR THERAPEUTIC MEASURES AND COMMENTS
SKIN/Bite (continued)				
Human — For bacteriology, see CID 37:1481, 2003	Viridans strep 100%, Staph epidermidis 53%, corynebacterium 41%, **Staph. aureus 29%, eikenella 15%**, bacteroides 82%, peptostrep 26%	**Early (not yet infected): AM-CL** 875/125 mg po bid times 5 days. **Later: Signs of infection (usually in 3-24 hrs): (AM-SB** 1.5 gm IV q8h or **cefoxitin** 2 gm IV q8h or **(TC-CL** 3.1 gm IV q6h or **(PIP-TZ** 3.375 gm IV q6h or 4 gm q8h or 4 gm q8h).** If penicillin/cephalosporin allergic: **Clinda** + **CIP** or **TMP-SMX**.		Cleaning, irrigation and debridement most important. For clenched fist injuries, x-rays should be obtained. Bites inflicted by hospitalized pts. consider aerobic Gm-neg. bacilli. **Eikenella resistant to clinda, nafcillin/oxacillin, metro, P Ceph 1, and erythro; susceptible to FQs and TMP-SMX.**
Pig (swine)	Polymicrobic: Gm-neg cocci & Gm-neg. bacilli, anaerobes, Pasteurella sp.	**AM-CL** 875/125 mg po bid	**P Ceph 3** or **TC-CL** or **AM-SB** or **IMP**	Information limited but infection is common and serious (Ln 348:888, 1996).
Prairie dog	Monkeypox	See Table 14A, page 137. No rx recommended		
Primate, non-human	Herpesvirus simiae	**Acyclovir** See Table 14B, page 137		CID 20:421, 1995
Rat	Spirillum minus & Streptobacillus moniformis		**Doxy**	Antirabies rx not indicated.
Seal	Marine mycoplasma	Tetracycline times 4 wks		Can take weeks to appear after bite (Ln 364:448, 2004).
Snake: pit viper (Ref: NEJM 347:347, 2002)	Pseudomonas sp., Enterobacteriaceae, Staph. epider, midis, Clostridium sp.			**Primary therapy is antivenom** (Ln 364:549, 2004) or **MRSA infection** (spider bite painful; arthrax not painful.) Ceftriaxone should be more effective vs organisms isolated. Ref: CID 43:1309, 2006.
Spider bite: Most necrotic ulcers attributed to spiders are probably due to another cause, e.g. cutaneous anthrax (Ln 364:549, 2004) or **MRSA infection** (spider bite painful; arthrax not painful.)				
Widow (Latrodectus)	Not infectious	None		May be community acquired. Tetanus prophylaxis indicated.
Brown recluse (Loxosceles) NEJM 352:700, 2005	Not infectious. Overdiagnosed! Spider distribution limited to S. Central & desert SW of US	Bite usually self-limited & self-healing. No therapy of proven efficacy.	**Dapsone** 50 mg po q24h often used despite marginal supportive data	Dapsone causes hemolysis (check for G6PD deficiency). Can cause hepatitis; baseline & weekly liver panels suggested.
Boils—Furunculosis—Subcutaneous abscesses in drug addicts ("skin poppers"). Carbuncles = multiple connecting furuncles				
Active lesions See Table 6, page 73 Community-acquired MRSA widespread. I&D mainstay of therapy. Ref: NEJM 355:666, 2006 & 357:380, 2007 & www.ccar-ccra.com/english/pdfs/CAMRS A-ExpMgtStrategies.pdf	Staph. aureus, both MSSA & community-acquired MRSA (See Comments)	**If afebrile & abscess <5 cm in diameter: I&D** & culture. No drugs. **If ≥5 cm in diameter: I&D**, culture, hot packs. **Doxy/mino** alternatives.	**Febrile, large &/or multiple abscesses; outpatient care: I&D** + culture abscess & maybe blood, hot packs + **TMP-SMX-DS** 1-2 tabs po bid + **RIF** 300 mg (adults) bid) times 5-10 days	Why: 1) 2) **TMP/SMX-DS?** See discussion Table 6 (MRSA). **TMP-SMX** activity vs streptococci uncertain. Usually clear clinical separation of strep "cellulitis" (erysipelas) from S. aureus abscess. If unclear or strep, use **clinda** or **TMP/SMX plus beta-lactam**. **Rifampin** Consider with severe infection after I&D and in combination with **TMP/SMX** (or other drugs). Few days of **TMP** alone first. Other options: 1) If compliance an issue, **dalbavancin** 1000 mg IV x 1 then, if necessary, 500mg IV on day 8, CID 41:1407, 2005); 2) **Linezolid** 600 mg po bid 10 days; 3) **Fusidic acid** (not available in US) 250-300 mg po q8-12h ± **RIF** (CID 42:394, 2006). 4) **FQs** only if in vitro susceptibility known.
To lessen number of recurrences	MSSA & MRSA	Guided by in vitro susceptibilities. **Diclox** 500mg po qid or **TMP-SMX-DS** 1-2 tabs po bid, all x 10 600mg po q24h, all x 10 days	**Bacitracin &** under fingernail treatment with **mupirocin ointment bid** (see comment)	Plus: Shower with Hibiclens q24h times 3 days & then 3 times per week. Mupirocin twice daily 5 days, povidone-iodine cream intranasal q6h times 5 days. Reports of S. aureus resistant to mupirocin. Triple antibiotic ointment active vs S.epidermidis and S.aureus (DMID 54:63, 2006) Mupirocin prophylaxis of non-surgical hosp. pts had no effect on S. aureus infection in placebo-controlled study (AnIM 140:419 & 484, 2004).

Abbreviations on page 2.   NOTE: All dosage recommendations are for adults (unless otherwise indicated) and assume normal renal function.

TABLE 1 (45)

ANATOMIC SITE/DIAGNOSIS/ MODIFYING CIRCUMSTANCES	ETIOLOGIES (usual)	SUGGESTED REGIMENS* PRIMARY	ALTERNATIVE†	ADJUNCT DIAGNOSTIC OR THERAPEUTIC MEASURES AND COMMENTS
SKIN/Boils—Furunculosis/Active Lesions (continued)				
Hidradenitis suppurativa	Lesions secondarily infected: S. aureus, Enterobacteriaceae, Pseudomonas, anaerobes. Not infected	Aspirate, base therapy on culture	Many lesions may require surgical excision.	Caused by keratinous plugging of apocrine glands of axillary and/or inguinal areas.
Burns. For overall management: NEJM 350:810, 2004—step-by-step case outlined & explained				
Initial burn wound care (CID 37:543, 2003& BMJ 332:649, 2006)	Not infected	Early excision & wound closure, shower hydrotherapy. Role of topical antimicrobics unclear.	Silver sulfadiazine cream, 1%, apply 1-2 times per day or 0.5% silver nitrate solution or mafenide acetate cream. Apply bid.	Marrow-induced neutropenia can occur during 1st wk of sulfadiazine but resolves when it is continued. Silver nitrate leaches electrolytes from wounds & stains everything. Mafenide inhibits carbonic anhydrase and can cause metabolic acidosis.
Burn wound sepsis	Strep. pyogenes, Enterobacter sp., S. aureus, S. epidermidis, E. faecalis, E. coli, P. aeruginosa. Fungi rare. Herpesvirus rare.	(Vanco 1 gm IV q12h) + (amikacin 10 mg per kg loading dose then 7.5 mg per kg IV q12h) + (PIP 4 gm IV q4h (give ½ q24h dose of piperacillin into subeschar tissues with surgical eschar removal within 12 hours)). Can use PIP-TZ if PIP not available.		Monitor serum levels; ½ of most antibiotics ↓. Staph. aureus tend to remain localized to burn wound; if toxic, consider toxic shock syndrome. Candida sp. colonize but seldom invade. Pneumonia is the major infectious complication. With staph. Complications include septic thrombophlebitis. Dapto (4 mg per kg IV q24h) alternative for vanco.
Cellulitis, erysipelas: Be wary of macrolides (erythro-resistant) & often TMP-SMX resistant group A strep & Staph. aureus			Review CID 44:705, 2007 & CID 41:1373, 2005.	diseases that masquerade as cellulitis (AnIM 142:47, 2005)
Extremities, non-diabetic For diabetes, see below	Group A strep, occ. Group B, C, G. Staph. aureus, including MRSA reported.	Pen G 1-2 million units q4h IV or (Nafcillin-IV- or oxacillin 2 gm IV q4h). If not severe: dicloxacillin 500 mg po qid or cefazolin 1 gm IV q8h. See Comment	Erythro 0.5 gm IV q6h or cefazolin or AM-CL or azithro or clarithro or tigecycline or dapto 4 mg/kg IV or ceftobiprole (CFB) 500 mg IV q12h. (Dosage, see footnote page 33 or Table 10C.)	"Spontaneous" erysipelas of leg in non-diabetic is usually due to strep, Gps A,B,C or G. Hence OK to start with IV pen G 1-2 million units q6h & observe for localized S. aureus infection. Look for tinea pedis with fissures, a common portal of entry, can often culture strep from between toes (CID 23:1162, 1996). For ½ of pts with hyperedema & recurrent erysipelas, see prophylaxis, Table 15. Reports of CA-MRSA presenting as erysipelas rather than furunculosis. If a concern, use empiric vanco, dapto or linezolid.
Facial, adult (erysipelas)	Group A strep, Staph. aureus (to include MRSA), S. pneumo	Vanco 1 gm IV q12h	Dapto 6 mg/kg IV q 24h or Linezolid 600 mg IV q12h	Choice of empiric therapy must have activity vs S. aureus. S. aureus erysipelas of face can mimic S. pyogenes erysipelas of a extremity. Forced to treat empirically for MRSA until in vitro susceptibilities available.
Diabetes mellitus and erysipelas (See Foot, "Diabetic", page 14)	Group A strep, Staph. aureus, Enterobacteriaceae; clostridia (rare)	Early mild: TMP-SMX-DS 2 tabs po bid + RIF 300 mg bid po. For severe disease: IMP or MER or ERTA IV + 4 mg/kg IV q24h). Dosage, see page 14, Diabetic foot		Prompt surgical debridement indicated to rule out necrotizing fasciitis and to obtain cultures. If septic, consider x-ray of extremity to demonstrate gas. Prognosis dependent on blood supply: assess arteries. See diabetic foot, page 14.
Erysipelas 2° to lymphedema (congenital = Milroy's disease) or post breast surgery with lymph node dissection	S. pyogenes, Groups A, C, G	Benzathine pen G 1.2 million units IM q4 wks (if minimal benefit in reducing recurrences of pts with underlying predisposing disease)	Benzathine pen G 1.2 million units IM q4 wks (if minimal benefit in reducing recurrences of pts with underlying predisposing disease)	Indicated only if pt is having frequent episodes of cellulitis. Pen V 250 mg po bid should be effective but not aware of clinical trials. In penicillin allergy, erythro 500 mg po q24h, azithro 500 mg q24h, or clarithro 500 mg po q24h.
Dandruff (seborrheic dermatitis)	Malassezia species	Ketoconazole shampoo 2% or selenium sulfide 2.5%		(see page 9, chronic external otitis)
Decubitus or venous stasis or arterial insufficiency ulcers: with sepsis	Polymicrobic: S. pyogenes (Gps A,C,G), enterococci, anaerobic strep, Enterobacteriaceae, Pseudomonas sp, Bacteroides sp., Staph. aureus	IMP or MER or TC-CL or PIP-TZ or ERTA Dosages, see footnotes pages 14, 22, 28, 55	CIP, Levo, or Moxi) + (clinda or metro)	Without sepsis or extensive cellulitis local care may be adequate. Debride as needed. Topical mafenide or silver sulfadiazine adjunctive. R/O underlying osteomyelitis. May need wound coverage with skin graft or skin substitute (JAMA 283:716, 2000).
Erythema multiforme	H. simplex type 1, mycoplasma, Strep. pyogenes, drugs (sulfonamides, phenytoin, penicillins)			Rx: Acyclovir if due to H. simplex

Abbreviations on page 2.   NOTE: All dosage recommendations are for adults (unless otherwise indicated) and assume normal renal function.

TABLE 1 (46)

ANATOMIC SITE/DIAGNOSIS/ MODIFYING CIRCUMSTANCES	ETIOLOGIES (usual)	SUGGESTED REGIMENS*		ADJUNCT DIAGNOSTIC OR THERAPEUTIC MEASURES AND COMMENTS
		PRIMARY	ALTERNATIVE[1]	
SKIN (continued)				
Erythema nodosum	Sarcoidosis, inflammatory bowel disease, M. tbc, coccidioidomycosis, yersinia, sulfonamides			**Rx: NSAIDs; glucocorticoids** if refractory.
Erythrasma	Corynebacterium minutissimum	**Erythro** 250 mg po q6h times 14 days		Coral red fluorescence with Wood's lamp. Alt: 2% aqueous clinda topically.
Folliculitis	Many etiologies: S. aureus, candida, P. aeruginosa, malassezia, demadex	See individual entities. See Whirlpool folliculitis, page 50.		
Furunculosis	Staph. aureus	See Boils, page 47		
Hemorrhagic bullous lesions Hx of sea water-contaminated abrasion or eating raw seafood, shock.	**Vibrio vulnificus, V. damsela** (CID 37:272, 2003)	**Ceftazidime** 2 gm IV q8h + **doxy** 100 mg IV/po bid	Either **cefotaxime** 2 gm IV q8h or **CIP** 750 mg po bid (or 400 mg IV bid)	¼ pts have chronic liver disease with mortality in 50% (NEJM 312:343, 1985). In Taiwan, where a number of cases are seen, the impression exists that ceftazidime is superior to tetracyclines (CID 15:271, 1992), hence both.
Herpes zoster (shingles). See Table 14				
Impetigo, ecthyma—usually children "Honey-crust" lesions (non-bullous)	**Group A strep impetigo:** crusted lesions can be Staph. aureus + strepto-cocci	Mupirocin ointment 2% tid or fusidic acid cream[NUS] 2% times 7-12 days or retapamulin ointment, 1% bid times 5 days For dosages, see Table 10C and Table 16, page 177 for children	**Azithro** or **clarithro** or **erythro** or **O Ceph 2**	In meta-analysis that combined strep & staph impetigo, mupirocin had higher cure rates than placebo. Mupirocin superior to oral erythro. Penicillin inferior to erythro. Few placebo-controlled trials. Ref.: Cochrane Database Systemic Reviews, 2004 (2): CD003261. 46% of USA-300 CA-MRSA isolates carry gene encoding resistance to mupirocin (Ln 367:731, 2006).
Bullous (if ruptured, thin "varnish-like" crust)	**Staph. aureus impetigo** MSSA & MRSA	For MSSA: po therapy with **dicloxacillin, oxacillin, cephalexin, AM-CL, azithro, clarithro,** or **mupirocin** ointment or **retapamulin** ointment	For MRSA: **Mupirocin** ointment, **TMP-SMX-DS,** minocycline	**Note**: While resistance to Mupirocin continues to evolve, over-the-counter triple antibiotic ointment (Neomycin, polymyxin B, Bacitracin) remains effective (DMID 54:63, 2006).
Infected wound, extremity—Post-trauma (for bites, see page 46; for post-operative, see below) **—Gram stain negative**				**Culture & sensitivity, check Gram stain. Tetanus toxoid if indicated.**
Mild to moderate, uncomplicated	Polymicrobic: S. aureus (MSSA & MRSA), Group A & anaerobic strep, Enterobac-teriaceae, Cl. Perfringens, Cl. tetani, if water exposure, Aeromonas sp.	**TMP-SMX-DS** 2 tabs po bid or **clinda** 300-450 mg po bid (see Comment)	**Minocycline** 100 mg po bid or **linezolid** 600 mg po bid (see Comment)	**Mild infection:** Suggested drugs focus on S. aureus & Strep species. If suspect Gm-neg, bacilli, add **AM-CL-ER** 1000/62.5 two tabs po bid. If MRSA is thought likely, minocycline may have inducible resistance to clinda.
Febrile with sepsis—hospitalized	Pseudomonas sp., Acinetobacter in soldiers in Iraq (EID 11:1218, 2005.	**AM-SB, TC-CL,** or **PIP-TZ** or **ERTA** (Dosage, page 22) + **vanco** 1 gm IV q12h	**Vanco** 1 gm IV q12h or **dapto** 6 mg/kg IV q24h or **ceftobiprole** 500 mg IV q8h (2-hr infusion) if mixed gm-neg & gm-pos; q12h over 1 hr (if only gm-pos)+ **CIP** or **Levo** IV—dose in Comment	**Fever—sepsis:** Another alternative is **linezolid** 600 mg IV/po q12h. If Gm-neg. bacilli & severe pen allergy, CIP 400 mg IV q12h or Levo 750 mg IV q24h. Why 1-2 TMP-SMX-DS? See discussion Table 6 (MRSA) **TMP-SMX** not predictably active vs strep species. Another option: **telavancin*** 10 mg/kg IV q24h if S. aureus a concern.

Abbreviations on page 2.   NOTE: All dosage recommendations are for adults (unless otherwise indicated) and assume normal renal function.

49

TABLE 1 (47)

ANATOMIC SITE/DIAGNOSIS/ MODIFYING CIRCUMSTANCES	ETIOLOGIES (usual)	SUGGESTED REGIMENS*		ADJUNCT DIAGNOSTIC OR THERAPEUTIC MEASURES AND COMMENTS
		PRIMARY	ALTERNATIVE†	
SKIN (continued)				
Infected wound, post-operative—Gram stain negative; for Gram stain positive cocci – see below				
Surgery not involving GI or female perineum (mild)	Staph. aureus, Group A, B, C or G strep	TMP-SMX-DS 1-2 tabs po bid	Clinda 300–450 mg po tid	Check Gram stain of exudate. If Gm-neg. bacilli **add** β-lactam/β-lactamase inhibitor: AM-CL-ER po or (ERTA or PIP-TZ or TC-CL) IV. Dosage on page 22. Why 1-2 **TMP/SMX-DS**? See discussion Table 10C (MRSA) TMP/SMX not predictably active vs strep species.
With sepsis (severe)		**Vanco** 1 gm IV q12h	**Dapto** 6 mg per kg IV q24h **or ceftobiprole** 500 Mg IV q24h (1-hr infusion)	
Surgery involving GI tract (includes oropharynx, esophagus) or female genital tract—fever, neutrophilia	MSSA/MRSA, coliforms, bacteroides & other anaerobes	[(PIP-TZ or P Ceph 3 + metro) or ERTA or IMP or MER] + (vanco 1 gm IV q12h or dapto 6 mg/kg IV q 24h) If severely ill. **Mild infection: AM-CL-ER** 1 gm po q 24h. Add **TMP-SMX-DS** 1-2 tabs po bid if Gm+ cocci on Gram stain. Dosages Table 10C & footnote		For all treatment options, see *Peritonitis, page 42*. Most important: Drain wound & get cultures. Can sub **linezolid** IV vs vanco. Can sub CIP or Levo for β-lactams. Why 2 **TMP-SMX-DS**? See discussion Table 10C (MRSA)
Meleney's synergistic gangrene	See *Necrotizing fasciitis, page 50*			
Infected wound, febrile patient—Gram-stain: Gram-positive cocci in clusters	S. aureus, possibly MRSA	**Do culture & sensitivity** Oral: **TMP-SMX-DS** 2 tabs po bid or **clinda** 300-450 mg po bid (see Comment)	Iv: **Vanco** 1 gm IV q12h or **dapto** 6 mg per kg IV q24h or 6 mg/kg q12h (expensive)[NEJM364:1,4] or **ceftobiprole** 500 mg IV q12h; or **dalbavancin**[FDA-A] 1gm IV, then 0.5gm IV day 8.	↑ in community-acquired MRSA (CA-MRSA). Need culture & sensitivity to verify. Other po options for CA-MRSA inc minocycline 100mg po q12h (inexpensive) & linezolid 600 mg po q12h (expensive). If MRSA clinda-sensitive but erythro-resistant, watch out for inducible clinda resistance. Another IV alternative: **tigecycline** 100 mg times 1 dose, then 50 mg IV q12h; **ceftobiprole** 500 mg IV q12h; **telavancin** 10 mg/kg IV q24h.
Necrotizing fasciitis ("flesh-eating bacteria") Post-surgery, trauma, streptococcal skin infections See *Gas gangrene, page 41, & Toxic shock, pages 56–56* Ref: CID 44:705, 2007	4 types: (1) Streptococci, Grp A, B, C, G. (2) Clostridia sp. (3) polymicrobic: aerobic + anaerobic (if S. aureus + anaerobic strep = Meleney's synergistic gangrene), (4) Community-acquired MRSA	For treatment of clostridia, see *Muscle, gas gangrene, page 41*. The terminology of polymicrobic wound infections is not precise: Meleney's synergistic gangrene, Fournier's gangrene, necrotizing fasciitis likely common pathophysiology. **All require prompt surgical debridement** of antibiotics. IV & surgical. Dx of necrotizing fasciitis req incision & probing. If no resistance to probing subcut (fascial plane), diagnosis = necrotizing fasciitis. **Need Gram stain/culture** to determine if etiology is strep, clostridia, polymicrobial, or S. aureus. **Treatment: Pen G** if strep or clostridia, **Dori**[FDA-A], **IMP** or **MER** if MRSA suspected. **NOTE:** If strep necrotizing fasciitis, reasonable to treat with penicillin G [strep] (SMJ 96:968, 2003); if clostridia ± gas gangrene, add clinda to penicillin (see footnote). MRSA ref: NEJM 352:1445, 2005		
Puncture wound—nail Through tennis shoe? P. aeruginosa	P. aeruginosa	Local debridement to remove foreign body & tetanus prophylaxis		Osteomyelitis evolves in only 1–2% of plantar puncture wounds.
Staphylococcal scalded skin syndrome	Toxin-producing S. aureus	**Nafcillin** or **oxacillin** 2 gm IV (children: 150 mg/kg/day div. q6h) x 5-7 days for MSSA. **vanco** 1 gm IV q12h (children 40–60 mg/kg/day div. q6h) for MRSA		Toxin causes intraepidermal split and positive Nikolsky sign. Drugs cause epidermal/dermal split, called **toxic epidermal necrolysis**—more serious (Ln 351:1417, 1998). Biopsy differentiates.
Ulcerated skin lesions	Consider anthrax, tularemia, P. aeruginosa (ecthyma gangrenosum), plague, blastomycosis, spider (rarely), mucormycosis, mycobacteria, leishmania, arterial insufficiency, venous stasis, amebiasis.			
Whirlpool (Hot Tub) folliculitis See *Folliculitis, page 49*	Pseudomonas aeruginosa	Usually self-limited, treatment not indicated		Decontaminate hot tub: drain and chlorinate. Also associated with exfoliative beauty aids (loofah sponges) (J Clin Micro 31:480, 1993).

Abbreviations on page 2. NOTE: All dosage recommendations are for adults (unless otherwise indicated) and assume normal renal function.

TABLE 1 (48)

ANATOMIC SITE/DIAGNOSIS/ MODIFYING CIRCUMSTANCES	ETIOLOGIES (usual)	SUGGESTED REGIMENS* PRIMARY	ALTERNATIVE†	ADJUNCT DIAGNOSTIC OR THERAPEUTIC MEASURES AND COMMENTS
SPLEEN. For post-splenectomy prophylaxis, see Table 1a, page 168; for Septic Shock Post-Splenectomy, see Table 1, pg 56.				
Splenic abscess				
Endocarditis, bacteremia	Staph. aureus, streptococci	**Nafcillin** or **oxacillin** 2 gm IV q4h if MSSA	**Vanco** 1 gm IV q12h if MRSA	Burkholderia (Pseudomonas) pseudomallei is common cause of splenic abscess in SE Asia.
Contiguous from intra-abdominal site	Polymicrobic	Treat as Peritonitis, secondary, page 42		
Immunocompromised	Candida sp.	**Amphotericin B** (Dosage, see Table 11, page 96)	**Fluconazole, caspofungin**	
SYSTEMIC FEBRILE SYNDROMES				
Spread by infected **TICK, FLEA, or LICE**				
Babesiosis: see CID 43:1089, 2006.	Etiol: B. microti et al. Vector: Ixodes ticks. Host: White-footed mouse & others	**Atovaquone** 750 mg po bid + **azithro** 500 mg po on day 1, then 250 mg po daily times 7 days) OR (**clinda** 1.2 gm IV bid or 600 mg po tid times 7 days + **quinine** 650 mg po tid times 7 days. **Ped. dosage:** Clinda 20–40 mg per kg per day and quinine 25 mg per kg per day plus **exchange transfusion**		Epidemiologic history crucial. **Babesiosis, Lyme disease, & granulocytic Ehrlichiosis** have same reservoir & tick vector. High % in coastal areas May to Sept. Can result from blood transfusion (JAMA 281:927, 1999). Usually subclinical. Illness likely in asplenic pts, pts with concomitant Lyme disease, older pts, pts with HIV. Dx: Giemsa-stained blood smear, antibody test available. PCR under study. **Rx: Exchange transfusions successful adjunct, used early, in severe disease.**
Asymptomatic bacteremia	B. quintana	**Doxy** 100 mg po/IV times 15 days		
Bartonella infections: CID 35:684, 2002; for B. Quintana – EID 12:217, 2006. Review EID 12:389, 2006				Can lead to endocarditis &/or trench fever; found in homeless, esp. if lice/leg pain.
Cat-scratch disease	B. henselae	**Azithro** 500 mg po x1 dose, then 250 mg po daily x4 more days	**Azithro** or symptomatic only—see page 41, usually lymphadenitis in immunocompetent pts	**Manifestations of Bartonella infections:** **Immunocompetent Patient:** Bartonella/endocarditis/FUO Cat scratch disease Encephalopathy
Bacillary angiomatosis; Peliosis hepatis—pts with AIDS	B. henselae, B. quintana	**Erythro** 500 mg po qid or **clarith** ER 1 gm po bid or **doxy** 100 mg po bid times 3 mos if severe, combination of **doxy** 100 mg po/IV bid + **RIF** 300 mg po bid	**Erythro** 500 mg po qid or **doxy** 100 mg po bid x 8 wks	**HIV/AIDS Patient:** Bacillary angiomatosis Bacillary peliosis Bacteremia/endocarditis/FUO
Bacteremia immunocompetent pts	Blood PCR for B. henselae	Mild illness: No treatment	Moderate illness: **Azithro**	Vertebral osteo Trench fever Parinaud's oculoglandular syndrome EID 13:938, 2007
Endocarditis (see page 25) (Circ 111:3167, 2005)	B. henselae, B. quintana	[**Ceftriaxone** 2 gm IV once daily x 6 wks + **Gentamicin** 1 mg/kg) IV q8h x 14 days] with or without **doxy** 100 mg IV/po bid x 6 wks		Hard to Dx with automated blood culture systems. Need lysis-centrifugation and/or blind subculture onto chocolate agar at 8–14 days. Diagnosis often by antibody titer ≥1:800. NOTE: Only aminoglycosides are bactericidal.
Oroya fever	B. bacilliformis	**CIP** IV or po—Dosage see Table 10C	**Chloro** 1 gm IV or po q6h	Oroya fever transmitted by sandfly bite in Andes Mtns. Related Bartonella (B. rochalimae) caused bacteremia, fever and splenomegaly (NEJM 356:2346 & 2381, 2007).
Trench fever (FUO)	B. quintana	**Doxy** 100 mg po bid (doxy alone if **no endocarditis**)		Person with arthropod & animal exposure: EID 13:938, 2007
SYSTEMIC FEBRILE SYNDROMES Spread by infected **TICK, FLEA or LICE** (continued)				
Ehrlichiosis: CDC def. is one of: (1) 4x ↑ IFA titer, (2) detection of Ehrlichia DNA in blood or CSF by PCR, (3) visible morulae in WBC and IFA ≥1:64 (MMWR 46(RR-10):1–55, 1997).				In endemic area (New York), high % of both adult ticks and nymphs were jointly infected with both HGE and B. burgdorferi (NEJM 337:49, 1997).
Human monocytic ehrlichiosis (HEM) (MMWR 55(RR-4), 2006; CID 43:1089, 2006)	Ehrlichia chaffeensis (Lone Star tick is vector)	**Doxy** 100 mg po/IV times 7–14 days	**Tetracycline** 500 mg po qid x 7–14d. No current rec. for children or pregnancy	History of outdoor activity and tick exposure April–Sept. Fever, rash (36%), leukopenia and thrombocytopenia. Blood smears no help. PCR for early dx.

* See Table 1, pg 56. † See footnotes. Abbreviations on page 2. NOTE: All dosage recommendations are for adults (unless otherwise indicated) and assume normal renal function.

TABLE 1 (49)

ANATOMIC SITE/DIAGNOSIS/ MODIFYING CIRCUMSTANCES	ETIOLOGIES (usual)	SUGGESTED REGIMENS*		ADJUNCT DIAGNOSTIC OR THERAPEUTIC MEASURES AND COMMENTS
		PRIMARY	ALTERNATIVE†	
SYSTEMIC FEBRILE SYNDROMES *(Ehrlichiosis continued)*				
Human granulocytic ehrlichiosis (HGE) *ISDA guideline CID 43:1089, 2006; CID 43:1089, 2006)*	Anaplasma (Ehrlichia) phagocytophilum (Ixodes sp. ticks also vector). Rarely + blood smear. Antibody test confirms. Ehrlichia ewingii (NEJM 341:148 & 195, 1999)	Doxy 100 mg po or IV times 7-14 days	Tetracycline 500 mg po qid times 7-14 days. Not in children (See Comment)	Upper Midwest. NE. West Coast & Europe. H/O tick exposure. April-Sept. Febrile flu-like illness after outdoor activity. No rash. Leukopenia/thrombocytopenia common. **Dx:** Up to 80% have + blood smear, antibody test confirms retrospectively. **Rx:** Tetracyclines in pregnancy (CID 27:213, 1998) but worry about resistance developing. Based on in vitro studies, no clear alternative Rx—Levo activity marginal (AAC 47:413, 2003).
Lyme Disease NOTE: Think about concomitant tick-borne disease—babesiosis (JAMA 275:1657, 1996) or ehrlichiosis. Lyme. Guideline CID 43:1089, 2006.	Borrelia burgdorferi ISDA guideline CID 43:1089, 2006			
Bite by Ixodes-infected tick in an endemic area		If endemic area & nymphal If not endemic area, not partially engorged deer tick: doxy 200 mg po times 1 partially engorged, not deer tick: No dose with food treatment		Prophylaxis study in endemic area: erythema migrans developed in 3% of control group and 0.4% doxy group (NEJM 345:79 & 133, 2001).
Early (erythema migrans) *See Comment*		Doxy 100 mg po bid, or amoxicillin 500 mg po bid or cefuroxime axetil 500 mg po bid qid. All regimens for 14-21 days. See Comment for peds doses	erythro 250 mg po qid. (10 days as good as 20: AnIM 138:697, 2003)	High rate of clinical failure with azithro & erythro (Drugs 57:157, 1999). **Peds** (all for 14-21 days): **Amox** 50 mg per kg per day in 3 div. doses or **cefuroxime axetil** 30 mg per kg per day in 2 div. doses or **erythro** 30 mg per kg per day in 3 div. doses. Lesions usually homogenous—not target-like (AnIM 136:423, 2002).
Carditis *See Comment*		(Ceftriaxone 2 gm IV q24h) or (cefotaxime 2 gm IV q4h) or (pen G 24 million units IV q4h) times 14-21 days	Doxy (see Comments) 100 mg po bid times 14-21 days or amoxicillin 500 mg po tid times 14-21 days.	First degree AV block: Oral regimen. High degree AV block (PR >0.3 sec.): IV therapy—permanent pacemaker not necessary.
Facial nerve paralysis (isolated finding, early)		Doxy 100 mg po bid or amoxicillin 500 mg po tid times 14-21 days		LP suggested to exclude neurologic disease. If LP neg, oral regimen OK. If abnormal or not done, suggest parenteral regimen.
Meningitis, encephalitis *For encephalopathy, see Comment*		Ceftriaxone 2 gm IV q24h times 14-21 days	Pen G 20 million units IV (ceftriaxone 2 gm IV q24h) q24h (in div. dose) or (cefotaxime 2 gm IV q8h) times 14-28 days	Encephalopathy, memory difficulty, depression, somnolence, or headache, CSF abnormalities. 89% had objective CSF abnormalities. 18/18 pts improved with ceftriaxone 2 gm per day times 30 days (JID 180:377, 1999). No compelling evidence that prolonged treatment has any benefit in post-Lyme syndrome (Neurology 69:1, 2007).
Arthritis		(Doxy 100 mg po bid) or (amoxicillin 500 mg po tid), both times 30- 60 days	(Ceftriaxone 2 gm IV q24h) or (pen G 20-24 million units IV per day IV) times 14-28 days	
		Choose should not include doxy; amoxicillin 500 mg po tid times 21 days.	If pen. allergic: azithro 500 mg po qd times 14-21 days	
Pregnant women		None indicated		
Asymptomatic seropositivity and symptoms post-tx				No benefit from treatment (NEJM 345:85, 2001)
Relapsing fever (EID 12:369, 2006)	Borrelia recurrentis B. hermsii, & other borrelia sp.	Doxy 100 mg po bid	Erythro 500 mg po qid	Jarisch-Herxheimer (fever, ↑ pulse, ↓ blood pressure) in most patients (occurs in ~2 hrs), not prevented by prior steroids. **Dx:** Examine peripheral blood smear during fever for spirochetes. Can relapse up to 10 times. Post-exposure doxy pre-emptive therapy highly effective (NEJM 355:148, 2006).

Abbreviations on page 2.

NOTE: All dosage recommendations are for adults (unless otherwise indicated) and assume normal renal function.

TABLE 1 (50)

ANATOMIC SITE/DIAGNOSIS/ MODIFYING CIRCUMSTANCES	ETIOLOGIES (usual)	SUGGESTED REGIMENS*		ADJUNCT DIAGNOSTIC OR THERAPEUTIC MEASURES AND COMMENTS
		PRIMARY	ALTERNATIVE†	
SYSTEMIC FEBRILE SYNDROMES—Review infected **TICK, FLEA or LICE/Relapsing fever** (continued)				
Rickettsial diseases. Review (CID 39:1493, 2004)	Spread by infected TICK, FLEA or LICE/Relapsing fever (continued)			
Spotted fevers (NOTE: Rickettsial pox not included)				
Rocky Mountain spotted fever (RMSF) (LnID 7:724, 2007 and MMWR 55 (RR-4), 2007)	R. rickettsii (Dermacentor ticks)	Doxy 100 mg po/IV bid times 1 day or 2 days after temp. normal	Chloro 100 mg po/IV bid times 7 days. NOTE: Chloro use found less safe factor for fatal RMSF (JID 184:1437, 2001)	Fever, rash (95%), petechiae 40–50%. **Rash spreads from distal extremities to trunk.** Dx: Immunohistochemistry on skin biopsy; or antibody titers. Highest incidence in Mid-Atlantic states; also seen in Oklahoma, S. Dakota, Montana. **NOTE: Only 3–18% of pts present with fever, rash, and hx of tick exposure; esp. in children many early deaths & empiric doxy reasonable** (MMWR 49: 888, 2000).
NOTE: Can mimic ehrlichiosis. Pattern of rash important—see Comment				
Other spotted fevers, e.g. Boutonneuse fever. R. africae review: LnID 3:557, 2003	6 species, e.g. R. conorii et al. (multiple ticks). In sub-Saharan Africa, R. africae	Doxy 100 mg po bid times 7 days	Chloro 500 mg po/IV qid times 7 days Children <8 y.o.: azithro or clarithro (see Comment)	Clarithro 7.5 mg per kg q12h & azithro 10 mg per kg per day times 1 or 3 days equally efficacious in children with Mediterranean spotted fever (CID 34:154, 2002). R. africae review: CID 36:1411, 2003. R. parkeri in U.S.: CID 38:805, 2004
Typhus group—Consider in returning travelers with fever				
Louse-borne	R. prowazekii (body louse)	Doxy 100 mg IV/po bid times 7 days	Chloro 500 mg IV/po qid times 7 days	**Brill-Zinsser disease** (Ln 357:1198, 2001) is a relapse of remote past infection, e.g. WW II. Truncal rash spreads centrifugally—opposite of RMSF. A winter disease.
Murine typhus (cat flea typhus similar)	R. typhi (rat reservoir and flea vector)	Doxy 100 mg IV/po bid times 7 days	Chloro 500 mg IV/po qid times 7 days	Most U.S. cases south Texas and southern Calif. Flu-like illness. Rash in ~50%. Dx based on suspicion; confirmed serologically.
Scrub typhus	O. tsutsugamushi (rodent reservoir, vector is larval stage of mites (chiggers))	Doxy 100 mg IV/po bid times 7 days	Chloro 500 mg IV/po qid times 7 days NOTE: Reports of doxy and chloro resistance from northern Thailand (Ln 348:86, 1996). In prospective random trial, single 500 mg dose of azithro as effective as doxy (AAC 51:3259, 2007)	Limited to Far East (Asia, India). Cases imported into U.S. Evidence of chigger bite, flu-like illness. Rash like louse-borne typhus. RIF alone reported 450 mg q12h times 7 days reported effective in (Ln 356:1057, 2000). Worry about RIF resistance.
Tularemia, typhoidal type Ref. bioterrorism: see Table 1B, page 60, & JAMA 285:2763, 2001	Francisella tularensis. (Vector depends on geography; ticks, biting flies, mosquitoes idsrael)	Gentamicin or tobra 5 mg per kg per day IV q8h IV times 7–14 days	Add severe if evidence of meningitis. CIP reported effective in 12 children (PIDJ 19:449, 2000)	Pneumonic form in 5–30% pts. No lymphadenopathy. Diarrhea, pneumonia common. Dx: blood cultures. Antibody confirmation. Rx: Jarisch-Herxheimer reaction may occur. Clinical failures with rx with P Ceph 3 (CID 17:976, 1993).
Other Zoonotic Systemic Bacterial Febrile illnesses: Obtain careful epidemiologic history				
Brucellosis Review: NEJM 352:2325, 2005				
Adult or child >8 years	Brucella sp. B. abortus—cattle B. suis—pigs B. melitensis—goats B. canis—dogs	[Doxy 100 mg po bid times 6 wks + gentamicin times 7 days (see Table 10C, page 90)] or [doxy times 6 wks + streptomycin 1 gm IM q24h times 2–3 wks] See Comment	[Doxy + RIF 600–900 mg po q24h; both times 6 wks] or [TMP-SMX 1 DS (160 mg TMP) po qid times 6 wks + gentamicin times 2 wks]	Clinical disease: Protean. Fever in 91%. Malodorous perspiration almost pathognomonic. Osteoarticular disease approx. 20%%; epididymitis/orchitis 6%. Lab: Mild hepatitis. Leukopenia & relative lymphocytosis. Dx: Serology; bone marrow culture; real-time PCR if available. Treatment: Drugs must penetrate macrophages & act in acidic milieu. Pregnancy: TMP-SMX-DS + RIF advised. Prospective random. Study documents doxy + 7 d of gent as effective as doxy + streptomycin. 1 d (CID 42:1075, 2006). Review of FQs in comb. therapy (AAC 50:22, 2006).
Child >8 years		TMP-SMX 5 mg per kg TMP po q12h times 6 wks + gentamicin or RIF 15 mg/kg/d po/IV		
Leptospirosis (CID 36:1507 & 1514, 2003; LnID 3:757, 2003)	Leptospira—in urine of domestic livestock, dogs, small rodents	Pen G 1.5 million units IV q6h or ceftriaxone 1 gm q24h. Duration: 7 days	Doxy 100 mg IV q12h or AMP 0.5–1 gm q6h	Severity varies. Two-stage mild anicteric illness to severe icteric disease (Weil's disease) with renal failure and myocarditis. Rx: Penicillin, doxy, & cefotaxime of equal efficacy in severe lepto (CID 39:1417, 2004).

Abbreviations on page 2.   NOTE: All dosage recommendations are for adults (unless otherwise indicated) and assume normal renal function.

TABLE 1 (51)

ANATOMIC SITE/DIAGNOSIS/ MODIFYING CIRCUMSTANCES	ETIOLOGIES (usual)	SUGGESTED REGIMENS*		ADJUNCT DIAGNOSTIC OR THERAPEUTIC MEASURES AND COMMENTS
		PRIMARY	ALTERNATIVE†	
SYSTEMIC FEBRILE SYNDROMES				
TICK, FLEA or LICE/Other Zoonotic Systemic Bacterial Febrile Illnesses (continued)				
Salmonella bacteremia (enteric fever most often caused by S. typhi)	Spread by infected. Salmonella enteritidis—a variety of serotypes	CIP 400 mg IV q12h times 14 days (switch to po when clinically possible)	Ceftriaxone 2 gm IV q24h times 14 days (switch to po CIP when possible)	Usual exposure is contaminated poultry and eggs. Many others. Myriad of complications to consider, e.g., mycotic aneurysm (10% of adults over age 50, AJM 110:60, 2001), septic arthritis, osteomyelitis, septic shock. Sporadic reports of response to CIP. Ref.: LnID 5:341, 2005
Miscellaneous Systemic Febrile Syndromes				
Kawasaki syndrome 6 weeks to 12 yrs of age, peak at 1 yr of age; 85% below age 5. (Ln 364:533, 2004)	Acute self-limited vasculitis with ↑ temp., rash, conjunctivitis, stomatitis, cervical adenitis, red hands/feet & coronary artery aneurysms (25%) at times 6–8 wks	IVIG 2 gm IV over 12 hrs + ASA 20-25 mg per kg qid THEN ASA 3-5 mg per kg per day to q24h times 6-8 wks	If still febrile after 1st dose of IVIG, some give 2nd dose (PIDJ 17:1144, 1998)	IV gamma globulin (2 gm over 10 hrs) in pts rx before 10th day of illness ↓ coronary artery lesions (Ln 347:1128, 1996) See Table 14B, page 91 for IVIG adverse effects and expense. Pulsed steroids of NO value: NEJM 356:659 & 663, 2007.
Rheumatic Fever, acute Ref.: Ln 366:155, 2005	Post–Group A strep pharyngitis (not Group B, C, or G) (see Pharyngitis, page 43)	ASA 80-100 mg per kg per day in children, 4-8 gm per day in adults. (2) Eradicate Group A strep: Pen times 10 days		(1) Symptom relief: ASA 80-100 mg per kg per day in children, 4-8 gm per day in adults. (2) Eradicate Group A strep: Pen times 10 days (see Pharyngitis, p. 43). (3) Start prophylaxis: see below
Prophylaxis Primary prophylaxis		Benzathine pen G 1.2 million units IM (see Pharyngitis, p. 43)	Penicillin for 10 days, prevents rheumatic fever even when started 7-9 days after onset of illness Alternative: Penicillin V 250mg po bid or sulfadiazine (sulfisoxazole) (gm po q24h or erythro 250mg po bid.	
Secondary prophylaxis (previous documented rheumatic fever)		Benzathine pen G 1.2 million units IM q3-4 wks	Duration? No carditis: 5 yr or age 21, whichever is longer; carditis without residual heart disease: 10 yr; carditis with residual valvular disease: 10 yr since last episode & at least age 40 (PEDS 96:758, 1995).	
Typhoid syndrome (typhoid fever, enteric fever) (Ln 366:749, 2005; LnID 5:623, 2005)	Salmonella typhi, S. paratyphi NOTE: In vitro resistance to nalidixic acid predicts clinical failure of CIP (FQs) (Ln 366:749, 2005)	(CIP 500 mg po bid times 10 days) or ceftriaxone 2 gm IV q24h times 14 days (See Comment) In children, CIP superior to ceftriaxone	Azithro 1 gm po day 1, then 500 mg po times 6 days (AAC 43: 1441, 1999) or 1 gm po q24h times 5 days (AAC 44:1855, 2000) (See Comment.)	Dexamethasone dose: 3 mg per kg then 1 mg per kg q6h times 8 doses ↓ mortality (NEJM 310:82, 1984). Complications: perforation of terminal ileum &/or cecum, osteo, septic arthritis, mycotic aneurysm (approx. 10% over age 50, AJM 110:60, 2001), meningitis. Other rx options: Controlled trial of CIP vs chloro. Efficacy equivalent. After 5 days, blood cultures positive: CIP 18%, chloro 36% (AAC 47:1727, 2003). Children & adolescents: Ceftriaxone (75 mg per kg per day in 2 divided doses) or azithro (20 mg per kg per day to 1 gm max.) equal efficacy. More relapses with ceftriaxone (CID 38:951, 2004).
Sepsis: Following suggested empiric therapy assumes pt is bacteremic; mimicked by viral, rickettsial infections and pancreatitis				
Neonatal—early onset <1 week old	Group B strep, E. coli, klebsiella, enterobacter, Staph. aureus (uncommon), Listeria (rare in U.S.)	AMP 25 mg per kg IV q8h + cefotaxime 50 mg per kg IV q12h	AMP + gent 2.5 mg per kg IV/IM q12h or (AMP + cefotaxime 50 mg per kg IV/IM q12h)	Blood cultures are key but only 5-10%. ↓ Discontinue antibiotics after 72 hrs if cultures and course do not support diagnosis. In Spain, listeria predominates; in S. America, salmonella.
Neonatal— late onset 1-4 weeks old	As above + H. influenzae & S. epidermidis	AMP 25 mg per kg IV q6h + cefotaxime 50 mg per kg q8h or (AMP + ceftriaxone 75 mg per kg q24h)	AMP + gent 2.5 mg per kg q8h IV or IM	
Child; not neutropenic	Strep. pneumoniae, meningococci, Staph. aureus (MSSA & MRSA), H. influenzae now rare	Cefotaxime 50 mg per kg q6h IV/IM or ceftriaxone 100 mg per kg IV (q24h) + vanco 15 mg per kg IV q8h	Aztreonam 7.5 mg per kg q8h + linezolid (see Table 16, page 177 for indiv.	If MSSA/MRSA a concern, add vanco. Major concerns are S. pneumoniae & community-acquired MRSA. "Coverage for Gm-neg. bacilli included but H. influenzae infection now rare. Meningococcemia mortality remains high (Ln 356:961, 2000).

Abbreviations on page 2.   NOTE: All dosage recommendations are for adults (unless otherwise indicated) and assume normal renal function.

TABLE 1 (52)

ANATOMIC SITE/DIAGNOSIS/ MODIFYING CIRCUMSTANCES	ETIOLOGIES (usual)	SUGGESTED REGIMENS*		ADJUNCT DIAGNOSTIC OR THERAPEUTIC MEASURES AND COMMENTS
		PRIMARY	ALTERNATIVE†	
SYSTEMIC FEBRILE SYNDROMES/Sepsis *(continued)*				
Adult; not neutropenic: NO HYPOTENSION but LIFE-THREATENING—For *Septic shock, see page 56*				
Source unclear—consider intra-abdominal or skin source. **Life-threatening.**	Aerobic Gm-neg. bacilli; S. aureus; streptococci; others	(**Dori** or **IMP** or **MER**) + **vanco**	(**Dapto** 6 mg per kg IV q24h) + (**P Ceph 3/4** or **PIP-TZ** or **TC-CL**).	Systemic inflammatory response syndrome (SIRS): 2 or more of the following: 1. Temperature >38°C or <36°C 2. Heart rate >90 beats per min. 3. Respiratory rate >20 breaths per min. 4. WBC >12,000 per mcL or >10% bands **Sepsis:** SIRS + a documented infection (+ culture) **Severe sepsis:** Sepsis + organ dysfunction or hypoperfusion abnormalities (lactic acidosis, oliguria, ↑ mental status) **Septic shock:** Sepsis-induced hypotension (systolic BP <90 mmHg) not responsive to 500 mL IV fluid challenge + peripheral hypoperfusion.
		Could substitute linezolid for vanco or dapto; however, linezolid bacteriostatic vs S. aureus.	*Dosages in footnote¹*	
If suspect biliary source *(see p.10)*	Enterococci + aerobic Gm-neg. bacilli	**AM-SB, PIP-TZ,** or **TC-CL**	**P Ceph 3 + metro; (CIP** or **Levo) + metro. Dosages—footnote¹**	
If illicit use IV drugs	S. aureus	**Vanco** if high prevalence of MRSA. Do NOT use empiric vanco + oxacillin pending organism ID. *Dosages—footnote¹*		In vitro nafcillin increased production of toxins by CA-MRSA (*JID 195:202, 2007*).
If suspect intra-abdominal source	Mixture aerobic & anaerobic Gm-neg. bacilli	*See secondary peritonitis, page 42*		
If petechial rash	Meningococcemia	**Ceftriaxone 2 gm IV q12h** (until sure no meningitis), consider Rocky Mountain spotted fever—*see page 53*		
If suspect urinary source	Aerobic Gm-neg. bacilli & enterococci	*See pyelonephritis, page 30*		
Neutropenia: Child or Adult (absolute PMN count <500 per mm3) in cancer and transplant patients. Guideline: CID 34:730, 2002				
Prophylaxis—afebrile Post-chemotherapy, impending neutropenia		**Levo** 500 mg po bid		Meta-analysis demonstrates substantive reduction in mortality (study using **Levo** 500 mg po bid q24h (*CID 40:1087 & 1094, 2005*). Also *NEJM 353:977, 988 & 1052, 2005*). Similar results in observational study using **Levo** 500 mg po bid.
Post-chemotherapy in AIDS patient.	pneumocystis (PCP)	**TMP-SMX-DS** po bid—adults; 10 mg per kg per day div bid po—children.		Need TMP-SMX to prevent PCP. Hard to predict which leukemia/lymphoma/solid tumor pt at ↑ risk of PCP.
Allogeneic hematopoietic stem-cell transplant	↑ risk pneumocystis, herpes viruses, candida	**TMP-SMX** as above + [either **acyclovir** or **ganciclovir**) + **fluconazole]**		Combined regimen justified by combined effect of neutropenia and immunosuppression.
Empiric therapy—febrile neutropenia (≥38.3°C x1 or ≥38°C for ≥1 hr)				
Low-risk adults Peds data pending *(Def. low risk in Comment)*	As above	**CIP** 750 mg po bid + **AM-CL** 875 mg po bid		Treat as outpatients with 24/7 access to inpatient care if: no focal findings, no hypotension, no COPD, no fungal infection, no dehydration, age <60 & >16.

¹ **P Ceph 3** (cefotaxime 2 gm IV q8h, use q4h if life-threatening; ceftizoxime 2 gm IV q8h; ceftriaxone 2 gm IV q24h), **AP Pen** (piperacillin 3 gm IV q12h), **AP Pen** (piperacillin 3 gm IV q4h, ticarcillin 3 gm IV q4h), **TC-CL** 3.1 gm IV q4h; **PIP-TZ** 3.375 gm IV q4h or 4-hr infusion of 3.375 gm IV q8h, **APAG** (see table 10D, page 100), **AMP** 30 mg (but IV q6h + a, **clinda** 900 mg IV q8h; **IMP** 0.5 gm IV q6h, **MER** 1 gm IV q8h, **Erta** 1 gm q24h, **Dori** 500 mg IV q8h (1-hr infusion), **P Ceph 4** (**CFP** 2 gm IV q12h), **CIP** 400 mg IV q12h, **levo** 750 mg IV q24h, **linezolid** 600 mg IV q12h.

3 **AP** (ceftazidime 2 gm IV q8h).

Abbreviations on page 2.

NOTE: All dosage recommendations are for adults (unless otherwise indicated) and assume normal renal function.

TABLE 1 (53)

ANATOMIC SITE/DIAGNOSIS/ MODIFYING CIRCUMSTANCES	ETIOLOGIES (usual)	SUGGESTED REGIMENS*		ADJUNCT DIAGNOSTIC OR THERAPEUTIC MEASURES AND COMMENTS
		PRIMARY	ALTERNATIVE†	
SYSTEMIC FEBRILE SYNDROMES Sepsis/Neutropenic: Child or Adult *(continued)*				
High-risk adults and children	Aerobic Gm-neg. bacilli; ceph-resistant viridans strep, MRSA	**Monotherapy:** ceftaz or IMP or MER or CFP or PIP-TZ *Dosages: Footnote 1 page 55 and Table 10.* Include empiric vanco if: suspect IV access infected; colonized with drug-resistant S. pneumo or MRSA; blood culture pos. for Gm+ cocci; pt hypotensive	**Combination therapy:** (Gent¹ or tobra) + (TC-CL or PIP-TZ)	Increasing resistance of viridans streptococci to penicillins, cephalosporins & FQs (CID 34:1469 & 1524, 2002; CID 31:1126, 2000; JAC 47:87, 2001). If **severe IgE-mediated β-lactam allergy?** No formal trials, but (aminoglycoside or CIP) + aztreonam) + vanco should work. In a meta-analysis of monotherapies, **cefepime** (CFP) associated with higher 30 d all cause mortality; individual pt assessments pending (LAC 57:176, 2006). PIP-TZ & CFP: Equal efficacy (JAC 43:447, 2006).
Persistent fever and neutropenia after 5 days of empiric antibacterial therapy—see CID 34:730, 2002—General guidelines				
	Candida species, aspergillus	Add either **caspofungin** 70 mg IV day 1, then 50 mg IV q24h, **OR voriconazole** 6 mg per kg IV q12h times 2 doses, then 3 mg per kg IV q12h		Conventional **ampho B** causes more fever & nephrotoxicity & lower efficacy than lipid-based ampho B; both **caspofungin & voriconazole** better tolerated & perhaps more efficacious than lipid-based ampho B (NEJM 346:225, 2002 & 351:1391 & 1445, 2005).
Shock syndromes				
Septic shock: Fever & hypotension Bacteremic shock, endotoxin shock Overall review: Ln 365:63, 2005 Antimicrobial therapy: CCM 32(Suppl.):S495, 2004 Surviving sepsis campaign: CCM 32:858, 2004 Low-dose steroids refs: JAMA 288:862 & 886, 2002; NEJM 355:1699, 2006; Critical Care 11:113, 2007.	Bacteremia with aerobic Gm-neg bacteria or Gm+ cocci	**Proven therapy: (1)** Replete intravascular volume, **(2)** correct, if possible, disease that allowed bloodstream invasion, **(3)** appropriate empiric antimicrobial rx, see suggestions under life-threatening sepsis, page 49 and Footnote 1 of empiric antimicrobial **activated Protein C** (drotrecogin) document below. **(5)** Low-dose steroids (if document relative adrenal insufficiency) (see Comment for criteria). Hydrocortisone 50 mg IV q6h + fludrocortisone (Florinef) 50 mcg po once q24h) times 7 days. **(6)** Low-dose **vasopressin** reported effective for catecholamine-resistant septic shock (Gem Resp Crit Care Med 25:705, 2004) **(6)** Blood glucose control: 80–110 mg per dL		**Activ. Protein C: Drotrecogin (Xigris):** In a double-blind placebo-controlled trial (DBPCT) (NEJM 344:699, 2001), 28-d. mortality ↓ from 31 to 25% in sickest pts. In less sick pts (APACHE II score <25) showed no benefit. Xigris not indicated in pts with single organ dysfunction, & low risk of death. In kids, no benefit & increased mortality (NEJM 353:1332 & 1398, 2005). **Hemorrhage** is major adverse event. **Dose** 24 mg per kg per hr over 96 hrs by continuous IV infusion. Stop 2 hrs before & restart 12 hrs after surgery. Approx. cost of drug for 4-day course: $8000. **Low-dose steroids:** In DBPCT, pts with low baseline cortisol (or <9 mcg response to 0.25 mg IV cosyntropin) had improved 28-d mortality with low doses steroids. Easier glucose control with 200 mg/day by continuos infusion. **Low-dose vasopressin:** Dose should not exceed 0.04 units per min. **Targeted glucose levels:** Tight plasma glucose control appears to reduce mortality (AnIM 164:2005, 2004).
Septic shock: postsplenectomy (asplenia)	S. pneumoniae, N. meningitidis, H. influenzae, Capnocytophaga (DF-2)	**Ceftriaxone** 2 gm IV q12h if meningitis Other management as per Septic shock, above	**Levo** 750 mg or **Moxi** 400 mg all once IV q24h	Howell-Jolly bodies in peripheral blood smear confirm absence of functional spleen. Often results in **symmetrical peripheral gangrene of digits** due to severe DIC. For prophylaxis, see Table 15A, page 167.
Toxic shock syndrome, Clostridium sordellii Post-partum, post-abortion, post-mifepristone, IVDUs CID 43:1436 & 1447, 2006	Clostridium sordellii Mortality 69%	Fluids, ac: **penicillin G** 18–20 million units per day div. q4–6h + **clindamycin** 900 mg IV q8h		Several deaths reported after use to abortifacient regimen (RU486) & misoprostol. Clinically; often abrupt onset, progressive, hypotension, edema, effusions, hemoconcentration, leukemoid reaction (WBCs~50,000) induced by neuraminidase (JID 195:1838, 2007).
Toxic shock syndrome, staphylococcal. Superantigen review: LnID 2:156, 2002 Colonization by toxin-producing Staph. aureus of: vagina (tampon-assoc.), surgical/traumatic wounds, endometrium, burns	Staph. aureus (toxic shock toxin-mediated)	(**Nafcillin** or **oxacillin** 2 gm IV q4h) or (if MRSA, **vanco** 1 gm IV q12h) + **IVIG**	**Cefazolin** 1–2 gm IV q8h) or (if MRSA, **vanco** 1 gm IV q12h OR **dapto** 6mg/kg IV q24h) + **IVIG**	**IVIG** 1 gm per kg day 1, then 0.5 gm per kg days 2 & 3—antitoxin antibodies present. (CID 42:729 2006). **Exposure of MRSA to nafcillin increased toxin production** in vitro (JID 195:202, 2007.

Abbreviations on page 2.   NOTE: All dosage recommendations are for adults (unless otherwise indicated) and assume normal renal function.

TABLE 1 (54)

ANATOMIC SITE/DIAGNOSIS/ MODIFYING CIRCUMSTANCES	ETIOLOGIES (usual)	SUGGESTED REGIMENS*		ADJUNCT DIAGNOSTIC OR THERAPEUTIC MEASURES AND COMMENTS
		PRIMARY	ALTERNATIVE†	
SYSTEMIC FEBRILE SYNDROMES/Shock syndromes (continued)				
Toxic shock syndrome, streptococcal [Ref.: *JID* 779(Suppl.2):S366–374, 1999]. NOTE: For Necrotizing fasciitis without toxic shock, see page 50. Associated with invasive disease, i.e., erysipelas, necrotizing fasciitis, secondary strep infection of varicella. Secondary cases TSS reported. [NEJM 335:547 & 590, 1996; CID 27:150, 1998].	Group A, B, C, & G Strep. pyogenes	**Pen G** 24 million units per day IV in div. doses) + **clinda** 900 mg IV q8h)	**Ceftriaxone** 2 gm IV q24h + **clinda** 900 mg IV q8h	Definition: Isolation of Group A strep, hypotension and ≥2 of: renal impairment, coagulopathy, liver involvement, ARDS, generalized rash, soft tissue necrosis [*JAMA* 269:390, 1993]. Associated with invasive disease. **Surgery usually required.** Mortality with fasciitis 30–50%, myositis 80% even with early rx (*CID* 14:2, 1992). Clinda ↓ toxin production. Use of NSAID may predispose to TSS. For reasons pen G may fail in fulminant S. pyogenes infections, see *JID* 167:1401, 1993).
		IVIG associated with ↓ in sepsis-related organ failure (*CID* 37:333 & 341, 2003). IVIG dose: 1 gm per kg day 1, then 0.5 gm per day on days 2 & 3. IVIG preps vary in neutralizing Antibody content (*CID* 43:743, 2006).		
Other Toxin-Mediated Syndromes—no fever unless complicated				
Botulism (*CID* 41:1167, 2005. As **biologic weapon**, *JAMA* 285:1059, 2001; Table 1B, page 59; www.bt.cdc.gov)	C. botulinum	For all types: Follow vital capacity, other supportive care. If no ileus, purge GI tract		
Food-borne Dyspnea at presentation bad sign (*CID* 43:1247, 2006).		Trivalent (types A, B, E) equine serum antitoxin—State Health Dept. or CDC (see Comment)	Trivalent (types A, B, E) equine antitoxin (see Comment)	**Equine antitoxin:** Obtain from State Health Depts. or CDC (404-639-2206 M-F OR 404-639-2888 evenings/weekends). Skin test first & desensitize if necessary. One vial IV and one vial IM.
Infant		No antibiotics; may ↑ type C. botulinum in gut and ↑ load of toxin		**Antimicrobials:** May make infant botulism worse. Untested in wound botulism. When used, pen G 10-20 million units per day usual dose. If complications (pneumonia, UTI) occur, avoid antimicrobials with assoc. neuromuscular blockade, i.e., aminoglycosides, tetracycline.
		Human botulinum immunoglobulin (BIG) IV, single dose. Call 510-540-2646. Do not use equine antitoxin.		**Differential dx:** Guillain-Barré, myasthenia gravis, tick paralysis, organophosphate toxicity, West Nile virus.
Wound		Débridement & anaerobic cultures. No proven value of local antitoxin. Role of antibiotics untested.	Trivalent equine antitoxin (see Comment)	Can result from spore contamination of tar heroin. Ref: *CID* 31:1018, 2000.
Tetanus	C. tetani	**Pen G** 24 million units per day in slow IV or **doxy** 100 mg IV q12h times 7–10 days	**Metro** 500 mg po q8h or 1 gm IV q12h times 7–10 days (See Comment)	Multifaceted treatment: Wound debridement; tetanus immunoglobulin (250–500 units IM), antimicrobics, & tetanus toxoid (tetanus does not confer immunity). Options for control of muscle spasms: continuous infusion of midazolam, IV propofol, and/or intrathecal baclofen (*CID* 38:321, 2004).
VASCULAR				
Cavernous sinus thrombosis (see below)	Staph. aureus, Group A strep, H. influenzae, aspergillus/mucor/rhizopus	**Vanco** 1 gm IV q12h + **ceftriaxone** 2 gm IV q24h.	(**Dapto** 6 mg per kg IV q24h)ᴬᴰᴸ or **linezolid** 600 mg IV q12h) + **ceftriaxone** 2 gm IV q24h	CT or MRI scan for diagnosis. Heparin controversial (*Ln* 338:597, 1991). If patient diabetic with ketoacidosis or post-desferrioxamine rx or neutropenic, consider fungal etiology: aspergillus, mucor, see Table 11A, pages 94 & 96.
IV line infection (see *LnID* 7:645, 2007): **Treatment:** [For Prevention, see below]		**Diagnosis of infected line** without removal of IV catheter? See CID 44:820 & 827, 2007.		

Abbreviations on page 2.   NOTE: All dosage recommendations are for adults (unless otherwise indicated) and assume normal renal function.

TABLE 1 (55)

ANATOMIC SITE/DIAGNOSIS/ MODIFYING CIRCUMSTANCES	ETIOLOGIES (usual)	SUGGESTED REGIMENS*		ADJUNCT DIAGNOSTIC OR THERAPEUTIC MEASURES AND COMMENTS
		PRIMARY	ALTERNATIVE[1]	
VASCULAR (continued)				
Heparin lock, midline catheter non-tunneled central venous catheter (subclavian, internal jugular), peripherally inserted central catheter (PICC) Avoid femoral vein if possible. ↑ risk of infection and/or thrombosis (*JAMA 286:700, 2001*)	Staph. epidermidis, Staph. aureus (MSSA/MRSA)	**Vanco** 1 gm IV q12h. **Linezolid alternative—see Comment.** Other rx and duration: **(1) If S. aureus**, remove catheter. Can use TEE result to determine rx (2 vs 4 wks of therapy) (*JAC 57:172, 2006*) **(2) If S. epidermidis** can try to "save" catheter. 80% cure after 7–10 days of therapy. If need to "salvage" the IV line can try to "lock" solution of 3 mg/mL of minocycline + 30 mg/mL of EDTA (in 25% ethanol). Use 2 mL per catheter lumen, dwell time minimum of 2 hrs (*AAC 51:78, 2007*). If IV minocycline not available, tigecycline should work.		If no response to, or intolerant of, **vanco** switch to **daptomycin** 6 mg per kg IV q24h. If no left-sided endocarditis or osteomyelitis, could use **linezolid** 600 mg IV/po bid. **Quinupristin-dalfopristin** an option. 7.5 mg per kg IV q8h via central line. **Dalbavancin** an option (if vanco cross-allergenic) (*1000 mg IV day 1, then 500 mg IV 8 days later if needed. See Table 6, page 73.* Culture removed catheter. With "roll" method, >15 colonies (*NEJM 312:1142, 1985*) suggests infection. Lines do not require "routine" changing when not infected. When infected, do not insert new catheter over a wire. Antimicrobial-impregnated catheters may ↓ infection risk; the debate is lively (*CID 37:65, 2003 & 38:1287, 2004 & 39:1829, 2004*).
Tunnel type indwelling venous catheters and ports (Broviac, Hickman, Groshong, Quinton), dual lumen hemodialysis catheters (Perma-cath)	Staph. epidermidis, Staph. aureus, (Candida sp.) Rarely, leuconostoc or lactobacillus—both resistant to vanco (*see Table 2, page 67*)			If subcutaneous tunnel infected, very low cure rates; need to remove catheter.
Impaired host (burn, neutropenic)	As above + Pseudomonas sp., Enterobacteriaceae, Corynebacterium jeikeium, aspergillus, rhizopus	(**Vanco + P Ceph 3 AP**) or (**vanco + AP Pen**) or **IMP** or **MER** (**P Ceph 3 + AFAPG**) (*Dosage, see page 55*)		Usually have associated septic thrombophlebitis. Biopsy of vein to rule out fungi. If fungal: surgical excision + amphotericin B. Surgical drainage, ligation or removal often indicated.
Hyperalimentation	As with tunnel + Candida sp. common (*see Table 11, resistant Candida species*)	If candida, **voriconazole** 3 mg per kg bid IV day 1, then 50 mg IV q24h **caspofungin** 70 mg IV day 1, then 50 mg IV q24h if clinically stable. **Fluconazole** 400 mg IV q24h		Remove venous catheter and discontinue antimicrobial agents if possible. Ophthalmologic consultation recommended. **Rx all patients with + blood cultures.** See Table 11A, Candidiasis, page 96.
Intravenous lipid emulsion	Staph. epidermidis Malassezia furfur	**Vanco** 1 gm IV q12h		Discontinue infusion. *AJM 90:129, 1991*
IV line infection: Prevention *NEJM 355:2725 & 2781, 2006; LnID 7:645, 2007*	To minimize risk of infection: Hand washing and **1.** Maximal sterile barrier precautions during catheter insertion **2.** Use 2% chlorhexidine for skin antisepsis **3.** If infection rate high despite #1 & 2, use either chlorhexidine/silver sulfadiazine or minocycline/rifampin-impregnated catheters. **4.** If possible, use subclavian vein, avoid femoral vessels			Collective data from in vitro & animal studies plus clinical trials support use of post-insertion flush lock solution of 30 mg/mL of minocycline + 30 mg/mL EDTA in 25% ethanol (*AAC 51:78, 2007*). Tigecycline should work in place of minocycline.
Septic pelvic vein thrombophlebitis (with or without septic pulmonary emboli) Postpartum or postabortion or postpelvic surgery	Streptococci, bacteroides, Enterobacteriaceae	**Metro + P Ceph 3**; **cefoxitin TC-CL, PIP-TZ**, or **AM-SB**	**IMP** or **MER** or **ERTA** or **(clinda** + **aztreonam** or **gent))**	Use heparin during antibiotic regimen. Continued oral anticoagulation not recommended. Cefotetan less active than cefoxitin vs non-fragilis bacteroides. Cefotetan has methyltetrazole side-chain which is associated with hypoprothrombinemia (prevent with vitamin K).
		Dosages: Table 10C, page 85		

Abbreviations on page 2.   *NOTE: All dosage recommendations are for adults (unless otherwise indicated) and assume normal renal function.*

TABLE 1B – PROPHYLAXIS AND TREATMENT OF ORGANISMS OF POTENTIAL USE AS BIOLOGICAL WEAPONS
(See page 2 for abbreviations)

DISEASE	ETIOLOGY	SUGGESTED EMPIRIC TREATMENT REGIMENS		SPECIFIC THERAPY AND COMMENTS
		PRIMARY	**ALTERNATIVE**	
Anthrax **Cutaneous, inhalational, gastrointestinal** Refs.: Ln 364:393 & 449, 2004; MMWR 50:909, 2001; NEJM 345:1607 & 1621, 2001; JAMA 286:2549, 2002; AnIM 144:270, 2006 or www.bt.cdc.gov Also see Table 1, pages 38 & 46 To report bioterrorism event: 770-488-7100 Rationale for CIP: CID 39:303, 2004	Bacillus anthracis Post-exposure **prophylaxis** Ref.: Ln 364:393 & 449, 2004; MMWR 50:909, 2001 Treatment—**Cutaneous anthrax** NEJM 345:1611, 2001. Skin lesions not painful	**Adults (including pregnancy):** (CIP) 500 mg po bid or **Levo** 500 mg po q24h) times 60 days **Children:** CIP 20–30 mg per kg per day div q12h times 60 days	**Adults (including pregnancy): Doxy** 100 mg po bid times 60 days **Children** (see **Comment**): **Doxy** >8 y/o & >45 kg: 100 mg po bid; >8 y/o & ≤45 kg: 2.2 mg per kg po bid; ≤8 y/o: 2.2 mg per kg po bid. All for 60 days.	1. Once organism shows susceptibility to penicillin, switch children to **amoxicillin** 80 mg per kg per day div q8h (max. 500 mg q8h); switch pregnant to **amoxicillin** 500 mg po tid. 2. Do **not** use cephalosporins or TMP-SMX. 3. Other **FQs** (Gati, Moxi) & clarithro should work but no clinical experience.
		Adults (including pregnancy): (CIP) 500 mg po bid or **Levo** 500 mg po q24h) times 60 days **Children:** CIP 20–30 mg per kg per day div q12h times 60 days	**Adults (including pregnancy): Doxy** 100 mg po bid or **Levo** **Children Doxy** >8 y/o & >45 kg: 100 mg po bid; >8 y/o & ≤45 kg: 2.2 mg per kg po bid; ≤8 y/o: 2.2 mg per kg po bid	1. If penicillin susceptible, then: **Adults: Amox** 500 mg po q8h times 60 days. **Children: Amox** 80 mg per kg per day div q8h (max. 500 mg q8h) 2. Usual treatment of cutaneous anthrax is 7–10 days; 60 days in setting of bioterrorism with presumed aerosol exposure 3. Other **FQs** (Gati, Moxi) should work based on in vitro susceptibility data
	Treatment— **Inhalational, gastrointestinal, or oropharyngeal** Characteristic signs & symptoms—**Present:** Rhinorrhea, Dyspnea, N/V; **Absent:** sore throat (AnIM 139:337, 2003)	**Adults (including pregnancy):** (CIP) 400 mg IV q12h or (**Levo** 500 mg IV q24h) or (**doxy** 100 mg IV q12h) + **RIF** 300 mg IV q12h. Switch to po when able & ↓ **CIP** to 500 mg po bid, **clinda** to 450 mg po bid, & **RIF** 300 mg po bid. Treat times 60 days. See Table 2, page 67 for other alternatives.	**Children:** (CIP 10 mg per kg IV q12h or 15 mg per kg po q12h) or (**Doxy** >8 y/o & >45 kg: 100 mg IV q12h; >8 y/o & ≤45 kg: 2.2 mg per kg IV q12h; ≤8 y/o: 2.2 mg per kg IV q12h) **plus clindamycin** 7.5 mg per kg IV q6h **plus RIF** 20 mg per kg per day IV (max. 600 mg) IV q.d. Treat times 60 days. See Table 16, page 177 for oral dosage.	1. Clinda may block toxin production. 2. Rifampin penetrates CSF & intracellular sites. 3. If isolate shown penicillin susceptible: a. **Adult: Pen G** 4 million units IV q4h b. **Child: Pen G** <12 y/o: 50,000 units per kg IV q6h; >12 y/o: 4 million units q4h c. Constitutive & inducible β-lactamases—do not use pen or AMP alone. 4. Do not use cephalosporins or TMP-SMX. 5. Erythro, azithro activity borderline; clarithro active. 6. No person-to-person spread.
Botulism: CID 41:1167, 2005; JAMA 285:1059, 2001 **Food-borne** See Table 1, page 57	Clostridium botulinum	Purge GI tract if no ileus. **Trivalent antitoxin** (types A, B, E): single 10 mL vial per pt. diluted in saline IV (slowly)	Antibiotics have no effect on toxin. Call state health dept for antitoxin.	Supportive care for all types. Follow vital capacity. Submit suspect food for toxin testing. Ref.: CID 39:357 & 363, 2004 & www.bt.cdc.gov
Hemorrhagic fever viruses Ebola, Lassa, Hanta, yellow fever, & others Ref.: JAMA 287:2391, 2002 See Table 14, page 135		Fluid/electrolyte balance. Optimize circulatory volume.	For Lassa & Hanta. **Ribavirin** dose same as Adults. Pregnancy. Children: LD 30 mg per kg IV (max. 2 gm) IV times 1, then 16 mg per kg IV (max. 1 gm per dose) q8h times 4 days, then 8 mg per kg IV (max. 500 mg) q8h times 6 days	Ribavirin active in vitro; not FDA-approved for this indication. NOTE: Ribavirin contraindicated in pregnancy. However, in this setting, the benefits outweigh the risks.
Plague Ref.: JAMA 283:2281, 2000 **Inhalation pneumonic plague** Both **gentamicin** and **doxy** alone efficacious (CID 42:614, 2006)	Yersinia pestis **Treatment** Post-exposure **prophylaxis**	**Gentamicin** 5 mg per kg IV q24h or **streptomycin** 15 mg per kg IV q12h Tobramycin should work. **Doxy** 100 mg po bid times 7 days	**Doxy** 200 mg IV times 1, & then 100 mg po bid (or **CIP** 400 mg IV q12h or **CIP** 500 mg po bid or 400 mg IV q12h) or **gentamicin plus doxy** Ref.: CID 38:663, 2004 **CIP** 500 mg po bid times 7 days	**Chloro** also active. 25 mg per kg IV qid. 1. In mass casualty situation, may have to treat po 2. Pediatric dose: see Table 16, page 177 3. Pregnancy: As for non-pregnant adults 4. Isolate during, first 48 hrs of treatment. 5. Pediatric doses: see Table 16, page 177 For community with pneumonic plague epidemic. Pediatric doses: see Table 16, page 177 Pregnancy: As for non-pregnant adults

TABLE 1B (2)

DISEASE	ETIOLOGY	SUGGESTED EMPIRIC TREATMENT REGIMENS		SPECIFIC THERAPY AND COMMENTS
		PRIMARY	ALTERNATIVE	
Smallpox Ref.: *NEJM* 346:1300, 2002 See Table 14, page 137	Variola virus	Smallpox vaccine up to 4 days after exposure; isolation; gloves, gown, & N95 respirator	Cidofovir protected mice against aerosol cowpox (*JID* 181:10, 2000)	***Immediately notify State Health Dept.*** & State notifies CDC (770-488-7100). Vaccinia immune globulin of no benefit. For vaccination complications, see *JAMA* 288:1901, 2002.
Tularemia **Inhalational tularemia** Ref.: *JAMA* 285:2763, 2001& www.bt.cdc.gov See Table 1, page 53 **Treatment**	Francisella tularemia	(**Streptomycin** 15 mg per kg IV bid) or **gentamicin** 5 mg per kg IV qd) times 10 days	**Doxy** 100 mg IV or po bid times 14–21 days or **CIP** 400 mg IV (or 750 mg po) bid times 14–21 days	For pediatric doses, see Table 16, page 177. Pregnancy: As for non-pregnant adults. **Tobramycin** should work.
Post-exposure prophylaxis		**Doxy** 100 mg po bid times 14 days	**CIP** 500 mg po bid times 14 days	For pediatric doses, see Table 16, page 177. Pregnancy: As for non-pregnant adults

TABLE 2 – RECOMMENDED ANTIMICROBIAL AGENTS AGAINST SELECTED BACTERIA

BACTERIAL SPECIES	ANTIMICROBIAL AGENT (See page 2 for abbreviations)		
	RECOMMENDED	ALTERNATIVE	ALSO EFFECTIVE[1] (COMMENTS)
Alcaligenes xylosoxidans (Achromobacter xylosoxidans)	IMP, MER, AP Pen	TMP-SMX. Some strains susc. to ceftaz (AAC 32: 276, 1988)	Resistant to APAG; P Ceph 1, 2, 3, 4; aztreonam; FQ (AAC 40:772, 1996)
Acinetobacter calcoaceticus—baumannii complex	IMP or MER or Dori or [FQ + (amikacin or ceftaz)]	AM-SB (CID 24:932, 1997; CID 34:1425, 2002). Sulbactam[NUS] also effective (JAC 42:793, 1998); colistin (CID 36:1111, 2003)	Up to 10% isolates resistant to IMP, MER; resistance to FQs, amikacin increasing. Doxy + amikacin effective in animal model (JAC 45: 493, 2000). (See Table 5, pg 72)
Actinomyces israelii	AMP or Pen G	Doxy, ceftriaxone	Clindamycin, erythro
Aeromonas hydrophila	FQ	TMP-SMX or (P Ceph 3, 4)	APAG; ERTA; IMP; MER; tetracycline (some resistant to carbapenems)
Arcanobacterium (C.) haemolyticum	Erythro	Benzathine Pen G	Sensitive to many drugs, resistant to TMP-SMX (AAC 38:142, 1994)
Bacillus anthracis (anthrax): inhalation	See Table 1B, page 59		
Bacillus cereus, B. subtilis	Vancomycin, clinda	FQ, IMP	
Bacteroides fragilis (ssp. fragilis)	Metronidazole	Cefoxitin, Dori, ERTA, IMP, MER, TC-CL, PIP-TZ, AM-SB, cefotetan, AM-CL	Resist to clindamycin, cefotetan limit utility against B.frag. (JAC 53(Suppl2):ii29, 2004; CID 35:5126, 2002).
"DOT" group of bacteroides			(not cefotetan)
Bartonella (Rochalimaea) henselae, quintana See Table 1, pg 41, 46, 51	Azithro, clarithro, CIP (bacillary angiomatosis), azithro (cat-scratch) (PIDJ 17:447, 1998; AAC 48:1921, 2004)	Erythro or doxy	Other drugs: TMP-SMX (IDC N.Amer 12: 137, 1998). Consider doxy + RIF for severe bacillary angiomatosis (IDC N.Amer 12: 137, 1998); doxy + gentamicin optimal for endocarditis (AAC 47:2204, 2003)
Bordetella pertussis	Erythro	TMP-SMX	An erythro-resistant strain reported in Arizona (MMWR 43:807, 1994)
Borrelia burgdorferi, B. afzelii, B. garinii	Ceftriaxone, cefuroxime axetil, doxy, amox (See Comments)	Penicillin G (HD), cefotaxime	Clarithro. Choice depends on stage of disease, Table 1, pg 54
Borrelia sp.	Doxy	Erythro	Penicillin G
Brucella sp.	Doxy + either gent or SM(IDCP 7, 2004; CID 42:1075, 2006)	(Doxy + RIF) or (TMP-SMX + gentamicin)	FQ + RIF (AAC 41:80,1997; EID 3: 213, 1997; CID 21:283,1995). Mino + RIF (J Chemother 15:248, 2003).
Burkholderia (Pseudomonas) cepacia	TMP-SMX or MER or CIP	Minocycline or chloramphenicol	(Usually resistant to APAG, AG, polymyxins) (AAC 37: 123, 1993 & 43:213, 1999; Inf Med 18:49, 2001) (Some resist to carba-penems). May need combo rx (AJRCCM 161:1206, 2000)
Burkholderia (Pseudomonas) pseudomallei See Table 1, pg 37, & Ln 361:1715, 2003	Initially, IV ceftaz or IMP (CID 29:381, 1999; CID 41:1105, 2005)	Then po TMP-SMX + doxy x 3 mo ± chloro (AAC 49:4020, 2005)	(Thai, 12-80% strains resist to TMP-SMX). FQ active in vitro. Combo chloro, TMP-SMX, doxy ↑ effective than doxy alone for maintenance (CID 29:375, 1999). MER also effective (AAC 48: 1763, 2004)
Campylobacter jejuni	Erythro	FQ (↑ resistance, NEJM 340:1525,1999)	Clindamycin, doxy, azithro, clarithro (see Table 5, pg 72) ...
Campylobacter fetus	Gentamicin	P Ceph 3	AMP, chloramphenicol, erythro
Capnocytophaga ochracea (DF-1) and	Clinda or AM-CL	CIP, Pen G	P Ceph 3, IMP, cefoxitin, FQ, (resist to APAG, TMP-SMX). C. haemolytica & C. granulosa oft resist to β-lactams & amino-glycosides [CID 35 (Suppl.1): S107, 2002].
canimorsus (DF-2)	AM-CL		
Chlamydophila pneumoniae	Doxy	Erythro, FQ	Azithro, clarithro
Chlamydia trachomatis	Doxy or azithro	Erythro or oflox	Levofloxacin
Chryseobacterium (Flavo-bacterium) meningo-septicum	Vancomycin ± RIF (CID 26:1169, 1998)	CIP, levofloxacin	In vitro susceptibilities may not correlate with clinical efficacy (AAC 41:1301, 1997; CID 26:1169, 1998)
Citrobacter diversus (koseri), C. freundii	AP Pen	FQ	APAG
Clostridium difficile	Metronidazole (po)	Vancomycin (po)	Bacitracin (po); nitazoxanide (CID 43:421, 2006; JAC 59:705, 2007). Rifaximin (CID 44:846, 2007).
Clostridium perfringens	Pen G + clindamycin	Doxy	Erythro, chloramphenicol, cefazolin, cefoxitin, AP Pen, CARB
Clostridium tetani	Metronidazole or Pen G	Doxy	AP Pen
Corynebacterium jeikeium	Vancomycin	Pen G + APAG	
C. diphtheriae	Erythro	Clindamycin	RIF. Penicillin reported effective (CID 27:845, 1998)
Coxiella burnetii (Q fever), acute disease	Doxy (see Table 1, page 27)	Erythro	In meningitis consider FQ (CID 20: 489, 1995). Endocarditis: doxy + hydroxy-chloroquine (JID 188:1322, 2003; LnID 3:709, 2003).
chronic disease	(CIP or doxy) + RIF	FQ + doxy x 3 yrs (CID 20:489, 1995)]	CQ + doxy (AAC 37:1773, 1993). ? gamma interferon (Ln 20:546, 2001)

BACTERIAL SPECIES	ANTIMICROBIAL AGENT (See page 2 for abbreviations)		
	RECOMMENDED	ALTERNATIVE	ALSO EFFECTIVE[1] (COMMENTS)
Ehrlichia chaffeensis, Ehrlichia ewubguum Anaplasma (Ehrlichia) phagocytophilium	Doxy	Tetracycline, RIF (CID 27:213, 1998)	CIP, oflox, chloramphenicol also active in vitro. Resist to clinda, TMP-SMX, IMP, AMP, erythro, & azithro (AAC 41:76, 1997).
Eikenella corrodens	Penicillin G or AMP or AM-CL	TMP-SMX, FQ	Doxy, cefoxitin, cefotaxime, IMP (Resistant to clinda, cephalexin, erythro, & metro)
Enterobacter species	Recommended agents vary with clinical setting. See Table 1 & Table 4		
Enterococcus faecalis	See Table 5, pg 71		
Enterococcus faecium, β-lactamase +, high-level aminoglycoside resist., vancomycin resist.: See Table 5, pg 71			
Erysipelothrix rhusiopathiae	Penicillin G or AMP	P Ceph 3, FQ	IMP, AP Pen (vancomycin, APAG, TMP-SMX resistant)
Escherichia coli	Recommended agents vary with clinical setting. See Table 1 & Table 4		
Francisella tularensis (tularemia) See Table 1B, pg 60	Gentamicin, tobramycin, or streptomycin	Doxy or CIP	Chloramphenicol, RIF. Doxy/chloro bacteriostatic → relapses
Gardnerella vaginalis (bacterial vaginosis)	Metronidazole	Clindamycin	See Table 1, pg 23 for dosage
Hafnia alvei	Same as Enterobacter spp.		
Helicobacter pylori	See Table 1, pg 18		Drugs effective in vitro often fail in vivo.
Haemophilus aphrophilus	[(Penicillin or AMP) + gentamicin] or [AM-SB + gentamicin]	P Ceph 2, 3 ± gentamicin	(Resistant to vancomycin, clindamycin, methicillin)
Haemophilus ducreyi (chancroid)	Azithro or ceftriaxone	Erythro, CIP	Most strains resistant to tetracycline, amox, TMP-SMX
Haemophilus influenzae Meningitis, epiglottitis & other life-threatening illness	Cefotaxime, ceftriaxone	TMP-SMX, AP Pen, FQs (AMP if β-lactamase neg) (US 25–30% AMP resist., Japan 35%)	Chloramphenicol (downgrade from 1st choice due to hematotoxicity). 9% US strains resist to TMP-SMX (AAC 41:292, 1997)
non-life threatening illness	AM-CL, O Ceph 2/3, TMP-SMX, AM-SB		Azithro, clarithro, telithro
Klebsiella ozaenae/ rhinoscleromatis	FQ	RIF + TMP-SMX	(Ln 342:122, 1993)
Klebsiella species	Recommended agents vary with clinical setting. See Table 1 & Table 4		
Lactobacillus species	(Pen G or AMP) ± gentamicin	Clindamycin, erythro	**May be resistant to vancomycin**
Legionella sp. (42 species & 60 serotypes recognized) (Sem Resp Inf 13:90, 1998)	FQ, or azithro, or (erythro ± RIF)	Clarithro	TMP-SMX, doxy. Most active FQs in vitro: Gemi, Levo, Moxi. See AnIM 129:328, 1998. Telithro active in vitro.
Leptospira interrogans	Penicillin G	Doxy	Ceftriaxone (CID 36:1507, 2003), cefotaxime (CID 39:1417, 2004)
Leuconostoc	Pen G or AMP	Clinda, erythro, minocycline	APAG. **NOTE: Resistant to vancomycin**
Listeria monocytogenes	AMP	TMP-SMX	Erythro, penicillin G (high dose), APAG may be synergistic with β-lactams. **Cephalosporin-resistant!**
Moraxella (Branhamella) catarrhalis	AM-CL or O Ceph 2/3, TMP-SMX	Azithro, clarithro, dirithromycin, telithro	Erythro, doxy, FQs
Morganella species	Recommended agents vary with clinical setting. See Table 1 & Table 4		
Mycoplasma pneumoniae	Erythro, azithro, clarithro, dirithro, FQ	Doxy	(Clindamycin & β lactams NOT effective)
Neisseria gonorrhoeae (gonococcus)	Ceftriaxone, cefixime, cefpodoxime	Ofloxacin & other FQs (Table 1, pg 20-21), spectinomycin, azith	Kanamycin (used in Asia). FQ resistance in Asia; rare in U.S., but ↑ (MMWR 47:405, 1998)
Neisseria meningitidis (meningococcus)	Penicillin G	Ceftriaxone, cefuroxime, cefotaxime	Sulfonamide (some strains), chloramphenicol. Chloro-resist strains in SE Asia (NEJM 339:868, 1998) (Prophylaxis: pg 8)
Nocardia asteroides	TMP-SMX, sulfonamides (high doses)	Minocycline	Amikacin + (IMP or ceftriaxone or cefuroxime) for brain abscess
Nocardia brasiliensis	TMP-SMX, sulfonamides (high doses)	AM-CL	Amikacin + ceftriaxone
Pasteurella multocida	Pen G, AMP, amox	Doxy, AM-CL	Ceftriaxone, cefpodoxime, FQ (active in vitro), azithro (active in vitro) (DMID 30:99, 1998; AAC 43:1475, 1999); resistant to cephalexin, oxacillin, clindamycin.
Plesiomonas shigelloides	CIP	TMP-SMX	AM-CL, P Ceph 1,2,3,4, IMP, MER, tetracycline, aztreonam
Proteus mirabilis (indole–)	AMP	TMP-SMX	Most agents except nafcillin/oxacillin. β-lactamase (including ESBL) production now being described in P. mirabilis (J Clin Micro 40:1549, 2002)
vulgaris (indole +)	P Ceph 3 or FQ	APAG	Aztreonam, BL/BLI, AP-Pen
Providencia sp.	Amikacin, P Ceph 3, FQ	TMP-SMX	AP-Pen + amikacin, IMP

TABLE 2 (3)

BACTERIAL SPECIES	ANTIMICROBIAL AGENT (See page 2 for abbreviations)		
	RECOMMENDED	ALTERNATIVE	ALSO EFFECTIVE[1] (COMMENTS)
Pseudomonas aeruginosa	AP Pen, AP Ceph 3, Dori, IMP, MER, tobramycin, CIP, aztreonam. For serious inf., use AP β-lactam + tobramycin or CIP (LnID 4:519, 2004)	For UTI, single drugs usually effective: AP Pen, AP Ceph 3, cefepime, IMP, MER, APAG, CIP, aztreonam	Resistance to β-lactams (IMP, ceftaz) may emerge during rx. β-lactam inhibitor adds nothing to activity of TC or PIP against P. aeruginosa. Clavulanic acid antag TC in vitro (AAC 43:882, 1999). (See also Table 5). Recommend combination therapy for serious infections, but value of combos controversial (LnID 5:192, 2005)
Rhodococcus (C. equi)	IMP, APAG, erythro, vanco, or RIF (Consider 2 agents)	CIP (variable)[resistant strains in SE Asia (CID 27:370, 1998)], TMP-SMX, tetra, or clinda	Vancomycin active in vitro but intracellular location of R. equi may impair efficacy (Sem Resp Inf 12:57, 1997; CID 34:1379, 2002)
Rickettsiae species	Doxy	Chloramphenicol	FQ: clari, azithro effective for Mediterranean spotted fever in children (CID 34:154, 2002).
Salmonella typhi	FQ, ceftriaxone	Chloramphenicol, amox, TMP-SMX, azithro (for uncomplicated disease: AAC 43:1441, 1999)	Multi drug resistant strains (chloramphenicol, AMP, TMP-SMX) common in many developing countries, seen in immigrants. FQ resistance now being reported (AJTMH 61:163, 1999).
Serratia marcescens	P Ceph 3, ERTA, IMP, MER, FQ	Aztreonam, gentamicin	TC-CL, PIP-TZ
Shigella sp.	FQ or azithro	TMP-SMX and AMP (resistance common in Middle East, Latin America). Azithro ref: AnIM 126:697, 1997	
Staph. aureus, methicillin-susceptible	Oxacillin/nafcillin	P Ceph 1, vanco, teicoplanin[NUS], clinda, dalbavancin	ERTA, IMP, MER, BL/BLI, FQ, erythro, clarithro, dirithromycin, azithro, telithro, quinu-dalfo, linezolid, dapto
Staph. aureus, methicillin-resistant (health-care associated)	Vancomycin	Teicoplanin[NUS], TMP-SMX (some strains resistant), quinu-dalfo, linezolid, daptomycin, dalbavancin	Fusidic acid[NUS], >60% CIP-resistant in U.S. (Fosfomycin + RIF), novobiocin. Partially vancomycin-resistant strains (GISA, VISA) & highly resistant strains now described—see Table 6, pg 73.
Staph. aureus, methicillin-resistant [community-acquired (CA-MRSA)]			CA-MRSA usually not multiply-resistant (Ln 359: 1819, 2002; JAMA 286: 1201, 2001). Oft resist. to erythro & variably to FQ. Vanco, teico[NUS], daptomycin or dalbavancin can be used in pts requiring hospitalization (see Table 6, pg 73).
Mild-moderate infection	TMP-SMX or doxy or mino) ± RIF (CID 40: 1429, 2005)	Clinda (D-test neg—see Table 5)	
Severe infection	Vanco or teico[NUS]	Linezolid or daptomycin or dalbavancin or televancin	
Staph. epidermidis	Vancomycin ± RIF	RIF + (TMP-SMX or FQ), dalbavancin, daptomycin or telavancin (AAC 51:3420, 2007)	Cephalothin or nafcillin/oxacillin if sensitive to nafcillin/oxacillin but 75% are resistant. FQs. (See Table 5)
Staph. haemolyticus	TMP-SMX, FQ, nitrofurantoin	Oral cephalosporin	Recommendations apply to UTI only.
Staph. lugdunensis	Oxacillin/nafcillin or penicillin G (if β-lactamase neg.) (Inf Dis Alert 22:193, 2003)	P Ceph 1 or vancomycin or teico[NUS]	Approx. 75% are penicillin-susceptible. Usually susceptible to gentamicin, RIF (AAC 32:2434, 1990).
Staph. saprophyticus (UTI)	Oral cephalosporin or AM-CL	FQ	Suscept to most agents used for UTI; occ. failure of sulfonamides, nitrofurantoin reported (JID 155:170, 1987). Resist to fosfomycin.
Stenotrophomonas (Xanthomonas, Pseudomonas) maltophilia	TMP-SMX	TC-CL or (aztreonam + TC-CL) (AAC 41:2612, 1997)	Minocycline, doxy, ceftaz. [In vitro synergy (TC-CL + TMP-SMX) & (TC-CL + CIP), AAC 39:2220, 1995; CMR 11:57, 1998]
Streptobacillus moniliformis	Penicillin G or doxy	Erythro, clindamycin	
Streptococcus, anaerobic (Peptostreptococcus)	Penicillin G	Clindamycin	Erythro, doxy, vancomycin
Streptococcus pneumoniae	Penicillin G	Multiple agents effective, e.g., amox	See footnote 2 pg 10
penicillin-susceptible			
penicillin-resistant (MIC ≥2.0)	(Vancomycin ± RIF) or Moxi See footnote 1 pg 7 and Table 5, pg 72	Gemi, Gati, Levo, or	For non-meningeal infec: P Ceph 3/4, AP Pen, quinu-dalfo, linezolid, telithro
Streptococcus pyogenes, Groups A, B, C, G, F, Strep. milleri (constellatus, intermedius, anginosus)	Penicillin G or V (some add genta for serious Group B infec & some add clinda for serious invasive Group A) (SMJ 96:968, 2003)	All β lactams, erythro, azithro, dirithromycin, clarithro, telithro	Macrolide resistance increasing.
Vibrio cholerae	Doxy, FQ	TMP-SMX	Strain 0139 is resistant to TMP-SMX
Vibrio parahemolyticus	Antibiotic rx does not ↓ course		Sensitive in vitro to FQ, doxy
Vibrio vulnificus, alginolyticus, damsela	Doxy + ceftaz	Cefotaxime, FQ (eg. levo, AAC 46:3580, 2002)	APAG often used in combo with ceftaz
Yersinia enterocolitica	TMP-SMX or FQ	P Ceph 3 or APAG	CID 19:655, 1994
Yersinia pestis (plague)	See Table 1B, pg 59		

[1] Agents are more variable in effectiveness than "Recommended" or "Alternative." Selection of "Alternative" or "Also Effective" based on in vitro susceptibility testing, pharmacokinetics, host factors such as auditory, renal, hepatic function, & cost.

TABLE 3 – SUGGESTED DURATION OF ANTIBIOTIC THERAPY IN IMMUNOCOMPETENT PATIENTS[1,2]

CLINICAL SITUATION		DURATION OF THERAPY
SITE	CLINICAL DIAGNOSIS	(Days)
Bacteremia	Bacteremia with removable focus (no endocarditis)	10–14 (CID 14:75, 1992) (See Table 1)
Bone	Osteomyelitis, adult; acute	42
	adult; chronic	Until ESR normal (often > 3 months)
	child; acute; staph. and enterobacteriaceae[3]	21
	child; acute; strep, meningococci, haemophilus[3]	14
Ear	Otitis media with effusion	<2 yr: 10 (or 1 dose ceftriaxone); ≥2yr: 5–7
	Recent meta-analysis suggests 3 days of azithro (JAC 52:469, 2003) or 5 days of "short-acting" antibiotics effective for uncomplicated otitis media (JAMA 279:1736, 1998), but may be inadequate for severe disease (NEJM 347:1169, 2002).	
Endocardium	Infective endocarditis, native valve	
	Viridans strep	14 or 28 (See Table 1, page 26)
	Enterococci	28 or 42 (See Table 1, page 26)
	Staph. aureus	14 (R-sided only) or 28 (See Table 1, page 26)
Gastrointestinal *Also see Table 1*	Bacillary dysentery (shigellosis)/traveler's diarrhea	3
	Typhoid fever (S. typhi): Azithro	5 (children/adolescents)
	Ceftriaxone	14*
	FQ	5–7
	Chloramphenicol	14
		*[Short course ↓ effective (AAC 44:450, 2000)]
	Helicobacter pylori	10–14
	Pseudomembranous enterocolitis (C. difficile)	10
Genital	Non-gonococcal urethritis or mucopurulent cervicitis	7 days doxy or single dose azithro
	Pelvic inflammatory disease	14
Heart	Pericarditis (purulent)	28
Joint	Septic arthritis (non-gonococcal) Adult	14–28 (Ln 351:197, 1998)
	Infant/child	Rx as osteomyelitis above
	Gonococcal arthritis/disseminated GC infection	7 (See Table 1, page 20)
Kidney	Cystitis (bladder bacteriuria)	3 (Single dose extended-release cipro also effective) (AAC 49:4137, 2005)
	Pyelonephritis	14 (7 days if CIP used)
	Recurrent (failure after 14 days rx)	42
Lung	Pneumonia, pneumococcal	Until afebrile 3–5 days (minimum 5 days)
	Community-acquired pneumonia	Minimum 5 days and afebrile for 2-3 days (CID 44:S55, 2007)
	Pneumonia, enterobacteriaceae or pseudomonal	21, often up to 42
	Pneumonia, staphylococcal	21–28
	Pneumocystis carinii, in AIDS;	21
	other immunocompromised	14
	Legionella, mycoplasma, chlamydia	7–14
	Lung abscess	Usually 28–42[4]
Meninges[5] (CID 39:1267, 2004)	N. meningitidis	7
	H. influenzae	7
	S. pneumoniae	10–14
	Listeria meningoencephalitis, gp B strep, coliforms	21 (longer in immunocompromised)
Multiple systems	Brucellosis (See Table 1, page 53)	42 (add SM or gent for 1st 7–14 days)
	Tularemia (See Table 1, pages 41, 53)	7–14
Muscle	Gas gangrene (clostridial)	10
Pharynx *Also see Pharyngitis, Table 1, page 43*	Group A strep pharyngitis	10
		O Ceph 2/3, azithromycin effective at 5 days (JAC 45, Topic TI 23, 2000). 3 days less effective (Inf Med 18:515, 2001)
	Diphtheria (membranous)	7–14
	Carrier	7
Prostate	Chronic prostatitis (TMP/SMX)	30–90
	(FQ)	28–42
Sinuses	Acute sinusitis	5–14[6]
Skin	Cellulitis	Until 3 days after acute inflamm disappears
Systemic	Lyme disease	See Table 1, page 52
	Rocky Mountain spotted fever (See Table 1, page 53)	Until afebrile 2 days

[1] It has been shown that early change from parenteral to oral regimens (about 72 hours) is cost-effective with many infections, i.e., intra-abdominal (AJM 91:462, 1991)

[2] The recommended duration is a minimum or average time and should not be construed as absolute

[3] These times are with proviso: sx & signs resolve within 7 days and ESR is normalized (J.D. Nelson, APID 6:59, 1991)

[4] After patient afebrile 4-5 days, change to oral therapy

[5] In children relapses seldom occur until 3 days or more after termination of rx. Practice of observing in hospital for 1 or 2 days after rx is expensive and non-productive. For meningitis in children, see Table 1, page 7.

[6] Duration of therapy dependent upon agent used and severity of infection. Longer duration (10-14 days) optimal for beta-lactams and patients with severe disease. For sinusitis of mild-moderate severity shorter courses of therapy (5-7 days) effective with "respiratory FQ's" (including gemifloxacin, levofloxacin 750mg), azithromycin. Courses as short as 3 days reported effective for TMP-SMX and azithro and one study reports effectiveness of single dose extended-release azithro. Authors feel such "super-short" courses should be restricted to patients with mild-mod disease (JAMA 273:1015, 1995; AAC 47:2770, 2003; Otolaryngol-Head Neck Surg 133:194, 2005; Otolaryngol-Head Neck Surg 127:1, 2002; Otolaryngol-Head Neck Surg 134:10, 2006).

TABLE 4 – COMPARISON OF ANTIMICROBIAL SPECTRA

(These are generalizations; major differences exist between countries/areas/hospitals depending on antibiotic usage—verify for individual location. See Table 5 for resistant bacteria)

Organisms	Penicillins – Penicillin G	Penicillin V	Antistaphylococcal Penicillins – Methicillin	Nafcillin/Oxacillin	Cloxacillin[NUS]/Diclox.	Amino-Penicillins – AMP/Amox	Amox/Clav	AMP-Sulb	Anti-Pseudomonal Penicillins – Ticarcillin	Ticar-Clav	Pip-Tazo	Piperacillin	Carbapenems – Doripenem	Ertapenem	Imipenem	Meropenem	Aztreonam	Fluoroquinolones – Ciprofloxacin	Ofloxacin	Pefloxacin[NUS]	Levofloxacin	Moxifloxacin	Gemifloxacin	Gatifloxacin
GRAM-POSITIVE:																								
Strep. Group A,B,C,G	+	+	+	+	+	+	+	+	+	+	+	+	+	+	+	+	0	±	±	0	+	+	+	+
Strep. pneumoniae	+	+	+	+	+	+	+	+	+	+	+	+	+	+	+	+	0	±	±	0	+	+	+	+
Viridans strep	+	±	±	±	±	+	+	+	±	+	+	±	+	+	+	+	0	0	0	0	+	+	+	+
Strep. milleri	+	+	+	+	+	+	+	+	+	+	+	+	+	+	+	+	0	0	0	0	+	+	+	+
Enterococcus faecalis	+	+	0	0	0	+	+	+	±	+	+	+	0	±	+	±	0	±	±	+	±	±	±	±
Enterococcus faecium	0	0	0	0	0	±	±	±	0	0	0	0	0	0	0	0	0	0	0	0	0	0	0	0
Staph. aureus (MSSA)	0	0	+	+	+	0	+	+	0	+	+	0	+	+	+	+	0	+	+	+	+	+	+	+
Staph. aureus (MRSA)	0	0	0	0	0	0	0	0	0	0	0	0	0	0	0	0	0	0	0	0	±	±	±	±
Staph. aureus (CA-MRSA)	0	0	0	0	0	0	0	0	0	0	0	0	0	0	0	0	0	+	+	+	+	+	+	+
Staph. epidermidis	0	0	0	0	0	0	0	0	0	0	0	0	0	±	0	±	0	±	±	+	±	±	±	±
C. jeikeium	+																							
L. monocytogenes	+	0	0	0	0	+	+	+	0	+	+	+	±	±	+	+	0	+	+	0	+	+	+	+
GRAM-NEGATIVE:																								
N. gonorrhoeae	0	0	0	0	0	0	+	+	+	+	+	+	+	+	+	+	+	±*	±*	±*	±*	±*		±*
N. meningitidis	+	0	0	0	0	+	+	+	+	+	+	+	+	+	+	+	+	+	+	+	+	+	+	+
M. catarrhalis	0	0	0	0	0	0	+	+	±	+	+	±	+	+	+	+	+	+	+	+	+	+	+	+
E. coli	0	0	0	0	0	±	+	+	+	+	+	+	+	+	+	+	+	+	+	+	+	+	+	+
E. coli/Klebs sp ESBL +	0	0	0	0	0	0	±	±	0	±	±	0	+	+	+	+	±	±	±	±	±	±		±
Enterobacter sp.	0	0	0	0	0	0	0	0	+	±	+	+	+	+	+	+	+	+	+	+	+	+	+	+
Serratia sp.	0	0	0	0	0	0	0	0	+	+	+	+	+	+	+	+	+	+	+	+	+	+	+	+
Salmonella sp.	0	0	0	0	0	+	+	+	+	+	+	+	+	+	+	+	+	+	+	+	+	+	+	+
Shigella sp.	0	0	0	0	0	+	+	+	+	+	+	+	+	+	+	+	+	+	+	+	+	+	+	+
Proteus mirabilis	0	0	0	0	0	+	+	+	+	+	+	+	+	+	+	+	+	+	+	+	+	+	+	+

+ = usually effective clinically or >60% susceptible; ± = clinical trials lacking or 30–60% susceptible; 0 = not effective clinically or <30% susceptible; blank = data not available

* Most strains ±, can be used in UTI, not in systemic infection

** Prevalence of quinolone-resistant GC varies worldwide from <1% to 30.9% in Europe and >90% in Taiwan. In US in 2006 it was 6.7% overall and as a result, CDC no longer recommends FQs for first line therapy of GC (MMWR 56:332, 2007; JAC 58:587, 2006; CID 40:188, 2005; AnIM 147:81, 2007).

TABLE 4 (2)

Organisms	Penicillins		Antistaphylococcal Penicillins			Amino-Penicillins			Anti-Pseudomonal Penicillins				Carbapenems				Aztreonam	Fluoroquinolones						
	Penicillin G	Penicillin V	Methicillin	Nafcillin/Oxacillin	Cloxacillin^NUS/Diclox.	AMP/Amox	Amox/Clav	AMP-Sulb	Ticarcillin	Ticar-Clav	Pip-Tazo	Piperacillin	Doripenem	Ertapenem	Imipenem	Meropenem	Aztreonam	Ciprofloxacin	Ofloxacin	Pefloxacin^NUS	Levofloxacin	Moxifloxacin	Gemifloxacin	Gatifloxacin
Proteus vulgaris	0	0	0	0	0	0	+	+	+	+	+	+	+	+	+	+	+	+	+	+	+	+	+	+
Providencia sp.	0	0	0	0	0	0	0	0	+	+	+	+	+	+	+	+	+	+	+	+	+	+	+	+
Morganella sp.	0	0	0	0	0	0	0	0	+	+	+	+	+	+	+	+	+	+	+	+	+	+		+
Citrobacter sp.	0	0	0	0	0	0	0	+	+	+	+	+	+	+	+	+	+	+	+	+	+	+		+
Aeromonas sp.	0	0	0	0	0	0	0	0	0	+	+	+	+	+	+	+	+	+	+	+	+	+		+
Acinetobacter sp.	0	0	0	0	0	0	0	±	0	+	±	0	±	0	+	±	0	±	±		±	±		±
Ps. aeruginosa	0	0	0	0	0	0	0	0	+	+	+	+	+	0	+	+	+	+	+	+	+	±		±
B. (Ps.) cepacia	0	0	0	0	0	0	0	0	+	+	0	±	0	0	0	0	0	0	0	0	±	0		0
S. (X.) maltophilia	0	0	0	0	0	0	0	0	0	+	0	0	0	0	0	0	0	0	0	0	0	0		0
Y. enterocolitica	0	0	0	0	0	0	+	±	+	+	+	0	+	+	+	+	+	+	+	+	+	+		+
Legionella sp.	+	+																+	+	+	+	+	+	+
P. multocida	+	+				+	+	+	+	+	+	+	+	+	+	+	0	+	+	+	+	+		+
H. ducreyi																	0	±	±		±	±		±
MISC:																								
Chlamydia sp.	0	0	0	0	0	0	0	0	0	0	0	0	0	0	0	0	0	±	±	0	+	+	+	+
M. pneumoniae	0	0	0	0	0	0	0	0	0	0	0	0	0	0	0	0	0	0	0	0	+	+	+	+
ANAEROBES:																								
Actinomyces	+	+				+	+	+	+	+	+	+	+	+	+	+	0	0	±	0	0	+		±
Bacteroides fragilis	0	0	0	0	0	0	+	+	+	+	+	+	+	+	+	+	0	0	0	0	0	+	+	+
P. melaninogenica	±	+	0	0	0	+	+	+	+	+	+	+	+	+	+	+	0	0	±	0	+	+		+
Clostridium (not difficile)	+^1	+^1				+	+	+	+	+	+	+	+	+	+	+	0	0	±	0	±	0		0
Clostridium (not difficile)	+	+				+	+	+	+	+	+	+	+	+	+	+	0	±	±	±	+	+	+	+
Peptostreptococcus sp.	+	+	+		+	+	+	+	+	+	+	+	+	+	+	+	0	±	±	±	+	+		+

+ = usually effective clinically or >60% susceptible; ± = clinical trials lacking or 30–60% susceptible; 0 = not effective clinically or <30% susceptible; blank = data not available
1 No clinical evidence that penicillins or fluoroquinolones are effective for C. difficile enterocolitis (but they may cover this organism in mixed intra-abdominal and pelvic infections)

TABLE 4 (3)

CEPHALOSPORINS

Organisms	1st Gene-ration: Cefazolin	2nd Generation: Cefotetan	2nd Generation: Cefoxitin	2nd Generation: Cefuroxime	3rd/4th Generation (including anti-MRSA): Cefotaxime	Ceftizoxime	Ceftriaxone	Ceftobiprole	Ceftazidime	Cefepime	Oral 1st Gen: Cefadroxil	Cephalexin	Oral 2nd Gen: Cefaclor/Loracarbef*	Cefprozil	Cefuroxime axetil	Oral 3rd Gen: Cefixime	Ceftibuten	Cefpodox/Cefdinir/Cefditoren
GRAM-POSITIVE:																		
Strep. Group A,B,C,G	+	+	+	+	+	+	+	+	+	+	+	+	+	+	+	+	+	+
Strep. pneumoniae†	+	+	+	+	+	+	+	+	±	+	+	+	±	+	+	±	±	+
Viridans strep	+	+	+	+	+	+	+	+	±	+	+	+	±	+	+	o	o	+
Enterococcus faecalis	o	o	o	o	o	o	o	o	o	o	o	o	o	o	o	o	o	o
Staph. aureus (MSSA)	+	+	+	+	+	+	+	+	+	+	+	+	+	+	+	o	o	±
Staph. aureus (MRSA)	o	o	o	o	o	o	o	+	o	o	o	o	o	o	o	o	o	o
Staph. aureus (CA-MRSA)	o	o	o	o	o	o	o	+	o	o	o	o	o	o	o	o	o	o
Staph. epidermidis	±	±	±	±	±	±	±	+	±	±	±	±	±	±	±	o	o	o
C. jeikeium	o	o	o	o	o	o	o		o	o	o	o	o	o	o	o	o	o
L. monocytogenes	o	o	o	o	o	o	o	o	o	o	o	o	o	o	o	o	o	o
GRAM-NEGATIVE																		
N. gonorrhoeae	+	o	±	+	+	+	+	+	+	+	o	o	+	+	+	+	+	+
N. meningitidis	±	±	±	+	+	+	+	+	+	+	±	±	+	+	+	+	+	+
M. catarrhalis	+	+	+	+	+	+	+	+	+	+	±	±	+	+	+	+	+	+
E. coli	o	o	o	+	+	+	+	+	+	+	o	o	±	±	+	+	+	+
H. influenzae	o	±	±	+	+	+	+	+	+	+	o	o	±	±	+	+	+	+
Klebsiella sp.	o	+	+	+	+	+	+	+	+	+	o	o	+	+	+	+	+	+
E.coli/Klebs sp ESBL +	o	o	o	o	o	o	o	o	o	o	o	o	o	o	o	o	o	o
Enterobacter sp.	o	o	o	o	±	±	±	+	±	+	o	o	o	o	o	o	o	±
Serratia sp.	o	o	o	o	+	+	+	+	+	+	o	o	o	o	o	o	o	o
Salmonella sp.	o	o	o	+	+	+	+	+	+	+	o	o	o	o	+	+	+	+
Shigella sp.	o	o	o	+	+	+	+	+	+	+	o	o	o	o	+	+	+	+
Proteus mirabilis	+	+	+	+	+	+	+	+	+	+	+	+	+	+	+	+	+	+
Proteus vulgaris	o	+	+	±	+	+	+	+	+	+	o	o	o	o	±	+	+	+
Providencia sp.	o	+	+	o	+	+	+	+	+	+	o	o	o	o	o	+	+	+
Morganella sp.	o	+	+	o	+	+	+	+	+	+	o	o	o	o	o	+	+	o

+ = **usually effective clinically or >60% susceptible**; ± = **clinical trials lacking or 30-60% susceptible**; o = not effective clinically or <30% susceptible; blank = data not available

* A 1-carbacephem best classified as a cephalosporin

† A. Cefaz 8-16 times less active than cefotax/ceftriax, effective only vs Pen-sens. strains (AAC 39:2193, 1995). Oral cefuroxime, cefprozil, cefpodoxime most active in vitro vs resistant S. pneumo (PIDJ 14:1037, 1995).

TABLE 4 (4)

CEPHALOSPORINS

Organisms	1st Generation	2nd Generation			3rd/4th Generation (including anti-MRSA)						Oral Agents — 1st Generation		Oral Agents — 2nd Generation			Oral Agents — 3rd Generation		
	Cefazolin	Cefotetan	Cefoxitin	Cefuroxime	Cefotaxime	Ceftizoxime	Ceftriaxone	Ceftobiprole	Ceftazidime	Cefepime	Cefadroxil	Cephalexin	Cefaclor/Loracarbef*	Cefprozil	Cefuroxime axetil	Cefixime	Ceftibuten	Cefpodox/Cefdinir/Cefditoren
C. freundii	0	0	±	0	+	+	+		0	+	0	0	0	0	0	0	0	0
C. diversus	0	±	±	±	+	+	+	+	+	+	0	0	±	0	±	+	+	+
Citrobacter sp.	0	±	±	±	+	+	+	+	+	+	0	0	0	0	0	+	+	0
Aeromonas sp.	0	0	0	0	+	+	+	+	+	+	0	0	0	0	0	0	0	0
Acinetobacter sp.	0	0	0	0	0	0	0	+	±	±	0	0	0	0	0	0	0	0
Ps. aeruginosa	0	0	0	0	0	0	0	+	+	+	0	0	0	0	0	0	0	0
B. (Ps.) cepacia	0	0	0	0	±	±	±		±	±	0	0	0	0	0	0	0	0
S. (X.) maltophilia	0	0	0	0	0	0	0	0	+	0	0	0	0	0	0	0	0	0
Y. enterocolitica	0	0	±	±	+	+	+	0	+	+	0	0	0	0	0	+	+	+
Legionella sp.																		
P. multocida		±	+	+	+	+	+		+	+						+	0	+
H. ducreyi			+	+	+	+	+		+	+			+		+	+		+
ANAEROBES:																		
Actinomyces	0	±[1]	+		+	+	+		0	+	0		0			0		0
Bacteroides fragilis		+	+	+	±	±	±		0	0			0					0
P. melaninogenica		0	+	+	+	+	+		+	+			+					
Clostridium difficile		+	+	+	+	+	+		+	+			+					
Clostridium (not difficile)		+	+	+	+	+	+		+	+			+					
Peptostreptococcus sp.	+	+	+	+	+	+	+	+	+	+	+		+	+	+			+

+ = **usually effective clinically or >60% susceptible**; ± = clinical trials lacking or 30–60% susceptible; 0 = not effective clinically or <30% susceptible; blank = data not available

* A 1-carbacephem best classified as a cephalosporin

† Cefotetan is less active against B. ovatus, B. distasonis, B. thetaiotamicron

TABLE 4 (5)

Gram-positive organisms

Class	Drug	Strep Group A,B,C,G	Strep. pneumoniae	Enterococcus faecalis	Enterococcus faecium	Staph.aureus (MSSA)	Staph.aureus (MRSA)	Staph.aureus (CA-MRSA)	Staph. epidermidis	C. jeikeium	L. monocytogenes
MISCELLANEOUS	Colistimethate (Colistin)	o	o	o	o	o	o	o	o	o	o
	Daptomycin	+	+[2]	+	+	+	+	+	+	+	±
	Linezolid	+	+	+	+	+	+	+	+	+	+
	Quinupristin-dalfopristin	+	+	o	+	+	+	+	+	+	+
	Metronidazole	o	o	o	o	o	o	o	o	o	o
	Rifampin	+	+	±	o	+	+	+	+	+	+
AGENTS URINARY TRACT	Fosfomycin		+	±							
	Nitrofurantoin	+	+	+	+	+	+				o
	TMP-SMX	±[1]	+	+[1]	o	+	+	+	±	+	o
	Trimethoprim	+	+	±	o	±	±	+	+	o	+
	Fusidic Acid[NUS]	±	±	+		+	+	+	+		
GLYCOPEPTIDES	Dalbavancin	+	+	+	±	+	+	+	+	+	+
	Telavancin	+	+	+	+	+	+	+	+	+	+
	Teicoplanin[NUS]	+	+	+	±	+	+	+	±	+	+
	Vancomycin	+	+	+	+	+	+	+	+	+	+
GLYCYL-CYCLINE	Tigecycline	+	+	+	+	+	+	+	+	+	+
TETRA-CYCLINES	Minocycline	+	+	o	o	±	±	+	o	o	+
	Doxycycline	±	+	o	o	±	±	+	o	o	+
KETOLIDE	Telithromycin	+	+	±	o	+	o	±	o	o	+
MACROLIDES	Clarithromycin	±	+	o	o	+	o	±	o	o	+
	Azithromycin	±	+	o	o	+	o	±	o	o	+
	Erythro/Dirithro	±	+	o	o	±	o	±	o	±	+
	Clindamycin	+	+	o	o	+	o	±	o	o	
	Chloramphenicol	+	+	±	±	±	o		o	o	+
AMINO-GLYCOSIDES	Amikacin	o	o	o	S	+	o		±	o	S
	Tobramycin	o	o	S	o	+	o		±	o	S
	Gentamicin	o	o	S		+	o		±	o	S

Gram-negative organisms

Class	Drug	N. gonorrhoeae	N. meningitidis	M. catarrhalis	H. influenzae	Aeromonas	E. coli	Klebsiella sp.	E.coli/Kleb sp ESBL+	Enterobacter sp.	Salmonella sp.	Shigella sp.	Serratia marcescens
MISCELLANEOUS	Colistimethate (Colistin)	o	o				+	+	+				o
	Daptomycin	o	o	o	o	o	o	o	o	o	o	o	o
	Linezolid	o	±	±	o	o	o	o	o	o	o	o	o
	Quinupristin-dalfopristin	+	o	±	o	o	o	o	o	o	o	o	o
	Metronidazole	o	o	o	o	o	o	o	o	o	o	o	o
	Rifampin	+	+	±	o	o	o	o	o	o	o	o	o
AGENTS URINARY TRACT	Fosfomycin	+			±	±							±
	Nitrofurantoin	+		±	±		+	±		±	+	+	o
	TMP-SMX	±	+	+	+	±	+	±	±	±	±	±	±
	Trimethoprim	o	±		+	±	+	±	±	±	±	±	o
	Fusidic Acid[NUS]	+	+		o	o	o	o	o	o	o	o	o
GLYCOPEPTIDES	Dalbavancin	o	o		o	o	o	o	o	o	o	o	o
	Telavancin	o	o		o	o	o	o	o	o	o	o	o
	Teicoplanin[NUS]	o	o		o	o	o	o	o	o	o	o	o
	Vancomycin	o	o		o	o	o	o	o	o	o	o	o
GLYCYL-CYCLINE	Tigecycline	+		+	+	+	+	+	+	+	+	+	+
TETRA-CYCLINES	Minocycline	±	+	+	+	+	+	±	o	+	±	+	o
	Doxycycline	±	+	+	+	+	+	±	o	+	±	+	o
KETOLIDE	Telithromycin	+	+	+	o	o	o	o	o	o	o	o	o
MACROLIDES	Clarithromycin	±	+	+	o	o	o	o	o	o	o	o	o
	Azithromycin	±	+	+	±	o	o	o	o	o	o	±	o
	Erythro/Dirithro	±	+	+	±	o	o	o	o	o	o	o	o
	Clindamycin	o	o	o		o	o	o	o	o	o	o	o
	Chloramphenicol	+	+	+	+	±	±	+	o	+	±	+	o
AMINO-GLYCOSIDES	Amikacin	o	o	+	+	+	+	+		+	+	+	+
	Tobramycin	o	o	+	+	+	+	+		+	+	+	+
	Gentamicin	o	o	+	o	+	+	+		+	+	+	+

+ = usually effective clinically or >60% susceptible; ± = clinical trials lacking or 30-60% susceptible; 0 = not effective clinically or <30% susceptible; S = synergistic with penicillins (ampicillin); blank = data not available. Antimicrobials such as azithromycin have high tissue penetration and some such as clarithromycin are metabolized to more active compounds, hence in vivo activity may exceed in vitro activity.

[1] Although active in vitro, TMP-SMX is not clinically effective for Group A strep pharyngitis or for infections due to E. faecalis.

[2] Although active in vitro, daptomycin is not clinically effective for pneumonia caused by strep pneumonia

TABLE 4 (6)

The following table lists antimicrobial activity against organisms (rows are antimicrobial agents grouped by class; columns are organisms). Symbol key is given in the footnotes.

Antibiotic	Proteus vulgaris	Acinetobacter sp.	Ps. aeruginosa	B.(Ps.) cepacia	S.(X.) maltophilia	Y. enterocolitica	F. tularensis	Brucella sp.	Legionella sp.	H. ducreyi	V. vulnificus	Chlamydophila sp.	M. pneumoniae	Rickettsia sp.	Mycobacterium avium	Actinomyces	Bacteroides fragilis	P. melaninogenica	Clostridium difficile	Clostridium (not difficile)**	Peptostreptococcus sp.
MISCELLANEOUS																					
Colistimethate (Colistin)	o	+	+	o	o	±															
Daptomycin	o	o	o	o	o	o	o	o	o	o	o										
Linezolid	o	o	o	o	o	o	o	o				+		o		±			±	+	+
Quinupristin-dalfopristin												o				+	+	o		+	+
Metronidazole	o	o	o	o	o	o	o	o	o	o	o	o	o	o	o	o	+	+	+	+	+
Rifampin	o	o	o	o				+	+						+						
AGENTS URINARY TRACT																					
Fosfomycin	±																				
Nitrofurantoin	o			o	o	o															
TMP-SMX	o	±	o	+	+	+	+	+	+	±	+				o						
Trimethoprim	o	o	o	+	o				+	+		o			+						
Fusidic Acid^NUS	o	o	o	o	o	o		±	o			o	o	o		+		+		+	+
GLYCOPEPTIDES																					
Dalbavancin	o	o	o	o					o						o	+	o	o	+	+	+
Telavancin	o	o	o	o					o						o	+	o	o	+	+	+
Teicoplanin^NUS	o	o	o	o					o						o				+	+	+
Vancomycin	o	o	o	o					o						o	+	o	o	+	+	+
GLYCYLCYCLINE																					
Tigecycline	±	±	o	±	+							+	+		o		+	+		+	+
TETRACYCLINES																					
Minocycline	o	o	o	±	o	o	+	+			+	+	+	+	o	+	±	+		+	+
Doxycycline	o	o	o	o	o	o	+	+			+	+	+	+	o	+	±	+		+	+
KETOLIDE																					
Telithromycin	o	o	o	o	o				o		+	+	+	+		+	+	+			
MACROLIDES																					
Clarithromycin	o	o	o	o	o	o			o		+	+	+		+	+	o	+		+	+
Azithromycin	o	o	o	o	o	o			o		+	+	+		+	+	o	+		+	+
Erythro/Dirithro	o	o	o	o	o	o			o		+	+	+	±		+	o			±	±
Clindamycin	o	o	o	o	o	o			o							±	o	+		±	+
Chloramphenicol	o	o	+	+	+	+	+				+	+		+	+	+	+	+	±	+	+
AMINOGLYCOSIDES																					
Amikacin	+	±	+	o	o	+					±			o	o	o	+	o	o	o	o
Tobramycin	+	o	+	o	o	+	+	+	+		±			o	o	o	o	o	o	o	o
Gentamicin	+	o	+	o	o	+	+	+			±			o	o	o	o	o	o	o	o

+ = usually effective clinically or >60% susceptible; ± = clinical trials lacking or 30-60% susceptible; o = not effective clinically or <30% susceptible; blank = data not available.

Antimicrobials such as azithromycin have high tissue penetration & some such as clarithromycin are metabolized to more active compounds, hence in vivo activity may exceed in vitro activity.

** Vancomycin, metronidazole given po active vs C. difficile; IV vancomycin not effective

TABLE 5 – TREATMENT OPTIONS FOR SELECTED HIGHLY RESISTANT BACTERIA
(See page 2 for abbreviations)

ORGANISM/RESISTANCE	THERAPEUTIC OPTIONS	COMMENT[1]
E. faecalis. Resistant to:		
Vanco + strep/gentamicin (MIC >500 mcg per mL), β-lactamase neg. (JAC 40:161, 1997).	Penicillin G or AMP (systemic infections). Nitrofurantoin, fosfomycin (UTI only). Usually resistant to Synercid.	AMP + ceftriaxone effective for endocarditis due to E. faecalis with high level AG resistance (no comparator treated with AMP alone) but no data for therapy of VRE (AnIM 146:574, 2007). Non BL+ strains of E. faecalis resistant to penicillin and AMP described in Spain, but unknown elsewhere (except BL+ strains) in U.S. and elsewhere (AAC 44:1349, 1996). Nitrofurantoin often effective in 60–70% of cases (AnIM 138:135, 2003). Cephalosporin, tigecycline active in vitro (JAC 59:209, 1996; JAC 62:123, 2003).
Penicillin (β-lactamase producers)	Vanco, AM-SB	Appear susceptible to AMP and penicillin by standard in vitro methods. Must use direct test for β-lactamase with chromogenic cephalosporin (nitrocefin) to identify. Rare since early 1990s. Ceftobiprole active in vitro (AAC 51:2043, 2007).
E. faecium. Resistant to:		
Vanco and high levels (MIC >500 mcg per mL) of streptomycin and gentamicin	Penicillin G or AMP (systemic infections). Fosfomycin, nitrofurantoin (UTI only)	For strains with pen/AMP MICs of ≥8 ≤64 mcg per mL, anecdotal evidence that high-dose (300 mg per kg per day) AMP Rx may be effective. Daptomycin, tigecycline active in vitro (JAC 52:123, 2003).
Penicillin, AMP, vanco, & high-level resist. to streptomycin and gentamicin (NEJM 342:710, 2000)	Linezolid 600 mg po or IV q12h and quino-dalfo 7.5 mg per kg IV q8h are bacteriostatic against most strains of E. faecium. Can try combinations of cell wall-active antibiotics with other agents (including FQ, chloramphenicol, RIF, or doxy). Chloramphenicol alone effective in some cases of bacteremia (Clin Micro Inf 7:17, 2001). Nitrofurantoin or fosfomycin may work for UTI.	For strains with Van B phenotype (vanco R, teico S), teicoplanin[AUS], preferably in combination with streptomycin or gentamicin (if not highly AG resistant), may be effective. Synercid roughly 70% effective in clinical trials (CID 30:790, 2000 & 33:1816, 2001). Linezolid shows similar efficacy. Comparable but somewhat lower (58% [linezolid, 43% QD] response rates in cancer pts (JAC 53:646, 2004). Emergence of resistance with therapeutic failure has occurred during monotherapy with either quinu-dalfo or linezolid (CID 30:790, 2000; Ln 357:1179, 2001). Nosocomial spread of linezolid-resistant E. faecium possible (NEJM 346:867, 2002). Daptomycin active in vitro against most strains (JAC 52:123, 2003). Tigecycline also active in vitro (Circulation 111:e394, 2005). **Infectious disease consultation imperative.**
S. aureus. Resistant to:		
Methicillin (health-care associated) (CID 32:108, 2001) **For community-acquired MRSA infections, see Table 6**	Vanco [For persistent bacteremia (≥7 days) on vanco or teicoplanin[AUS], see Table 6]	Alternatives: teicoplanin[AUS], daptomycin (AAC 49:770, 2005; NEJM 355:653, 2006), linezolid (Chest 124:1789, 2003), dalbavancin (EMID 48:137, 2004), TMP-SMX (best susceptibility test), minocycline & doxy (some strains)(NEJM 357:380, 2007). Tigecycline (CID 41(Suppl 5):S303, 2005), or quinu-dalfo (CID 34:1481, 2002). Fusidic acid[AUS], fosfomycin. RIF may be active; use only in combination to prevent in vivo emergence of resistance. Staphylococci (incl. CA-MRSA) with inducible MLS₈ resistance may appear susceptible to clindamycin in vitro. Clinda therapy may result in therapeutic failure (CID 37:1257, 2003). Test for inducible resistance (double-disc "D test") before treating with clinda (J Clin Micro 42:2777, 2004). Investigational drugs with activity against MRSA include oritavancin (LY333328), telavancin, ceftobiprole, ceftaroline.
Vanco, methicillin (VISA & VRSA) (NEJM 339:520, 1998; CID 32:108, 2001; MMWR 51:902, 2002; NEJM 348:1342, 2003)	Unknown, but even high-dose vanco may fail. Linezolid, quinu-dalfo, daptomycin active in vitro.	VISA/GISA: Vanco-intermediate resistance of MRSA with MICs of ≤16 mcg/mL. Anecdotal data on treatment regimens. Most susceptible to TMP-SMX, minocycline, doxycycline, RIF and AGs (CID 32:108, 2001). RIF should always be combined with a 2nd therapeutic agent to prevent emergence of RIF resistance during therapy. VRSA: only 6 clinical isolates of truly vancomycin-resistant strains described. Organisms still susceptible to TMP-SMX, chloro, linezolid, minocycline, quinu-dalfo (MMWR 51:902, 2002; NEJM 348:1342, 2003).
S. epidermidis. Resistant to:		
Methicillin	Vanco (± RIF and gentamicin for prosthetic valve endocarditis)	Vanco more active than teicoplanin[AUS] (Clin Micro Rev 8:585, 1995). New FQs (levofloxacin, gatifloxacin, moxifloxacin) active in vitro, but development of resistance is a potential problem.
Methicillin & glycopeptides (AAC 49: 770, 2005)	Quinu-dalfo (see comments on E. faecium) generally active in vitro, as are linezolid, daptomycin, & dalbavancin	

[1] Guideline on prevention of resistance: CID 25:584, 1997

TABLE 5 (2)

ORGANISM/RESISTANCE	THERAPEUTIC OPTIONS	COMMENT[1]
S. pneumoniae. Resistant to: Penicillin G (MIC > 0.1 ≤ 2.0)	Ceftriaxone or cefotaxime. High-dose penicillin (≥ 10 million units per day) or AMP (amox) likely effective for nonmeningeal sites of infection (e.g., pneumonia); telithro	IMP, ERTA, cefepime, cefpodoxime, cefuroxime also active (IDCP 3:75, 1994). MER less active than IMP (AAC 38:898, 1994). Gemi, moxi, levo also have good activity (AAC 38:898, 1994; DMID 31:45, 1998; Exp Opin Invest Drugs 8:123, 1999). High-dose cefotaxime (300 mg per kg per day, max. 24 gm per day) effective in meningitis due to strains with cefotaxime MICs as high as 2 mcg per mL (AAC 40:218, 1996). Review (Ln 352:Suppl 2):S21, 1997.
Penicillin G (MIC ≥ 4.0)	(Vanco ± RIF). Alternatives if non-meningeal infection: ceftriaxone/cefotax, high-dose AMP, ERTA, IMP, MER, or an active FQ (Gemi, moxi, levo), telithro	Note new CLSI breakpoints for penicillin susceptibilities. Meningeal isolates ≤0.06 = S, 0.12:1.0 = I, ≥2.0 = R. For non-meningeal isolates ≤2.0 = S, 4.0 = I, ≥8.0 = R.
Penicillin, erythro, tetracycline, chloramphenicol, TMP-SMX	Vanco ± RIF. (Gemi, moxi, or levo); telithro (non-meningeal infections)	60–80% of strains susceptible to clindamycin (DMID 25:261, 1996).
Acinetobacter baumannii. Resistant to: IMP, P Ceph 3 AP, AP Pen, APAG, FQ (see page 2 for abbreviations)	AM-SB (CID 34:1425, 2002). Sulbactam alone is active against some A. baumannii (JAC 42:793, 1998). Colistin effective most multi-resistant strains (CID 36:1111, 2003; JAC 54:1083, 2004; CID 43:589, 2006).	6/8 patients with A. baumannii meningitis (7 organisms resistant to IMP) cured with AM-SB (CID 24: 932, 1997). Various combinations of FQs and AGs, IMP and AGs or RIF, or AP Pens or P Ceph 3 APs with AGs may show activity against **some** multiresistant strains (CID 36:1268, 2003). MER + sulbactam active in vitro in vivo (JAC 53:393, 2004). Active in vitro: triple drug combinations of polymyxin B, IMP & RIF (AAC 48:753, 2004), other colistin-containing combination regimens (CID 43:595, 2006; AAC 51:1621, 2007) & tigecycline (CID 41:S315, 2005), but several studies document borderline activity of tigecycline against acinetobacter (AAC 59:772, 2007; AAC 51: 376, 2007).
Campylobacter jejuni. Resistant to: FQs	Erythro, azithro, clarithro, doxy, clindamycin	Resistance to **both** FQs & macrolides reported (CID 22:868, 1996; EID 7:24, 2002; AAC 47:2358, 2003).
Klebsiella pneumoniae (producing ESBL) Resistant to: Ceftazidime & other 3rd generation cephalosporins (see Table 10C), aztreonam	IMP, MER. (CID 39:31, 2004) (See Comment)	P Ceph 4, TC-CL, PIP-TZ show in vitro activity, but not proven entirely effective in animal models (IJAA 8:37, 1997); some strains which hyperproduce ESBLs are primarily resistant to TC-CL and PIP-TZ (J Clin Micro 34:358, 1996). Note: there are strains of ESBL-producing klebsiella sensitive in vitro to P Ceph 2, 3 but resistant to ceftazidime; infections with such strains do not respond to P Ceph 2 or 3 (J Clin Micro 39:2206, 2001). FQ may be effective if susceptible but many strains resistant. Note Klebsiella sp. with carbapenem resistance due to class A carbapenemase. Some of these organisms resistant to all antimicrobials except colistin (CID 39:55, 2004). Tigecycline active in vitro (AAC 50:3166, 2006).
Resistant to: Carbapenems, 2nd & 3rd generation cephalosporins due to KPC enzymes	Colistin (AAC 48:4793, 2004)	
Pseudomonas aeruginosa. Resistant to: IMP, MER	CIP (check susceptibility), APAG (check susceptibility), Colistin effective for multiresistant strains (CID 28:1008, 1999; CMN 13:560, 2007)	Many strains remain susceptible to aztreonam & ceftazidime or (AP Pen & APAG) or (AP Ceph 3 + APAG) may show in vitro activity (AAC 39:2411, 1995). Combinations of AP Pen & APAG) or (AP Ceph 3 + APAG) may show in vitro activity (AAC 39:2411, 1995).

[1] Guideline on prevention of resistance: CID 25:584, 1997

TABLE 6 - SUGGESTED MANAGEMENT OF SUSPECTED OR CULTURE-POSITIVE COMMUNITY-ACQUIRED PHENOTYPE OF METHICILLIN-RESISTANT S. AUREUS (CA-MRSA) INFECTIONS

In the absence of definitive comparative efficacy studies, the Editors have generated the following guidelines. With the magnitude of the clinical problem and a number of new drugs, it is likely new data will require frequent revisions of the regimens suggested. (See page 2 for abbreviations). All doses below.

CLINICAL ILLNESS	ABSCESS, AFEBRILE; & IMMUNOCOMPETENT: OUTPATIENT CARE	ABSCESS(ES) WITH FEVER: OUTPATIENT CARE	VENTILATOR-ASSOCIATED PNEUMONIA	BACTEREMIA OR POSSIBLE ENDOCARDITIS OR BACTEREMIC SHOCK	BLOOD CULTURES DRAWN ON DAY 7 OF THERAPY ARE POSITIVE (See footnote)
Management (for drug doses, see footnote)	**TMP-SMX-DS or doxycycline or minocycline** (CID 40:1429, 2005 & AAC 51:3298, 2007). **NOTE:** for abscesses <5 cm diameter, **I&D** sufficient (PIDJ 23:123, 2004).	(**TMP-SMX-DS ± rifampin**) or **linezolid** or 1 dose of **dalbavancin IV**	**Vanco or teico**[NUS] IV or **linezolid** IV Ref. Chest 124:1632, 2003	**Vanco or teico**[NUS] IV or **dapto** IV. **Dapto** not inferior to **vanco** in bacteremia trial (NEJM 355:653, 2006). Add **clinda** if clinical picture of toxic shock syndrome.	**Dapto for vanco** or vice versa. **Dapto** therapy reported after **vanco** exposure & prior to **dapto** therapy (CID 45:601, 2007) (See footnote 2). **Dapto** dose safely increased to 12 mg/kg/d (AAC 50:3245, 2006). **Quinupristin-dalfopristin (Q-D)** 2nd choice ± **vanco.** Linezolid ~70% effective in compassionate use trial (JAC 50:1017, 2002)
Comments	Culture abscess: **I&D** Hot packs. Close follow-up. Ref. NEJM 357:380, 2007.	Culture abscess & maybe blood. **I&D** Hot packs. Close follow-up. / Effective dose of **TMP-SMX-DS** is unclear IV dose is 8-10 mg/kg/d; roughly equivalent to 2 tabs po bid. Two small studies report failure with 1 tab bid (refs in footnote below). Anecdotally, most pts respond to **I&D** and 1 tab bid. **Clinda** also not listed due to geographic "pockets" of inducible resistance (CID 40:280, 2005).[3]	Need quant. cultures for diagnosis; e.g., protected specimen brush / **Linezolid** superior to **vanco** in retrospective subset analysis; prospective study in progress.	**Vanco** MIC≥1.5: disproportionate failure in MCS (CID 42:513, 2006 & 44:1208, 2007). Ideal **vanco** trough level unclear. More nephrotoxicity with higher troughs (Curr Ther 29:107, 2007). If **vanco** MIC≥2 ug/mL, consider alternative therapy. ID consultation suggested. / Efficacy of **TMP-SMX** vs. **vanco** uncertain. If **TMP-SMX** was inferior to **vanco** vs bacteremic MSSA. **Dapto** failures associated with development of **dapto** resistance (NEJM 355:653, 2006)	If MRSA resistant to **erythro**, likely that Q-D will have bacteriostatic, & not bactericidal activity. Interest in Q-D + **vanco**, but no data. Do not add **linezolid** to **vanco** - no benefit & may be antagonistic (AAC 47:3002, 2003). Linezolid successful in compassionate use (JAC 50:1017, 2002) & in pts with reduced **vanco** in vitro suscept. (CID 38:521, 2004). New **dapto** likely available in 2008: ceftobiprole, ceftaroline and telavancin.

Clindamycin: 300 mg po qid. **Daptomycin:** 6 mg per kg per IV q24h. **Doxycycline or minocycline** 100 mg po bid. **Linezolid** 600 mg po/IV q12h. however, frequency of nausea justifies dosing 600 mg q24h. **Rifampin:** Long serum half-life justifies loading dose 600 mg q24h. **TMP-SMX-DS:** Standard dose 8-10 mg per kg per day TMP. For 70 kg person = 700 mg TMP component per day. Longer duration of bacteremia, greater likelihood of endocarditis. **Dalbavancin** 1000 mg IV, then 500 mg IV 8 days later. **Quinupristin-dalfopristin (Q-D):** 7.5 mg per kg IV q8h via central line. **Nafcillin or oxacillin** 2 gm IV q4h. **V-K, Clinda or Fusidic acid** use other options. TMP-SMX-DS contains 160 mg TMP. Hence, suggest **2 TMP-SMX-DS po bid**; small studies report failures with one TMP-SMX-DS po bid. Increased dapto MICs (J Am Acad Derm 50:854, 2004 & AAC 51:2628, 2007). **Vancomycin:** 1 gm IV q12h.

1 Bacteremia may persist 7 days after starting vanco (AnIM 115:674, 1991). Longer duration of bacteremia, greater likelihood of endocarditis (JID 190:1140, 2004).

2 Before switching, look for undrained abscess(es) &/or infected foreign body. Recheck vanco and dapto MICs to exclude increases that may have developed during therapy. reported in some isolates after vanco exposure in vitro; clinical significance to be determined (CID 45:601, 2007).

3 To date, no data that inducible clinda resistance has led to clinical treatment failure.

TABLE 7 - METHODS FOR PENICILLIN DESENSITIZATION (CID 35:26, 2002)

(See Table 10C, page 92, for TMP/SMX desensitization)

Perform in ICU setting. Discontinue all β-adrenergic antagonists. Have IV line, ECG and spirometer (CCT/D 13:131, 1993). Once desensitized, rx must not lapse or risk of allergic reactions ↑. A history of Stevens-Johnson syndrome, exfoliative dermatitis, erythroderma are nearly absolute contraindications to desensitization and are only as an approach to IgE sensitivity

Oral Route: If oral prep available and pt has functional GI tract, oral route is preferred. 1/3 pts will develop transient reaction during desensitization or treatment, usually mild.

Step *	1	2	3	4	5	6	7	8	9	10	11	12	13	14
Drug (mg per mL)	0.5	0.5	0.5	0.5	0.5	0.5	0.5	5.0	5.0	5.0	50	50	50	50
Amount (mL)	0.1	0.2	0.4	0.8	1.6	3.2	6.4	1.2	2.4	4.8	1.0	2.0	4.0	8.0

* Interval between doses: 15 min. After Step 14, observe for 30 minutes, then 1.0 gm IV

Parenteral Route:

Step **	1	2	3	4	5	6	7	8	9	10	11	12	13	14	15	16	17
Drug (mg per mL)	0.1	0.1	0.1	0.1	0.1	1.0	1.0	1.0	10	10	100	100	100	100	1000	1000	1000
Amount (mL)	0.1	0.2	0.4	0.8	1.6	0.16	0.32	0.64	0.24	0.48	0.1	0.2	0.4	0.8	0.16	0.32	0.64

** Interval between doses: 15 min. After Step 17, observe for 30 minutes, then 1.0 gm IV [Adapted from Sullivan, TJ, in Allergy: Principles and Practice, C.V. Mosby, 1993, p. 1726, with permission.]

TABLE 8 - RISK CATEGORIES OF ANTIMICROBICS IN PREGNANCY

Antibacterial Agents

DRUG	FDA CATEGORIES*
Aminoglycosides:	
Amikacin, gentamicin, isepamicin[NUS]	D
netilmicin[NUS], streptomycin & tobramycin	D
Beta-lactams:	
Penicillins, pens + BLI; cephalosporins, aztreonam	B
Imipenem/cilastatin	C
Meropenem, ertapenem, doripenem	B
Chloramphenicol	C
Ciprofloxacin, oflox, levoflox, gatiflox, gemiflox, moxiflox	C
Clindamycin	B
Colistin	C
Dalbavancin	C
Daptomycin	B
Fosfomycin	B
Fusidic acid[†]	see Footnote 1
Linezolid	C
Macrolides:	
Erythromycins/azithromycin	B
Clarithromycin	C
Metronidazole	B
Nitrofurantoin	B
Rifaximin	C
Sulfonamides/trimethoprim	C
Telithromycin	C

Antibacterial Agents (continued)

DRUG	FDA CATEGORIES
Tetracyclines, tigecycline	D
Tinidazole	C
Vancomycin	C
Antifungal Agents: (CID 27:1151, 1998)	
Amphotericin B preparations	B
Anidulafungin	C
Caspofungin	C
Fluconazole, itraconazole, ketoconazole	C
flucytosine	C
Micafungin	C
Posaconazole	C
Terbinafine	B
Voriconazole	D
Antiparasitic Agents:	
Albendazole/mebendazole	C
Atovaquone/proguanil; atovaquone alone	C
Chloroquine	C
Eflornithine	C
Ivermectin	C
Mefloquine	C
Miltefosine	B
Nitazoxanide	B
Pentamidine	C
Praziquantel	B
Pyrimethamine/pyrisulfadoxine	C
Quinidine	C

Antimycobacterial Agents

DRUG	FDA CATEGORIES
Quinine	X
Clofazimine	C
Clofazimine/cycloserine	C
Dapsone	C
Ethambutol	B "avoid"
Ethionamide	C
INH, pyrazinamide	C
Rifabutin	B "safe"
Rifampin	C
Thalidomide	X "do not use"
Antiviral Agents:	
Abacavir	C
Acyclovir	B
Adefovir	C
Amantadine	C
Atazanavir	B
Cidofovir	C
Darunavir	B
Delavirdine	C
Didanosine (ddl)	B
Efavirenz	**D** / X
Emtricitabine	B
Enfuvirtide	B
Entecavir	C
Famciclovir	B
Fosamprenavir	C

Antiviral Agents (continued)

DRUG	FDA CATEGORIES
Foscarnet	C
Ganciclovir	C
Indinavir	C
Interferons	C
Lamivudine	C
Lopinavir/ritonavir	C
Maraviroc	B
Nelfinavir	B
Nevirapine	C
Oseltamivir	C
Raltegravir	C
Ribavirin	X
Rimantadine	C
Ritonavir	B
Saquinavir	B
Stavudine	C
Telbivudine	B
Tenofovir	B
Tipranavir	C
Valacyclovir	B
Valganciclovir	C
Zalcitabine	C
Zanamivir	C
Zidovudine	C

* **FDA Pregnancy Categories: A**—studies in pregnant women, no risk; **B**—animal studies no risk, but human studies inadequate or animal toxicity but human studies no risk; **C**—animal studies show toxicity, human studies inadequate but benefit of use may exceed risk; **D**—evidence of human risk, but benefits may exceed risk; **X**—fetal abnormalities in humans, risk > benefit

1 Fusidic acid: no problems reported

TABLE 9A – SELECTED PHARMACOLOGIC FEATURES OF ANTIMICROBIAL AGENTS (Footnotes at end of table)

DRUG	DOSE, ROUTE OF ADMINISTRATION	FOR PO DOSING—Take Drug[7] WITH FOOD	WITHOUT FOOD[6]	WITH OR WITHOUT FOOD	% AB[5]	PEAK SERUM LEVEL mcg per mL[3]	PROTEIN BINDING, %	SERUM T½, HOURS[2]	BILIARY EXCRETION, %	CSF/ BLOOD, %	CSF LEVEL POTENTIALLY THERAPEUTIC[4]
PENICILLINS: Natural											
Benzathine Pen G	1.2 million units IM					0.15					
Penicillin G	2 million units IV		X			20	65		500	5-10	Yes for Pen-sens. S. pneumo
Penicillin V	500 mg po				60-73	5-6	65	0.5			
PENASE-RESISTANT PENICILLINS											
Clox/Diclox	500 mg po		X		50	10-15	95-98	0.5			
Nafcillin/Oxacillin	500 mg IV		X		Erratic	10-15	90-94	0.5			Yes-high-dose IV therapy
AMINOPENICILLINS											
Amoxicillin	250 mg po			X	75	4-5	17	1.2	100-3000	13-14	
AM-CL	875/125 mg po	X				11.6/2.2	20/30	1.4/1.1	100-3000		
AM-CL-ER						17/2.1	18/25	1.3/1.0			
Ampicillin	2 gm IV					47	18-22	1.2	100-3000	13-14	Yes
AM-SB	3 gm IV					109-150	28/38	1.2			
ANTIPSEUDOMONAL PENICILLINS											
Indanyl carb.	382 mg po			X	35	6.5	50	1.0	3000-6000	30	Not for P. aeruginosa; marginal for coliforms
Piperacillin	4 gm IV					400	16-48	1.0			
PIP-TZ	3/.375 gm IV					209	16-48	1.0	>100	40	Not for P. aeruginosa; marginal for coliforms
Ticarcillin	3 gm IV					260	45	1.2			
TC-CL	3.1 gm IV					330	45/25	1.1			
CEPHALOSPORINS—1st Generation											
Cefadroxil	500 mg po			X	90	16	20	1.5	22	1-4	No
Cefazolin	1 gm IV					188	73-87	1.9	29-300		
Cephalexin	500 mg po			X	90	18-38	5-15	1.0	216		
CEPHALOSPORINS—2nd Generation											
Cefaclor	500 mg po			X	93	9.3	22-25	0.8	≥60		
Cefaclor-CD	500 mg po		X			8.4	22-25	0.8	≥60		
Cefotetan	1 gm IV					124	78-91	4.2	2-21		
Cefoxitin	1 gm IV					110	65-79	0.8	280		
Cefprozil	500 mg po			X	95	10.5	36	1.5			
Cefuroxime	1.5 gm IV					100	33-50	1.3	35-80	3	±
Cefuroxime axetil	250 mg po	X			52	4.1	50	1.5		17-88	Yes
Loracarbef			X		90	8	25	1.2			
CEPHALOSPORINS—3rd Generation											
Cefdinir	300 mg po				25	1.6	60-70	1.7			
Cefditoren pivoxil	400 mg po	X			16	4	88	1.6			
Cefixime	400 mg po			X	50	3-5	65	3.1	800		
Cefotaxime	1 gm IV					100	30-51	1.5	15-75	10	Yes
Cefpodoxime proxetil	200 mg po	X			46	2.9	40	2.3	115		
Ceftazidime	1 gm IV					60	<10	1.9	13-54	20-40	Yes
Ceftibuten	400 mg po		X		80	15	65	2.4			

See page 79 for all footnotes; see page 2 for abbreviations

TABLE 9A (2) (Footnotes at the end of table)

DRUG	DOSE, ROUTE OF ADMINISTRATION	FOR PO DOSING—Take Drug			% AB	PEAK SERUM LEVEL mcg per mL	PROTEIN BINDING, %	SERUM T½, HOURS	BILIARY EXCRETION, %	CSF/BLOOD, %	CSF LEVEL POTENTIALLY THERAPEUTIC
		WITH FOOD	WITHOUT FOOD	WITH OR WITHOUT FOOD							
CEPHALOSPORINS—3rd Generation (continued)											
Ceftizoxime	1 gm IV					132	30	1.7	34-82	8-16	
Ceftriaxone	1 gm IV					150	85-95	8	200-500	8-16	Yes
CEPHALOSPORIN—4th Generation											
Cefepime	2 gm IV					193	20	2.0	∝ 5	10	Yes
Ceftobiprole	500 mg IV					29-44	16	3-4			
CARBAPENEMS											
Doripenem	500 mg IV					23	8.1	1			
Ertapenem	1 gm IV					154	95	4	10	8.5	+
Imipenem	500 mg IV					40	15-25	1	minimal	Approx 2	+
Meropenem	1 gm IV					49	2	1	3-300		±
MONOBACTAM											
Aztreonam	1 gm IV					125	56	2	115-405	3-52	No; intrathecal: 5-10 mg
AMINOGLYCOSIDES											
Amikacin, gentamicin, kanamycin, tobramycin—see Table 10D, page 93, for dose & serum levels											
Neomycin	po				<3	0	0-10	2.5	10-60	0-30	
FLUOROQUINOLONES											
Ciprofloxacin	750 mg po / 400 mg IV			X / X	70	1.8-2.8 / 4.6	20-40 / 20-40	4 / 4	2800-4500 / 2800-4500	26	1 mcg per mL: Inadequate for Strep. species (CID 31:1131, 2000)
	500 mg ER po / 1000 mg ER po			X / X		1.6 / 3.1	26-40 / 26-40	6.6 / 6.3			
Gatifloxacin	400 mg po/IV			X	96	4.2-4.6	20	7-8		36	
Gemifloxacin	320 mg po			X	71	0.7-2.6	55-73	7			
Levofloxacin	500 mg po/IV / 750 mg po/IV			X	98 / 99	5.7 / 8.6	24-38 / 24-38	7 / 7		30-50	
Moxifloxacin	400 mg po/IV			X	89	4.5	30-50	10-14			
Ofloxacin	400 mg po/IV			X	98	4.6/6.2	32	9			
MACROLIDES, AZALIDES, LINCOSAMIDES, KETOLIDES											
Azithromycin	500 mg po / 500 mg IV			X	37	0.4 / 3.6	7-51	68	High		
Azithromycin-ER	2 gm po		X		∝ 30	0.8	7-50	12/68	High		
Clarithromycin	500 mg po / 500 mg IV			X	50	3-4 / 2-3	65-70	59	High		
Dirithromycin	ER—500 mg po		X		∝ 50	2-3	65-70	5-7	7000		
Erythromycin	500 mg po				10	0.4	15-30	8			
Erythromycin Oral (various) Lacto/gluco	500 mg po / 500 mg po	X / X			18-45	0.1-1.2 / 3-4	70-74 / 76-74	2-4 / 2-4	7	2-13	
Telithromycin	800 mg po				57	2.3	60-70	10			No
Clindamycin	150 mg po / 600 mg IV			X	90	2.5 / 10	85-94 / 85-94	2.4 / 2.4	250-300 / 250-300	No	No

TABLE 9A (3) (Footnotes at the end of table)

Food columns (WITH FOOD / WITHOUT FOOD / WITH OR WITHOUT FOOD) fall under the grouped header **FOR PO DOSING — Take Drug***.

DRUG	DOSE, ROUTE OF ADMINISTRATION	WITH FOOD	WITHOUT FOOD	WITH OR WITHOUT FOOD	% AB[1]	PEAK SERUM LEVEL mcg per mL	PROTEIN BINDING, %	SERUM T½, HOURS[2]	BILIARY EXCRETION, %[3]	CSF[4]/BLOOD, %	CSF LEVEL POTENTIALLY THERAPEUTIC[6]
MISCELLANEOUS ANTIBACTERIALS											
Chloramphenicol	1 gm IV			X	High	11–18	25–50	4.1		45–89	Yes
Colistin	150 mg					5–7.5		2–3			No
Dalbavancin	1 gm, then 0.5 gm IV on day 8					240	93	168	0		
Daptomycin	4–6 mg per kg IV					58–99	92	8–9			
Doxycycline	100 mg po		X			1.5–2.1	93	18	200–3200		No (26%)
Fosfomycin	3 gm po		X			26	<10	5.7			
Fusidic acid	500 mg p.o.		X			30	95–99	5–15			
Linezolid	600 mg po/IV			X	91	15–20	31	5		60–70	
Metronidazole	500 mg po/IV			X	100	20–25	20	6–14	100	45–89	
Minocycline	200 mg po			X		2.0–3.5	76	16	200–3200		No
Polymyxin B	20,000 units per kg IV					1–8		4.3–6			
Rifampin	600 mg po		X			4–32	80	1.5	10,000		
Rifaximin	200 mg po				<0.4	0.004–0.01		2–5			
Sulfamethoxazole (SMX)	2 gm po				70–90	50–120		7–12			
Tetracycline	250 mg po		X			1.5–2.2		6–12	200–3200		
Telavancin	10 mg/kg q24h					87.5	90	7–8			No (7%)
Tigecycline	50 mg IV q12h					0.63	71–89	42	Low		
Trimethoprim (TMP)	100 mg po	X			80	1		8–15	138		No
TMP-SMX-DS	160/800 mg po				85	1–2/40–60				50/40	Most meningococci resistant. Static vs coliforms. See Meningitis, Table 1, page 6
Vancomycin	1 gm IV			X		20–50	<10–55	4–6	100–200	7–14	Need high doses. See Meningitis, Table 1, page 6
ANTIFUNGALS											
Amphotericin B											
Standard	0.4–0.7 mg per kg IV					0.5–3.5		24			
Ampho B lipid complex (ABLC)	5 mg per kg IV					1–2.5		173			
Ampho B cholesteryl complex	4 mg per kg IV					2.9		39			
Liposomal ampho B	5 mg per kg IV					83		6.8 ± 2.1			
Azoles											
Fluconazole	400 mg po/IV			X	90	6.7	11	20–50		50–94	Yes
Itraconazole	800 mg po/IV	X			90	Approx. 14	99.8	20–50		0	
Itraconazole, oral soln	Oral soln 200 mg po		X			0.3–0.7		35			
Posaconazole	200 mg po/IV	X			Low	0.21–1.0	98–99	20–66		0	Yes CID 37:728, 2003
Voriconazole	200 mg IV x 1, then 100 mg po q24h		X		96	3	58	6		22–100	Yes JAC 56:745, 2005
Anidulafungin	200 mg IV x 1, then 100 mg IV q24h					7.2	84	26.5			No
Caspofungin	70 mg IV x 1, then 50 mg IV qd					9.9	97	9–11			No
Flucytosine	2.5 gm po			X	78–90	30–40		3–6		60–100	Yes
Micafungin	150 mg IV		X			16.4	>99	15–17			No

See page 79 for all footnotes; see page 2 for abbreviations

TABLE 9A (4) (Footnotes at the end of table)

DRUG	DOSE, ROUTE OF ADMINISTRATION	FOR PO DOSING—Take Drug			% AB[1]	PEAK SERUM LEVEL mcg per mL	PROTEIN BINDING, %	SERUM T½, HOURS[2]	BILIARY EXCRETION, %[3]	CSF/ BLOOD, %	CSF LEVEL POTENTIALLY THERAPEUTIC[5]
		WITH FOOD	WITHOUT FOOD[4]	WITH OR WITHOUT FOOD							
ANTIMYCOBACTERIALS											
Ethambutol	25 mg per kg po	X			80	2-6	10-30	4		25-50	No
Isoniazid	300 mg po		X		100	3-5		0.7-4		90	Yes
Pyrazinamide	20-25 mg per kg po			X	95	30-50	5-10	10-16		100	Yes
Rifampin	600 mg po		X		70-90	4-32	80	1.5-5	10,000	7-56	Yes
Streptomycin	1 gm IV (see Table 10D, page 93)					25-50	0-10	2.5	10-60	0-30	No. Intrathecal: 5-10 mg
ANTIPARASITICS											
Albendazole	400 mg po	X			80						
Atovaquone suspension	750 mg po	X			47	0.5-1.6	70	67		<1	No
Dapsone	100 mg po			X	100	1.1	99.9	10-50			
Ivermectin	12 mg po	X				0.05-0.08	98	10-50			
Mefloquine	1.25 gm po	X				0.5-1.2	99	13-24 days			
Nitazoxanide	500 mg po	X				3	75				
Proguanil					"High"		75				
Pyrimethamine	25 mg po			X		0.1-0.3	87	96			
Praziquantel	20 mg per kg po	X			80	0.2-2.0		0.8-1.5			
Tinidazole	2 gm po			X	48	13	12	13	Chemically similar to metronidazole		
ANTIVIRAL DRUGS—NOT HIV											
Acyclovir	400 mg po			X	10-20	1.21	9-33	2.5-3.5			
Adefovir	10 mg po			X	59	0.02	≤4	7.5			
Entecavir	0.5 mg po		X		100	4.2 ng/mL	13	128-149			
Famciclovir	500 mg po			X	77	3-4	<20	2-3			
Foscarnet	60 mg per kg IV					155		4		<1	No
Ganciclovir	5 mg per kg IV					8.3	1-2	3.5			
Oseltamivir	75 mg po			X	75	0.065/3.5[13]	3	1-3			
Ribavirin	600 mg po	X			64	0.8		44			
Rimantadine	100 mg po			X		0.1-0.4	3.3	25			
Telbivudine	600 mg po			X				40-49			
Valacyclovir	1000 mg po			X	55	5.6	13-18	3			
Valganciclovir	900 mg po	X			59	5.6	1-2	4			

DRUG	DOSE, ROUTE OF ADMINISTRATION	FOR PO DOSING—Take Drug			% AB[1]	PEAK SERUM LEVEL mcg per mL	PROTEIN BINDING, %	INTRACELLULAR T½, HOURS[2]	SERUM T½, HOURS[2]	CYTOCHROME P450
		WITH FOOD	WITHOUT FOOD	WITH OR WITHOUT FOOD						
ANTI-HIV VIRAL DRUGS										
Abacavir	600 mg po			X	83	3.0	50	12-26	1.5	
Atazanavir	400 mg po	X			"Good"	2.3	86		7	
Darunavir	600 mg with 100 mg ritonavir	X			82	3.5	95		15	Inhibitor
Delavirdine	400 mg po			X	85	19 ± 11	98		5.8	Inhibitor
Didanosine	400 mg EC[14] po		X		30-40	?	<5	25-40	1.4	
Efavirenz	600 mg po		X		42	13 mcM[11]	99		52-76	Inducer/inhibitor

See page 79 for all footnotes; see page 2 for abbreviations

TABLE 9A (5) (Footnotes at the end of table)

DRUG	DOSE, ROUTE OF ADMINISTRATION	WITHOUT FOOD[7]	WITH FOOD	WITH OR WITHOUT FOOD[7]	% AB[1]	PEAK SERUM LEVEL mcg per mL[2]	PROTEIN BINDING, %	INTRACELLULAR T½, HOURS[2]	SERUM T½, HOURS[2]	CYTOCHROME P450
ANTI-HIV VIRAL DRUGS *(continued)*										
Emtricitabine	200 mg po			X	93	18	<4	39	10	
Enfuvirtide	90 mg sc				84	5	92		4	
Fosamprenavir	1400 mg po+RTV			X	No data	6	90	No data	7.7	Inducer/inhibitor
Indinavir	800 mg po	X			65	12.6 mcM[14]	60		1.2-2	Inhibitor
Lamivudine	300 mg po			X	86	2.6	<36	18-22	5-7	
Lopinavir	400 mg po		X		No data	9.6	98-99		5-6	Inhibitor
Maraviroc	300 mg po			X	33	3-9	76		14-18	
Nelfinavir	1250 mg po		X		20-80	3-4	98		3.5-5	Inhibitor
Nevirapine	200 mg po			X	>90	2	60		25-30	Inducer
Raltegravir	400 mg po			X	?		83	alpha 1/beta 9	3-5	
Ritonavir	300 mg po		X		65	7.8	98-99		3-5	Potent inhibitor
Saquinavir	1000 mg po (with 100 mg ritonavir)		X		4	3.1	97		1-2	Inhibitor
Stavudine	40 mg			X	86	1.4	<5	7.5	1	
Tenofovir	300 mg po			X	25	0.3	<1-7	>60	17	
Tipranavir	500 mg + 200 mg ritonavir		X			78-86 mcM[14]	99.9		5.5-6	
Zalcitabine	0.75 mg po			X	85	0.03	<4	Unknown	1.2	
Zidovudine	300 mg po			X	60	1-2	<38	11	0.5-3	

FOOTNOTES:

1 % absorbed under optimal conditions
2 Assumes CrCl >80 mL per min.
3 Peak concentration in bile/peak concentration in serum x 100. If blank, no data.
4 CSF levels with inflammation
5 Judgment based on drug dose & organ susceptibility. CSF concentration ideally ≥10 above MIC.

7 Total drug; adjust for protein binding to determine free drug concentration
7 For adult oral preps; not applicable for peds suspensions.
8 Food decreases rate and/or extent of absorption.
9 Concern over seizure potential: see Table 1D

10 Take all po FQs 2-4 hours before sucralfate or any multivalent cations: Ca⁺⁺, Fe⁺⁺, Zn⁺⁺
11 Given with atovaquone as Malarone for malaria prophylaxis.
12 Oseltamivir/oseltamivir carboxylate
13 EC = enteric coated
14 mcM=micromolar

TABLE 9B – PHARMACODYNAMICS OF ANTIBACTERIALS*

BACTERIAL KILLING/PERSISTENT EFFECT	DRUGS	THERAPY GOAL	PK/PD MEASUREMENT
Concentration-dependent/Prolonged persistent effect	Aminoglycosides; daptomycin; ketolides; quinolones; metro	High peak serum concentration	24-hr AUC¹/MIC
Time-dependent/No persistent effect	Penicillins; cephalosporins; carbapenems; monobactams	Long duration of exposure	Time above MIC
Time-dependent/Moderate to long persistent effect	Clindamycin; erythro/azithro/clarithro; linezolid; tetracyclines; vancomycin	Enhanced amount of drug	24-hr AUC/MIC

* Adapted from Craig, W.A. IDC No. Amer 17:479, 2003 & Drusano, G.L. CID 44:79, 2007   ¹ AUC = area under drug concentration curve

TABLE 10A – SELECTED ANTIBACTERIAL AGENTS—ADVERSE REACTIONS—OVERVIEW

Adverse reactions in individual patients represent all-or-none occurrences, even if rare. After selection of an agent, the physician should read the manufacturer's package insert [statements in the product labeling (package insert) must be approved by the FDA]

Numbers = frequency of occurrence (%); + = occurs, incidence not available; 0 = not reported; R = rare, defined as <1%; ++ = significant adverse reaction. NOTE: Important reactions in bold print. A blank means no data found.

ADVERSE REACTIONS	Penicillin G,V	Dicloxacillin	Nafcillin	Oxacillin	Amoxicillin	Amox-Clav	Ampicillin	Amp-Sulb	Piperacillin	Pip-Taz	Ticarcillin	Ticar-Clav	Doripenem	Ertapenem	Imipenem	Meropenem	Aztreonam	Aminoglycosides	Linezolid	Telithromycin
Rx stopped due to AE					2–4.4			3	3.2	3.2		3	3.4	4	3	1.2	<1			
Local phlebitis																	4			
Hypersensitivity																				
Fever	+		+	+	+	+						+	+	+	+					+
Rash	**3**	4	4	4	**5**	3	**5**	**2**	4	2	**3**	**2**	+	+	+	+	+	+		2
Photosensitivity					0	**0**	0	0												+
Anaphylaxis	R	R	R	R	0	R	R	R	+	+	+	+					R			
Serum sickness	4																			
Hematologic																				
+ Coombs	3	0	R	R	0	+	0	+	+	+			1	2			R			
Neutropenia	R	0	R	R	+	+	6	6	+	+	+	+			2		R			1.1
Eosinophilia	+	+	22	22	2	22	2	22	+	+	+	+	+	+	+	+	8			
Thrombocytopenia	R	0	R	R	R	R	R	R	+	+	+	R					R			
↑ PT/PTT									+	+	+	+					R			
GI																				
Nausea/vomiting	+	0	0		2	3	2	3	+	7	2	+	1	+	3	2	4		3/1	7/2
Diarrhea	+	0	0		**5**	**9**	**5**	**9**	2	11	3	+	+	6	2	5	+		4	10
C. difficile colitis	+	R	R	R	+	+	+	+	+	+	+	+	+	+	+	+	+			
Hepatic LFTs	0	R	+	+	R	R	6	R	6	4	4	2	+	+	+	+	0		+	+
Hepatic failure	0	R	R	R	R	R	R	R									0			1.3
Renal ↑ BUN, Cr	R	0	+	+	R	R	0	0	0	0	0	0					0	**5–25**[1]		+
CNS																				
Headache	R	0	0		+	+			R	+		+		R	R		3		2	2
Confusion	R	R	R		0	R	R	R	R	R	R	R					R			+
Seizures	R			+	R	R	R	R	R	R	R	+	See footnote[2]	See footnote[2]	See footnote[2]	See footnote[2]	+		2	2

Aminoglycosides column = Amikacin, Gentamicin, Kanamycin, Netilmicin[NUS], Tobramycin.
Misc. column = Linezolid, Telithromycin.

[1] Varies with criteria used

[2] **All β-lactams in high concentration can cause seizures** (JAC 45:5, 2000). In rabbit, IMP 10x more neurotoxic than benzylpenicillin (JAC 22:687, 1988). In clinical trial of IMP for ped meningitis, trial stopped due to seizures in 7/25 IMP recipients; hard to interpret as purulent meningitis causes seizures (PIDJ 10:122, 1991). Risk with IMP ↓ with careful attention to dosage (Epilepsia 42:1590, 2001).
Postulated mechanism: Drug binding to $GABA_A$ receptor. IMP binds with greater affinity than MER.
Package insert, percent seizures: ERTA 0.5, IMP 0.4, MER 0.7. However, in 3 clinical trials of MER for bacterial meningitis, no drug-related seizures (Scand J Inf Dis 31:3, 1999; Drug Safety 22:191, 2000).
In febrile neutropenic cancer pts. IMP-related seizures reported at 2% (CID 32:381, 2001; Peds Hem Onc 17:585, 2000).

TABLE 10A (2)

PENICILLINS, CARBAPENEMS, MONOBACTAMS, AMINOGLYCOSIDES

ADVERSE REACTIONS	Penicillin G,V	Dicloxacillin	Nafcillin	Oxacillin	Amoxicillin	Amox-Clav	Ampicillin	Amp-Sulb	Piperacillin	Pip-Taz	Ticarcillin	Ticar-Clav	Doripenem	Ertapenem	Imipenem	Meropenem	Aztreonam	Aminoglycosides (Amikacin, Gentamicin, Kanamycin, Netilmicin[NUS], Tobramycin)	Linezolid	Telithromycin
Special Senses																				
Ototoxicity	0	0	0	0	0	0	0	0	0	0	0	0			R		0	3–14[1]		
Vestibular	0	0	0	0	0	0	0	0	0	0	0	0					0	4–6[1]		
Cardiac																				
Dysrhythmias	R	0	0	0	0	0	0	0	0	0	0	0			0		+			
Miscellaneous, Unique (Table 10C)	+	+	+	+	+	+	+	+	+	+	+	+		+	+		+		++	++
Drug/drug interactions, common (Table 22)	0	0	0	0	0	0	0	0	0	+	0	0			0		0	+	+	+

CEPHALOSPORINS/CEPHAMYCINS

ADVERSE REACTIONS	Cefazolin	Cefotetan	Cefoxitin	Cefuroxime	Cefotaxime	Ceftazidime	Ceftizoxime	Ceftriaxone	Cefepime	Ceftobiprole	Cefaclor/Cef.ER[1]/Loracarb	Cefadroxil	Cefdinir	Cefixime	Cefpodoxime	Cefprozil	Ceftibuten	Cefditoren pivoxil	Cefuroxime axetil	Cephalexin
Rx stopped due to AE		3		2	5	4		2	1.5	3			3	3	2.7	2	2	2	2.2	
Local phlebitis	+	1	R	R	2	1	2	4	+	2										
Hypersensitivity																				
Fever	+	+							+	+	+					+				
Rash				2	2	2	2	2	2		+	+	R	R	R	1	R	R	R	
Photosensitivity	R			0	R	R	0	2			+			1	1			R	R	
Anaphylaxis											R									
Serum sickness											R²	+			R	R		R		
Hematologic																				
+ Coombs	+	2							14		+		R	R	R	R	R		R	
Neutropenia		2							1				R	R		R	R	R		

[1] Cefaclor extended release tablets

[2] Serum sickness requires biotransformation of parent drug plus inherited defect in metabolism of reactive intermediates (Ped Pharm & Therap 125:805, 1994)

* See note at head of table, page 80

TABLE 10A (3)

CEPHALOSPORINS/CEPHAMYCINS

ADVERSE REACTIONS	Cephalexin	Cefuroxime axetil	Cefditoren pivoxil	Ceftibuten	Cefprozil	Cefpodoxime	Cefixime	Cefdinir	Cefadroxil	Cefaclor/Cef.ER¹/Loracarb	Ceftobiprole	Cefepime	Ceftriaxone	Ceftizoxime	Ceftazidime	Cefotaxime	Cefuroxime	Cefoxitin	Cefotetan	Cefazolin
Eosinophilia	9	1	R	5	2	3	R	R		3		1	6	4	8	1	7	3	+	
Thrombocytopenia				R	+	R	R					+	+	+	+	+		+	++	+
↑ PT/PTT												+	+		+	+			++	
GI																				
Nausea/vomiting			6/1	6/2	4	4	13/7	3		3/2		1	R		1	1	R	1	1	
Diarrhea	2	3	1.4	3	3	7	16	15		1-4		1	3	3	1	1	R			
C. difficile colitis	+	+	+	+	+	+	+	+	+	+	+	+	+	+	+	+	+	+	+	+
Hepatic ↑ LFTs	+	4	R	3	2	4	R	1	+	3		+	3	4	6	1	4	3	1	
Hepatic failure			R	R		+	R	R				0	3	0	4	0	0	0	0	
Renal ↑ BUN, Cr	+	R	R	R	0	0	R			+		+	1	0	R	0	0	3	0	+
CNS																				
Headache	+	R	2	R	R	4	+	2		3		2	R		1					
Confusion	+		2			1				+		+								
Seizures																				
Special Senses																				
Ototoxicity	0	0		0	0	0	0	0	0	0		0	0	0	0	0	0	0	0	0
Vestibular	0	0		R	R	0	0	0	0	0		0		0	0	0	0	0	0	0
Cardiac																				
Dysrhythmias	0	0	+	0	0	0	0	0	0	0		0	0	0	0	0	0	0	0	0
Miscellaneous, Unique (Table 10C)	0	0	+	+	R	0	0	+	0	+²	+	+	+	0	0	0	0	0	0	0
Drug/drug interactions, common (table 22)	0	0		0	0	0	0	0	0	0		0	0	0	0	0	0	0	0	0

¹ Cefaclor extended release tablets
² Serum sickness requires biotransformation of parent drug plus inherited defect in metabolism of reactive intermediates (Ped Pharm & Therapy 125:805; 1994)
* See note at head of table, page 80

TABLE 10A (4)

ADVERSE REACTIONS (AE)	MACROLIDES			QUINOLONES						OTHER AGENTS											
	Azithromycin, Reg. & ER[1]	Clarithromycin, Reg. & ER[1]	Erythromycin	Ciprofloxacin/Cipro XR	Gatifloxacin[NUS]	Gemifloxacin	Levofloxacin	Moxifloxacin	Ofloxacin	Chloramphenicol	Clindamycin	Colistimethate (Colistin)	Dalbavancin	Daptomycin	Metronidazole	Quinupristin-dalfopristin	Rifampin	Tetracycline/Doxy/Mino	Tigecycline	TMP-SMX	Vancomycin
Rx stopped due to AE	1	3		3.5	2.9	2.2	4	3.8	4					2.8					5		13
Local: phlebitis														6		++				8	8
Hypersensitivity																					
Fever										+	+			+				+	+	++	
Rash	R	R		R	R	1-22[2]	1.7	R	R	+	+		1.8	4		R	1	+	R	++	3
Photosensitivity				R	R	R	R	R	R									+	+		0
Anaphylaxis				R	R	R	R	R	R		+						R			+	R
Serum sickness				R							+										
Hematologic																					
Neutropenia	R			R	R				1	+	+			+		2	R	+		+	2
Eosinophilia				R					1		+							+		+	
Thrombocytopenia	R	R		R						+	+					2	+	+	+	+	0
↑ PT/PTT		1									+										
GI																					
Nausea/vomiting	3	3[3]	++	5	8/<3	2.7	7/2	7/2	7	+	+		3/2	6.3	**12**	2	+	+	30/20	3	0
Diarrhea	5	3-6	**8**	2	4	3.6	5	5	4	+	**7**		2.5	5	+	+	+	+	13	+	+
C. difficile colitis		+		**R**	**R**	**R**	**R**	**R**	**R**	+	++				R		R	+		+	
Hepatic																					
Hepatic: LFTs	0	+	+	2	R	1.5	+	2	2	+	+			R	R	2	+	+	4	+	0
Hepatic failure	0	0				+														+	
Renal																					
↑ BUN, Cr				1								+		R							5
CNS																					
Dizziness, light headedness	R			2	3	0.8		2	3				2	R	++				2	+	5
Headache	R	2		1	4	1.2	5.4	2	4	+	+		5	5			+	+	3.5	+	
Confusion				+	+				+	+	+				+					+	
Seizures				R	R			2	R	R	+					2	+		R	R	

[1] Regular and extended-release formulations
[2] **Highest frequency:** females <40 years of age after 14 days of rx, with 5 days or less of Gemi; incidence of rash <1.5%
[3] Less GI upset/abnormal taste with ER formulation

* See note at head of table, page 80

TABLE 10A (5)

ADVERSE REACTIONS (AE)	MACROLIDES			QUINOLONES						OTHER AGENTS											
	Azithromycin, Reg. & ER[1]	Clarithromycin, Reg. & ER[1]	Erythromycin	Ciprofloxacin/Cipro XR	Gatifloxacin[NUS]	Gemifloxacin	Levofloxacin	Moxifloxacin	Ofloxacin	Chloramphenicol	Clindamycin	Colistimethate (Colistin)	Dalbavancin	Daptomycin	Metronidazole	Quinupristin-dalfopristin	Rifampin	Tetracycline/Doxy/Mino	Tigecycline	TMP-SMX	Vancomycin
Special senses																					
Ototoxicity	+		+	O					O												R
Vestibular																		21[1]			
Cardiac																					
Dysrhythmias	±	±	+	R	+[2]	+[2]	+[2]	+[2]	O		R										O
Miscellaneous, Unique (Table 10C)					+[2]	+[2]	+[2]	+[2]	+				+	+			+		+		
Drug/drug interactions, common (Table 22)	+	+	+	+	+	+	+	+	+	+					+	++	+	+	+	+	+

[1] Minocycline has 21% vestibular toxicity
[2] Fluoroquinolones as class assoc. **with QTc prolongation.** Ref.: *CID 34:861, 2002.*

TABLE 10B – ANTIMICROBIAL AGENTS ASSOCIATED WITH PHOTOSENSITIVITY

The following drugs are known to cause photosensitivity in some individuals. There is no intent to indicate relative frequency or severity of reactions.
Source: 2007 Red Book, Thomson Healthcare, Inc. Listed in alphabetical order:

Azithromycin, benzafibrate, ciprofloxacin, dapsone, doxycycline, erythromycin ethyl succinate, flucytosine, ganciclovir gatifloxacin, gemifloxacin, griseofulvin, interferons, lomefloxacin, ofloxacin, pyrazinamide, saquinavir, sulfonamides, tetracyclines, tigecycline, tretinoins, voriconazole

* See note at head of table, page 80

TABLE 10C – SUMMARY OF CURRENT ANTIBIOTIC DOSAGE,* SIDE-EFFECTS, AND COST

CLASS, AGENT, GENERIC NAME (TRADE NAME)	USUAL ADULT DOSAGE* (Cost)	ADVERSE REACTIONS, COMMENTS (See Table 10A for Summary)
NATURAL PENICILLINS		**Most common adverse reactions are hypersensitivity.** Anaphylaxis in up to 0.05%, 5–10% fatal. Commercially available skin test antigen (penicilloyl polylysine) does not predict anaphylactic reactions. Hematologic, renal, CNS (seizures) reactions usually seen with high dose (>20 million units per day) and renal failure. With procaine pen G and benzathine pen G, an immediate but transient (5–30min. after injection) toxic reaction with bizarre behavior & neurologic reactions (Hoigne syndrome). Coombs test positive hemolytic anemia's are rare but typically severe; in contrast, the Coombs test is often + with cephalosporin therapy, but clinically significant hemolysis is rare. Penicillin allergy ref.: JAMA 278:1895, 1997
Benzathine penicillin G (Bicillin L-A)	600,000–1.2 million units IM q2–4 wks Cost: 600,000 units $28	
Penicillin G	**Low: 600,000–1.2 million units IM per day** **High: 220 million units IV q24h (=12gm)** Cost: 5 million units $42	
Penicillin V	0.25–0.5gm po bid, tid, qid before meals & at bedtime Cost: 500 mg G $0.36	
PENICILLINASE-RESISTANT PENICILLINS		
Dicloxacillin (Dynapen)	0.125–0.5gm po q6h ac. Cost: 500mg G $0.20	Blood levels ~2 times greater than cloxacillin. Acute hemorrhagic cystitis reported. Acute abdominal pain with GI bleeding without antibiotic-associated colitis also reported.
Flucloxacillin[NUS] (Floxapen, Lutgen, Staphol)	0.25–0.5gm po q6h	In Australia, cholestatic hepatitis (women predominate, age >65, rx mean 2 weeks; onset 3 weeks from starting rx (Ln 339:679, 1992). 16 deaths since 1980; recommendation: use only in severe infection (Ln 344:676, 1994).
Nafcillin (Unipen, Nafcil)	1–2gm IV/IM q4h. Cost: 2 gm IV $20.00	Extravasation can result in tissue necrosis. With dosages of 200–300 mg per kg per day hypokalemia may occur.
Oxacillin (Prostaphlin)	1–2gm IV/IM q4h. Cost: 2 gm IV $20.11	**Reversible neutropenia (over 10% with ≥21-day rx, occasionally WBC <1000 per mm³).** **Hepatic dysfunction with ≥12 gm per day (esp. if ↑ LFTs usually after start of rx, reversible. In children, more rash and liver toxicity with oxacillin as compared to nafcillin (CID 34:50, 2002).
AMINOPENICILLINS		
Amoxicillin (Amoxil, Polymox)	250mg–1gm po tid Cost: 500 mg G $0.13, NB $0.55	IV available in UK, Europe. IV amoxicillin rapidly converted to ampicillin. Rash with infectious mono—see Ampicillin.
Amoxicillin-clavulanate (Augmentin) AM-CL extra-strength peds suspension (ES-600) AM-CL-extended release adult tabs	Peds ES susp.: 600/42.9 per 5mL. Dose: Cost 75 mL $50. For adult formulations, see Comments	With bid regimen, less diarrhea & less clavulanate. Clavulanate assoc. with rare reversible cholestatic hepatitis, esp. men >60 yrs. on rx >2 weeks (ArIM 156:1327, 1996). 2 cases anaphylactic reaction to clavulanic acid (J All Clin Immun 95:748, 1995). **Comparison adult Augmentin product dosage regimens:** Cost for 10 days rx:
		Augmentin 500/125 1 tab po tid $145 NB $97 G
		Augmentin 875/125 1 tab po bid $187 NB $160 G
		Augmentin-XR 1000/62.5 2 tabs po bid $36
IV amox-clav available in Europe		
Ampicillin (Principen)	0.25–0.5gm po q6h. Cost: 500mg G po $0.30 150–200mg/kg IV/day. Cost: 1gm IV G $7.38	Maculopapular rash occurs (not urticaria), **not true penicillin allergy** in 65–100% pts with infectious mono, 90% with chronic lymphatic leukemia, and 15–20% with allopurinol therapy.
Ampicillin-sulbactam (Unasyn)	1.5–3gm IV q6h. Cost: 3gm NB $15.00 (see Comment)	Supplied in vials: ampicillin 1 gm, sulbactam 0.5 gm or amp 2 gm, sulbactam 1 gm. Antibiotic is not active vs pseudomonas. Total daily dose sulbactam ≤4 gm
ANTIPSEUDOMONAL PENICILLINS NOTE: Platelet dysfunction may occur with any of the antipseudomonal penicillins, esp. in renal failure patients.		
Piperacillin (Pipracil) (Canada only)	3–4gm IV q4–6h (200–300 mg per kg per day up to 500 mg per kg per day). For urinary tract infection: 2 gm IV q6h. Cost: 4gm NB $12.62	1.85 mEq Na⁺ per gm. See PIP-TZ comment on extended infusion.
Piperacillin-tazobactam (Zosyn)	3.375gm IV q6h. Cost: 3.375gm NB $19 4.5gm NB $24 For P. aeruginosa: 4.5gm IV q6h + tobra	Supplied as: piperacillin 3 gm + tazobactam (TZ) 0.375 gm. TZ more active than sulbactam as β-lactamase inhibitor. PIP-TZ 3.375 gm IV q6h a common reason for serious pseudomonas infections. PIP-TZ can also be given as an extended infusion of 3.375 gm IV for 4 hrs & then repeated every 8 hrs (CID 44:357, 2007). For adding P. aeruginosa infection, tobra or CIP is added to the PIP-TZ. Piperacillin can cause false-pos. serum antigen test for galactomannan—a test for invasive aspergillosis.

---

* NOTE: all dosage recommendations are for adults (unless otherwise indicated) & assume normal renal function.
§ Cost = average wholesale price from 2007 RED BOOK, Thomson Healthcare, Inc.
(See page 2 for abbreviations)

TABLE 10C (2)

CLASS, AGENT GENERIC NAME (TRADE NAME)	USUAL ADULT DOSAGE* (Cost*)	ADVERSE REACTIONS, COMMENTS (See Table 10A for Summary)
ANTIPSEUDOMONAL PENICILLINS (continued)		
Ticarcillin disodium (Ticar)	3gm IV q4-6h. Cost: 3.0 gm NB $12.38	Coagulation abnormalities common with large doses, interferes with platelet function. ↑ bleeding times; may be clinically significant in pts with renal failure. (4.5 mEq/L Na⁺ per gm).
Ticarcillin-clavulanate (Timentin)	3.1 gm IV q4-6h. Cost: 3.1 gm IV $16	Supplied in vials: ticarcillin 3 gm, clavulanate 0.1 gm per vial. 4.5–5 mEq/L Na⁺ per gm. Diarrhea due to clavulanate. Rare reversible cholestatic hepatitis secondary to clavulanate (AHM 156:1327, 1996).
CARBAPENEMS. NOTE: In pts with pen allergy, 11% had allergic reaction after imipenem or meropenem (CID 38:1102, 2004); 9% in a 2ⁿᵈ study (JAC 54:1155, 2004); and 0% in 2 other studies (NEJM 354:2835, 2006; AnIM 146:266, 2007).		
Doripenem	500 mg IV q8h (infusion duration varies with indication). Cost: 500 mg $46.76	Most common adverse reactions (≥5%): Headache, nausea, diarrhea, rash & phlebitis. Can lower serum valproic acid levels. Adjust dose if renal impairment.
Ertapenem (Invanz)	1gm IV/IM q24h. Cost: 1gm NB $59.80	Lidocaine diluent for IM use; ask about lidocaine allergy. Standard dosage may be inadequate in obesity (BMI ≥40) (AAC 90:1222, 2006).
Imipenem + cilastatin (Primaxin) Ref: JAC 58:916, 2005	0.5gm IV q6h, for P. aeruginosa 1gm q6-8h (see Comment). Cost: 500mg NB $39	For moderate or severe infection due to P. aeruginosa, dosage can be increased to 3 or 4 gm per day div. q6h or q8h. Pharmacokinetic studies suggest that continuous infusion of carbapenems may be more efficacious & safer (J Clin Pharm 43:1116, 2003; AAC 49:1881, 2005). For seizure comment, see footnote, Table 10A, page 80.
Meropenem (Merrem)	0.5–1 gm IV q8h. Up to 2 gm IV q8h for meningitis. Cost: 1gm NB $68	Comments: Does not require a dehydropeptidase inhibitor (cilastatin). ↑ activity vs aerobic gm-neg. slightly ↑ over IMP, activity vs staph & strep slightly ↓, anaerobes — to IMP. B. ovatus, B. distasonis more resistant to meropenem.
MONOBACTAMS		
Aztreonam (Azactam)	1gm q8h–2gm IV q6h. Cost: 1gm $30	Can be used in pts with allergy to penicillins/cephalosporins. Animal data and a letter raise concern about cross-reactivity with ceftazidime (Rev Inf Dis 7:613, 1985), side-chains of aztreonam and ceftazidime are identical.
CEPHALOSPORINS (1st parenteral, then oral drugs).	**NOTE:** Prospective data demonstrate correlation between use of cephalosporins (esp. 3ʳᵈ generation) and ↑ risk of C. difficile toxin-induced diarrhea. May also ↑ risk of colonization with vancomycin-resistant enterococci. **For cross-allergenicity, see Oral, on page 87.**	
1ˢᵗ Generation, Parenteral Cefazolin (Ancef, Kefzol)	0.25gm q8h–1.5gm IV/IM q6h. Cost: 1gm G $260	Do not give into lateral ventricles—seizures!
2ⁿᵈ Generation, Parenteral Cefotetan (Cefotan)	1–3gm IV/IM q12h. (Max. dose not >6gm q24h) Cost: 1gm NB $13.50	Increasing resistance of B. fragilis, Prevotella bivius, Prevotella disiens (most common in pelvic infections). Ref. CID 35 (Suppl 1):S126, 2002. Methylthiotetrazole (MTT) side chain can inhibit vitamin K activation.
Cefoxitin (Mefoxin)	1–2gm IV/IM q6-8h. 2gm IV/IM q4h. Cost: 1gm G $13.70, NB $15.29	In vitro may induce ↑ β-lactamase, esp. in Enterobacter sp.
Cefuroxime (Kefurox, Ceftin, Zinacef)	0.75–1.5gm IV/IM q8h. Cost: 1.5gm IV G $13.46	More stable vs staphylococcal β-lactamase than cefazolin
3ʳᵈ Generation, Parenteral—Use of 3 P. Ceph 3 drugs correlates with incidence of C. difficile toxin diarrhea, perhaps due to cephalosporin resistance of C. difficile (CID 38:646, 2004).		
Cefoperazone-sulbactam⁰ˢ (Sulperazon)	Usual dose 1–2gm IV q12h; if severe infection should use 2–3gm IV q6h	In SE Asia & elsewhere, used to treat intra-abdominal, biliary, & gyn. infections. Other uses due to broad spectrum of activity. Possible clotting problem due to side-chain. For dose logic: JAC 15:196, 1985
Cefotaxime (Claforan)	1gm q8-12h to 2gm IV q4h. Cost: 2gm G $18. NB $26.98	
Ceftazidime (Fortaz, Tazicef)	1–2gm IV/IM q8-12h. Cost: 2gm NB $21-28.93	May result in ↑ incidence of C. difficile-assoc. diarrhea and/or selection of vancomycin-resistant E. faecium. Ceftaz is susceptible to extended-spectrum cephalosporinases (CID 27:76 & 81, 1998).
Ceftizoxime (Cefizox)	1gm q8-12h to 4gm IV q8h. Cost: 2gm NB $23.74	Maximum daily dose: 12 gm

---

* NOTE: all dosage recommendations are for adults (unless otherwise indicated) & assume normal renal function.
* Cost = average wholesale price from 2007 Red Book, Thomson Healthcare, Inc.
(See page 2 for abbreviations)

TABLE 10C (3)

CLASS, AGENT, GENERIC NAME (TRADE NAME)	USUAL ADULT DOSAGE* (Cost#)	ADVERSE REACTIONS, COMMENTS (See Table 10A for Summary)
CEPHALOSPORINS/3rd Generation, Parenteral (continued)		
Ceftriaxone (Rocephin)	**1 gm once daily** IV dosage in adults: **Purulent meningitis: 2gm q12h.** Can give IM in 1% lidocaine. Cost: 1gm NB $51.16, G $6.60	**"Pseudocholelithiasis"** 2° to sludge in gallbladder by ultrasound (50%), symptomatic (9%) (NEJM 322:1821, 1990). More likely with ≥2 gm per day with pt on total parenteral nutrition and not eating (AnIM 115:712, 1991). Clinical significance still unclear but has led to cholecystectomy (JID 173:356, 1996) and gallstone pancreatitis (JJ 17:662, 1998). In pilot study, 2 gm once daily by continuous infusion superior to 2 gm bolus once daily (JAC 59:285, 2007).
Other Generation, Parenteral		
Cefepime (Maxipime)	1–2gm IV q12h. Cost: 2gm NB $36.59	Active vs P. aeruginosa and many strains of Enterobacter, serratia, C. freundii resistant to ceftazidime, cefotaxime, aztreonam (LInID 7:338, 2007). More active vs S. aureus than 3rd generation cephalosporins.
*Cefpirome*Adv/c (HR 810)	1–2gm IV q12h	Similar to cefepime: ↑ activity vs enterobacteriaceae, P. aeruginosa, Gm + organisms. Anaérobes: less active than cefoxitin, more active than cefotax or ceftaz.
Ceftobiprole*Adv/Adv [investigational]	**0.5 gm IV q8h for mixed gm-neg & gm-pos infections. 0.5 gm IV q12h for gm-pos infections**	Infuse over 2 hrs for q8h dosing, over 1 hr for q12h dosing. Associated with caramel-like taste disturbance. Ref.: Clin Microbiol Infections 13(Supp2):17 & 25, 2007.
Cephalosporins, Oral 1st Generation, Oral		
Cefadroxil (Duricef)	0.5–1gm po q12h. Cost: 0.5gm G $3.50, NB $4.60	**Cross-Allergenicity: Patients with a history of IgE-mediated allergic reactions to a penicillin (e.g., anaphylaxis, angioneurotic edema, immediate urticaria) should not receive a cephalosporin.** If the history is a "measles-like" rash to a penicillin, available data suggest a 5–10% risk of rash in such patients; there is no enhanced risk of anaphylaxis. Cephalosporin skin tests, if available, predictive of reaction (AnIM 141:16, 2004).
Cephalexin (Keflex, Keftab, generic)	0.25–0.5gm po q6h. Cost: 0.5gm G $0.36, NB $3.45	Any of the cephalosporins can result in **C. difficile toxin-mediated diarrhea/enterocolitis.** The reported frequency of nausea/vomiting and non-C. difficile toxin diarrhea is summarized in Table 10A.
2nd Generation, Oral		
Cefaclor (Ceclor)	0.25–0.5 gm po q8h. Cost: 0.25 gm G $1, NB $2	There are few drug-specific adverse effects, e.g.:
Cefaclor-ER (Ceclor CD)	0.375–0.5 gm po q12h. Cost: 0.5 gm G $3.90	**Cefaclor:** Serum sickness-like reaction 0.1–0.5%—arthralgia, rash, erythema multiforme but no adenopathy, proteinuria or demonstrable immune complexes. Reported in children with repeated exposure. Appear due to mixture of drug, biotransformation and genetic susceptibility (Ped Pharm & Therap 125:805, 1994).
Cefprozil (Cefzil)	0.25–0.5 gm po q12h. Cost: 0.5 gm NB $9.50	**Cefdinir:** Drug-iron complex causes red stools in roughly 1% of pts.
Cefuroxime axetil po (Ceftin)	0.125–0.5 gm po q12h. Cost: 0.5 gm G $7.40, NB $15	**Cefditoren pivoxil:** Hydrolysis yields pivalate. Pivalate absorbed (70%) & becomes pivaloylcarnitine which is renally excreted, 39–63% ↓ in serum carnitine concentrations. Carnitine involved in fatty acid (FA) metabolism & FA transport into mitochondria. Effect transient & reversible. No clinical events documented to date (Med Lett 44:5, 2002). Also contains caseinate (milk protein); **avoid if milk allergy** not same as lactose intolerance). Need gastric acid for optimal absorption.
3rd Generation, Oral		
Cefdinir (Omnicef)	**300 mg po q12h or 600 mg q24h** Cost: 300 mg $5.41	**Cefpodoxime:** Now available from Lupin Pharmaceuticals.
Cefditoren pivoxil [Spectracef]	**200–400 mg po bid** Cost: 200 mg $2.70	**Cefixime:** Can cause false-neg. urine dipstick test for leukocytes.
Cefixime [Suprax]	0.4 gm po q12–24h. Cost: 0.4 gm NB $10.26	**Cephalexin:** There are rare reports of acute liver injury, bloody diarrhea, pulmonary infiltrates with eosinophilia.
Cefpodoxime proxetil (Vantin)	0.1–0.2 gm po q12h. Cost: 0.2 gm G $4.20, NB $9.90	
Ceftibuten (Cedax)	0.4 gm po q24h. Cost: 0.4 gm NB $11	

* **NOTE:** all dosage recommendations are for adults (unless otherwise indicated) & assume normal renal function.
# Cost = average wholesale price from 2007 RED BOOK, Thomson Healthcare, Inc.
(See page 2 for abbreviations)

TABLE 10C (4)

CLASS, AGENT, GENERIC NAME (TRADE NAME)	USUAL ADULT DOSAGE* (Cost*)	ADVERSE REACTIONS, COMMENTS (See Table 10A for Summary)
AMINOGLYCOSIDES AND RELATED ANTIBIOTICS—See Table 10D, page 93, and Table 17A, page 178		
GLYCOPEPTIDES		
Dalbavancin[NUS & NDF] (Zeven)	1gm IV, then 0.5gm IV on day 8. No cost data	Semi-synthetic lipoglycopeptide with very long serum half-life. So far, 2 published clinical trials (CID 40:374, 2005 & 37:1298, 2003). No serious AEs.
Telcoplanin[NUS] (Targocid)	**For septic arthritis—maintenance dose** 12mg/kg per day; S. aureus endocarditis—trough serum levels >20mg/mL required (12mg/kg q12hr times 3 loading dose, then 12mg/kg q24hr)	Hypersensitivity: fever (at 3mg/kg 2.2%, at 24 mg per kg 8.2%); skin reactions 2.4%. Marked ↓ platelets (high dose ≥15 mg per kg per day). Red neck syndrome less common than with vancomycin.
Vancomycin (Vancocin) Ref. on obesity: Pharmacotherapy 27:1081, 2007.	**Normal weight pt:** 15mg/kg IV q12h. If critically ill, consider loading dose of 25–30 mg/kg IV. **Morbidly obese (90% over ideal body weight):** use actual body weight and dose as above. **P.O. for C. diff colitis:** 125mg po q6h. For intrathecal – see comment Cost: 1 gm IV G $7.75, NB $34.50; 125mg po $17.65	**Measure serum levels** if ↑ planned dose ≥2gm per day, rapidly changing renal function, chronic renal failure, or on hemodialysis. Target levels: peak 20–50mcg/mL, trough 5–10mcg/mL. Vanco serum levels overestimated in renal failure patients if fluorescence or immunoassay method used; need monoclonal enzyme immunoassay (EMIT). Rapid infusion (over <1hr) can cause non-specific histamine release manifest as angioneurotic edema, flushed skin ("Red neck syndrome") or hypotension. Can continue vanco but infuse over 1–2hrs. **Ototoxicity & nephrotoxicity now rare** unless vanco given with an aminoglycoside, amplifies the risk of nephrotoxicity. Neutropenia, rash occur. Rarely, associated with linear IgA bullous dermatosis (CID 38:442, 2004). **Intrathecal** vanco used for meningitis &/or ventriculitis/shunt infections. **Initial** dosing ranges from 5–10mg/day (infants) to 10–20mg/day (children/adults) adjusted to achieve trough CSF conc. of 10–20mcg/mL. (AnPharmacotherapy 27:912, 1993). Gray baby syndrome in premature infants, anaphylactoid reactions, optic atrophy or neuropathy (very rare), digital paresthesias, minor disulfiram-like reactions.
CHLORAMPHENICOL, CLINDAMYCIN, OXAZOLIDINONES, QUINUPRISTIN-DALFOPRISTIN (SYNERCID)		
Chloramphenicol (Chloromycetin)	No oral drug available in U.S. Hematologic (↓ RBC – ⅓ pts, aplastic anemia 1:21,600 courses).	
Clindamycin (Cleocin)	**0.15–0.45 gm** po q6h. 600–900 mg Cost: 1 gm IV G $22.75; po $6.60 **IV/IM** q6h Cost: 300 mg po NB $6.62, G $3.86 600 mg IV NB $9.24, G $4.16	0.6 gm IV/IM q8h. Cost: 600 mg IV $10.51 Based on number of exposed pts, these drugs are the most frequent cause of **C. difficile toxin-mediated diarrhea** & the most severe form can cause **pseudomembranous colitis (toxic megacolon)**.
Erythromycin Group (Review drug interactions before use)		
Azithromycin (Zithromax) Azithromycin ER (ZMax)	**po preps:** Tabs 250 & 600mg; Peds suspension: **to 4gm** 250 & 600mg per-5mL. Adult ER suspension: 2gm. Media varies with indication; see Table 1. Acute otitis media (page 9); acute exac. chronic bronchitis (page 33); pneumonia (pages 35–36), & sinusitis (page 44). Cost: azithro 250 mg G $7.77, NB $39.23; Z-PAK $9.22; Z-MAX $65	**Motilin** is a gastric hormone that activates duodenal/jejunal receptors to initiate peristalsis. Erythro (E) and E esters, both po and IV activate motilin receptors and cause uncoordinated peristalsis with resultant 20–25% incidence of anorexia, nausea or vomiting (Gut 33:397, 1992). Less binding and GI distress with azithromycin/clarithromycin. Systemic reports in 1st 2 wks of life associated with **infantile hypertrophic pyloric stenosis** (J Ped 139:380, 2001). **Frequent drug-drug interactions:** see Table 22, page 198. Major concern is prolonged QTc interval on EKG. **Prolonged QTc:** Mutations in 6 genes (LQT 1–6) produce abnormal cardiac Na channels. Variable penetrance: no symptoms, repeated syncope or sudden death. Several drugs and drug interactions (see FQs page 90 for list). Can result in torsades de pointes (ventricular tachycardia) and/or cardiac arrest. Refs.: CID 43:1603, 2006; www.qtdrugs.org & www.torsades.org. Transient reversible tinnitus or deafness with >4 gm per day of erythro IV in pts with renal or hepatic impairment. Reported with ≥600 mg/day of azithro (CID 24:76, 1997).
Base and esters (Erythromb, Ilosone) IV name: E. lactobionate	**IV** 0.5gm IV q6h. Cost: $33. **0.25gm q6h–0.5 gm po/IV q6h: 15–20mg/kg up to 4gm q24h. Infuse over 30+ min.** Cost: 250mg base G $0.18, stearate $0.24, estolate $0.31, ESS 400 $0.23. IV 1 gm NB $16.72.	Dosages of oral erythro preparations expressed as base equivalents. With differences in absorption/biotransformation, variable amounts of active erythro required to achieve same free erythro serum level, e.g. 400 mg E ethyl succinate = 250 mg base.
Clarithromycin (Biaxin) clarithro extended release (Biaxin XL)	**0.5 gm po q12h.** Cost: 500 mg $3 **Extended release: Two 0.5 gm tabs po per day.** Cost: 500 mg ER $5.70; 500mg G $5.42	

---

* NOTE: all dosage recommendations are for adults (unless otherwise indicated) & assume normal renal function.

† Cost = average wholesale price from 2007 Red Book, Thomson Healthcare, Inc.

(See page 2 for abbreviations)

TABLE 10C (5)

CLASS, AGENT, GENERIC NAME (TRADE NAME)	USUAL ADULT DOSAGE* (Cost†)	ADVERSE REACTIONS, COMMENTS (See Table 10A for Summary)
CHLORAMPHENICOL, CLINDAMYCIN(S), ERYTHROMYCIN GROUP, KETOLIDES, OXAZOLIDINONES, QUINUPRISTIN-DALFOPRISTIN *(continued)*		
Ketolide Telithromycin (Ketek) *(Med Lett 46:66, 2004)*	Two 400 mg tabs po q24h. 400 mg tabs. Cost: 400 mg $5.76 300 mg tabs available	As of 9/06, 2 cases acute liver failure & 23 cases serious liver injury reported, or 23 cases per 10 million prescriptions. Occurred during or immediately after treatment. *(AnIM 144:415, 447, 2006)*. **Uncommon: blurred vision** 2° slow accommodation; may cause exacerbation of **myasthenia gravis (Black Box Warning)**. Potential QT₋ prolongation. Several **drug-drug interactions** *(Table 22, pages 198–199)*. *(NEJM 355:2260, 2006)*
Linezolid (Zyvox)	**PO or IV dose: 600 mg q12h.** Available as 600 mg tabs, oral suspension (100 mg per 5 mL), & IV solution. 600 mg po $65; 600 mg IV $82.	**Reversible myelosuppression:** thrombocytopenia, anemia, & neutropenia reported. Most often after >2 wks of therapy, incidence of thrombocytopenia after 2 wks of rx 7/20 osteomyelitic pts; 5/7 pts treated with vanco & then linezolid. Refs. *CID 37:1609, 2003 & 38:1058 & 1065, 2004.* 6-fold increased risk in pts with ESRD *(CID 42:66, 2006)* and dose-dependent inhibition of mitochondrial protein synthesis *(CID 42:1111, 2006; AAC 50:2042, 2006; Pharmacotherapy 27:771, 2007)*. **Lactic acidosis; peripheral neuropathy, optic neuropathy.** After 4 or more wks of therapy. Data supports time and dose-dependent inhibition of mitochondrial protein synthesis *(CID 42:1578 and 43:180, 2006)*. **Inhibitor of monoamine oxidase:** risk of severe hypertension if taken with foods rich in tyramine. Avoid concomitant pseudoephedrine, phenylpropanolamine, and caution with SSRIs = **Serotonin syndrome** (fever, agitation, mental status changes, tremors) risk with concomitant SSRIs.
Quinupristin + dalfopristin (Synercid) *(CID 36:473, 2003)*	**7.5 mg per kg IV q8h via central line** Cost: 350 mg–150 mg $150	Venous irritation (5%); none with central venous line. Asymptomatic ↑ unconjugated bilirubin. **Arthralgia** 2%–50% *(CID 36:476, 2003)*. **Drug-drug interactions:** Cyclosporine, nifedipine, midazolam, many more—see Table 22.
TETRACYCLINES *(Mayo Clin Proc 74:727, 1999)*		Similar to other tetracyclines. ↑ nausea on empty stomach. Erosive esophagitis, esp. if taken at bedtime. Phototoxicity + but less than with tetracycline. Deposition in teeth less. Can be used in patients with renal failure. **Comments:** Effective in treatment and prophylaxis for malaria, leptospirosis, typhus fevers
Doxycycline (Vibramycin, Doryx, Monodox, Adoxa, Periostat)	**0.1 gm po/IV q12h.** Cost: 100 mg po $0.08–0.11, NB $5.66; 100 mg IV NB $14.75	
Minocycline (Minocin, Dynacin)	**0.1 gm po q12h.** Cost: 100 mg $3.40, NB $10 IV minocycline no longer available.	Similar to other tetracyclines. **Vestibular symptoms** (30-90% in some groups, none in others): vertigo 33%, ataxia 43%, nausea 50%, vomiting 3%, women more frequently than men. Hypersensitivity pneumonitis, reversible, ~34 cases reported *(BMJ 310:1520, 1995)*. **Comments:** More effective than other tetracyclines vs staph and in prophylaxis of meningococcal disease. P. acnes many resistant to other tetracyclines, not to mino. Active vs Nocardia asteroides, Mycobacterium marinum.
Tetracycline, Oxytetracycline (Sumycin) *(CID 36:462, 2003)*	**0.25–0.5 gm po q6h, 0.5–1 gm IV q12h.** Cost: 250 mg po $0.06	GI (oral 19%, tetra 4), anaphylactoid reaction (rare), deposition in teeth, negative N balance. Hepatotoxicity, enamel hypoplasia, pseudotumor cerebri (encephalopathy). Outdated drug: Fanconi syndrome. See drug-drug interactions, Table 22. **Contraindicated in pregnancy, hepatotoxicity in mother, transplacental to fetus.**
Tigecycline (Tygacil)	**100 mg IV initially, then 50 mg IV q12h with po food, if possible to decrease risk of nausea.** Cost: 50 mg $57	Derivative of tetracycline. High incidence of nausea (25%) & vomiting (20%) but only 1% of pts discontinued therapy due to an adverse event. Pregnancy Category D. Do not use in children under age 18. Like other tetracyclines, may cause photosensitivity, pseudotumor cerebri, pancreatitis, a catabolic state (elevated BUN) and maybe hyperpigmentation *(CID 45:136, 2007)*. **Comments:** IV dosage over 2.0 gm per day may be associated with fatal hepatotoxicity. False-neg. urine dipstick for leukocytes.

* **SSRI** = selective serotonin reuptake inhibitors; e.g., fluoxetine (Prozac).
* NOTE: all dosage recommendations are for adults (unless otherwise indicated) & assume normal renal function.
* Cost = average wholesale price from 2007 Red Book, Thomson Healthcare, Inc.
  (See page 2 for abbreviations)

TABLE 10C (6)

CLASS, AGENT, GENERIC NAME (TRADE NAME)	USUAL ADULT DOSAGE* (Cost)	ADVERSE REACTIONS, COMMENTS (See Table 10A for Summary)
FLUOROQUINOLONES (FQs):	All can cause false-positive urine drug screen for opiates (Pharmacother 26:435, 2006)	
Ciprofloxacin (Cipro) and Ciprofloxacin-extended release (Cipro XR, Proquin XR)	**500–750 mg po bid. Urinary tract infection: 250 mg bid po or Cipro XR 500 mg q24h Parenteral** rx 200–400 mg IV q12h. Cost: 500 mg po $3.30; NB $6.00, Cipro XR 500 mg $8.32; Proquin XR 500 mg $10.80. **Cipro 400 mg IV** $30.00; **Ophthalmic solution** $47.30 for 5 mL.	**Children:** No FQ approved for use under age 16 based on joint cartilage injury in immature animals. Articular SEs in children est. at 2–3% (LnID 3:537, 2003). **CNS toxicity:** Poorly understood. Varies from mild (lightheadedness) to moderate (confusion) to severe (seizures). May be aggravated by NSAIDs. **Gemi skin rash:** Macular rash after 8–10 d. of rx. Incidence of rash with ≤5 d of therapy only 1.5%. Frequency highest females, < age 40, treated 14 d. (22.6%). In men, < age 40, frequency 7.7%. Mechanism unclear. Indication to DC therapy.
Gatifloxacin (Tequin)[4,5] See comments	**200–400 mg IV/po q24h** (See comment) Ophthalmic solution (Zymar) $62 for 5 mL.	**Hypoglycemia/hyperglycemia** Due to documented hypo and hyperglycemic reactions (NEJM 354:1352, 2006), US distribution of Gati ceased in 6/2006. Gati ophthalmic solution remains available.
Gemifloxacin (Factive)	**320 mg q24h** Cost: 320 mg $22.40	**Opiate screen false-positive:** FQs can cause false-positive urine assay for opiates (JAMA 286:3115, 2001; AnPharmacotherapy 38:1525, 2004). **Photosensitivity:** See Table 10B, page 84 **QT₀ (corrected QT) interval prolongation:** ↑ QT₀ (>500msec or >60msec from baseline) is considered possible with any FQ. ↑ QT₀ can lead to torsades de pointes and ventricular fibrillation. Risk low with current marketed drugs). Risk ↑ in women. ↓ K⁺, ↓ Mg²⁺: bradycardia. (Refs: CID 43:1603, 2006). Major problem is ↑ risk with concomitant drugs.
Levofloxacin (Levaquin)	**250–750 mg po/IV q24h** Cost: 750 mg po $22; 750 mg IV $58; ophthal solution (Quixin) $57 for 5 mL.	**Avoid concomitant drugs with potential to prolong QT₀:**

<table>
<thead>
<tr><th>Anti-arrhythmics:</th><th>Anti-Infectives:</th><th>CNS Drugs</th><th>Misc.</th></tr>
</thead>
<tbody>
<tr><td>Amiodarone</td><td>Azoles (not posa)</td><td>Fluoxetine</td><td>Salmeterol</td></tr>
<tr><td>Disopyramide</td><td>Clarithro/erythro</td><td>Sertraline</td><td>Naratriptan</td></tr>
<tr><td>Dofetilide</td><td>FQs (not CIP)</td><td>Tricyclics</td><td>Sumatriptan</td></tr>
<tr><td>Flecainide</td><td>Halofantrine</td><td>Venlafaxine</td><td>Dolasetron</td></tr>
<tr><td>Ibutilide</td><td>NNRTIs</td><td>Haloperidol</td><td>Droperidol</td></tr>
<tr><td>Procainamide</td><td>Protease Inhibitors</td><td>Phenothiazines</td><td>Fosphenytoin</td></tr>
<tr><td>Quinidine</td><td>Pentamidine</td><td>Pimozide</td><td>Indapamide</td></tr>
<tr><td>Sotalol</td><td>Telithromycin</td><td>Quetiapine</td><td>Tamoxifen</td></tr>
<tr><td></td><td></td><td>Ziprasidone</td><td>Tizanidine</td></tr>
<tr><td></td><td></td><td>Risperidone</td><td></td></tr>
<tr><td colspan="2">**Anti-Hypertensives:**</td><td></td><td></td></tr>
<tr><td>Bepridil</td><td></td><td></td><td></td></tr>
<tr><td>Isradipine</td><td></td><td></td><td></td></tr>
<tr><td>Nicardipine</td><td></td><td></td><td></td></tr>
<tr><td>Moexipril</td><td></td><td></td><td></td></tr>
</tbody>
</table>

Updates online: www.qtdrugs.org; www.torsades.org

Moxifloxacin (Avelox)	**400 mg po/IV q24h** Cost: 400 mg po $12, IV $42 Ophthalmic solution (Vigamox) $62 for 3 mL.	**Tendinopathy:** Over age 60, approx. 2–6% of all Achilles tendon ruptures attributable to use of FQ (ArIM 163:1801, 2003). Risk with concomitant steroid or renal disease (CID 36:1404, 2003). Overall incidence is low (Eur J Clin Pharm 63:499, 2007).
Ofloxacin (Floxin)	**200–400 mg po bid** Cost: 400 mg po $6 Ophthalmic solution (Ocuflox) $41 for 5 mL.	
POLYMYXINS		
Polymyxin B (Poly-Rx)	**15,000–25,000 units/kg/day divided q12h** Cost 500,000 units $15.20	Also used as/for: bladder irrigation, intrathecal, ophthalmic preps. Source: Bedford Labs, Bedford, OH. Differs from colistin by one amino acid.

* NOTE: all dosage recommendations are for adults (unless otherwise indicated) & assume normal renal function.
† Cost = average wholesale price from 2007 Red Book, Thomson Healthcare, Inc. (See page 2 for abbreviations)

TABLE 10C (7)

CLASS, AGENT GENERIC NAME (TRADE NAME)	USUAL ADULT DOSAGE* (Cost*)	ADVERSE REACTIONS, COMMENTS (See Table 10A for Summary)
POLYMYXINS (continued)		
Colistin (=Polymyxin E) (LnID 6:589, 2006) Don't confuse dose calc for the "base" vs the "salt": 10,000 units = 1 mg base 2.4 mg colistimethate sodium salt in US; label refers to mgs of base. See AAC 50:2274 & 4231, 2006	**Parenterals:** In US: **Colymycin-M** 2.5-5 mg/kg per day divided into 2-4 doses = 6.7-13.3 mg/kg per day of colistimethate sodium (max 800 mg/day). Cost: 150mg $55. **Elsewhere: Colomycin** daily, 50,000-75,000 IU/kg per day IV in 3 divided doses (=4-6mg/kg per day of colistimethate sodium). >60kg: 1-2 mill IU IV t/d	**Intrathecal** 10 mg/day and **Intraventricular** 1.6 mg/day reported successful. **Inhalation:** In cystic fibrosis pts (mucous breakdown and others) CID 41:1754, 2005). Combination therapy. Few studies. Manufacturer reports of efficacy of colistin & rifampin vs A. baumannii and P. aeruginosa (VAP 2) in cystic fibrosis pts. attempts at eradication of P. aeruginosa containing p.o cipro + nebulized colistimethate sodium. **Topical & oral:** Colistin sulfate used. **Nephrotoxicity:** Reversible tubular necrosis. Exact frequency unclear. **Neurotoxicity:** Frequency vertigo, facial paresthesia, abnormal vision, confusion, ataxia, & neuromuscular blockade → respiratory arrest all dose-dependent. In cystic fibrosis pts, 29% experienced paresthesia, ataxia or both. **Other:** Maybe hyperpigmentation
MISCELLANEOUS AGENTS		
Daptomycin (Cubicin) (Ref on resistance: CID 45:601, 2007)	**Skin/soft tissue:** 4 mg per kg IV q24h **Bacteremia/right-sided endocarditis: 6 mg per kg IV q24h** **Morbid obesity:** base dose on total body weight (J Clin Pharm 45:48, 2005) Cost: 500 mg $206.	**Potential muscle toxicity:** At 4 mg per kg per day, ↑ CPK in 2.8% dapto pts & 1.8% comparator-treated pts. Suggest weekly CPK. DC dapto if CPK exceeds 10x normal level or if symptoms of myopathy and CPK > 1,000. Manufacturer suggests stopping statins during dapto rx. Selected reagents (Hemosil, Hemoclane, Hemoliance Recombiplastin), can falsely prolong PT & INR (4/12/06 Dear Doctor letter). **NOTE:** Dapto well-tolerated in healthy volunteers at doses up to 12 mg/kg q24h x 14d (AAC 50:3245, 2006). Resistance of S. aureus reported during dapto therapy, post-vanco therapy & de novo.
Fosfomycin (Monurol)	**3 gm with water po times 1 dose.** Cost $41	Diarrhea in 9% compared to 6% of pts given nitrofurantoin and 2.3% given TMP-SMX.
Fusidic acid** (Fucidin)	**500 mg po/IV tid (Denmark & Canada)**	Jaundice (17% with IV use; 6% with po). CID 42:394, 2006.
Methenamine hippurate (Hiprex, Urex)	**1 gm po bid** Cost: 1 gm $1.23 1 gm = 480 mg methenamine	Nausea and vomiting, skin rash or dysuria. Overall ~3%. Methenamine requires (pH <5) urine to liberate formaldehyde. Useful in suppression therapy after infecting organisms cleared; do not use for pyelonephritis. Comment: Do not force fluids; may dilute formaldehyde. Of no value in pts with chronic Foley. If urine (pH >5.0, co-administer ascorbic acid (1-2 gm q4h) to acidify the urine; cranberry juice (1200-4000 mL per day) has been used, results ±
Methenamine mandelate (Mandelamine)	**1 gm po q6h (480 mg methenamine).** Cost: 1 gm N$ $0.29	
Metronidazole (Flagyl) Ref: Activity vs. B. fragilis AAC 51:1649, 2007.	**Anaerobic infections:** usually IV, 7.5 mg per kg (~500 mg) q6h (not to exceed 4 gm q24h). **With long T½, can use IV at 15 mg per kg q12h.** If life-threatening, give loading dose of IV 15 mg per kg. **Oral Dose: 500 mg qid.** Cost: 500 mg tab $ S$0.14, 500 mg IV $32.75; 70 gm[?] vaginal gel N$ $5. vaginal gel $76.54. Extended release tabs 750 mg $10.50.	Absorbed into serum from vaginal gel. **Neurol.:** headache, rare paresthesias or peripheral neuropathy; ataxia, seizures, aseptic meningitis; report of reversible MRI-induced cerebellar lesions (NEJM 346:68, 2002). **Avoid alcohol during & 48 hrs after (disulfiram-like reaction).** Very dark urine (common but harmless). Skin: urticaria. Mutagenic in Ames test. Tumorigenic in animals (high dose over lifetime). No evidence of risk in man. No teratogenicity.
Nitrofurantoin macrocrystals (Macrodantin, Furadantin)	**100 mg po q6h.** Cost: 100 mg G $1.21, NB $2.50 **Dose for long-term UTI suppression: 50-100 mg at bedtime**	Absorption ↑ with meals. Increased activity in acid urine, much reduced at pH 8 or over. Not effective in endstage renal disease (JAC 33[Suppl. A]:121, 1994). Nausea and vomiting, hypersensitivity, peripheral neuropathy. Pulmonary reactions (with chronic rx): acute ARDS type, **chronic desquamative interstitial pneumonia with fibrosis.** Intrahepatic cholestasis & **hepatitis** similar to chronic active hepatitis. Hemolytic anemia in G6PD deficiency. **Contraindicated in renal failure.** Should not be used in infants <1 month of age.
monohydrate/macrocrystals (Macrobid)	**100 mg po bid** Cost: 100 mg $2.54	Efficacy of Macrobid 100 mg bid = Macrodantin 50 mg qid. Adverse effects 5.6% less nausea than with Macrodantin.
Rifaximin (Xifaxan)	**200 mg po tid times 3 days.** Cost: 200 mg $4.16	For traveler's diarrhea, adverse events equal to or less than placebo.

* NOTE: all dosage recommendations are for adults (unless otherwise indicated) & assume normal renal function.
† NOTE: = average wholesale price from 2007 RED Book, Thomson Healthcare, Inc.
(See page 2 for abbreviations)

TABLE 10C (8)

CLASS, AGENT, GENERIC NAME (TRADE NAME)	USUAL ADULT DOSAGE* (Cost†)	ADVERSE REACTIONS, COMMENTS (See Table 10A for Summary)
MISCELLANEOUS AGENTS (continued)		
Sulfonamides (e.g., sulfisoxazole (Gantrisin), sulfamethoxazole (Gantanol), (Truxazole))	Dose varies with indications. Cost 500 mg: $0.09	**Short-acting are best:** high urine concentration and good solubility at acid pH. More active in alkaline urine. **Allergic reactions:** skin rash, drug fever, pruritus, photosensitization. Periarteritis nodosa & SLE. Stevens-Johnson syndrome, serum sickness syndrome, mycocarditis. **Neurotoxicity** (psychosis, neuritis). **Hepatic toxicity.** Blood dyscrasias, usually agranulocytosis. Crystalluria. Nausea & vomiting, headache, dizziness, malaise, mental depression, acidosis, sulfhemoglobin. Hemolytic anemia in G6PD deficient & unstable hemoglobin pts. Avoid sulfa in newborn infants or in women near term, frequency & toxicity enhanced (binds to albumin, blocking binding of bilirubin to albumin)
Tinidazole (Tindamax)	**Tabs 250, 500 mg.** Dose for giardiasis: 2 gm po times 1 with food. Cost: 500 mg $4.56	**Adverse reactions:** metallic taste 3.7%, nausea 3.2%, anorexia/vomiting 1.5%. All higher with multi-day dosing.
Trimethoprim (Trimpex, Proloprim, and others)	100 mg po q12h or 200 mg po q24h. Cost: 100 mg NB $0.90, G $0.15	Frequent side-effects are rash and pruritus. Rash in 3% at 100 mg bid; 6.7% at 200 mg q24h. Rare reports of photosensitivity, exfoliative dermatitis, Stevens-Johnson syndrome, toxic epidermal necrosis, and aseptic meningitis (CID 19:431, 1994). Check drug interaction with phenytoin. Increases serum K⁺ (see TMP-SMX Comments). TMP can ↑ homocysteine blood levels (Ln 352:1827, 1998)
Trimethoprim (TMP)– Sulfamethoxazole (SMX) (Bactrim, Septra, Sulfatrim, Cotrimoxazole) Single-strength (SS) is 80 TMP/400 SMX, double-strength (DS) 160 TMP/800 SMX Ref.: AHM 163:402, 2003	**Standard po rx (UTI, otitis media): 1 DS tab bid. P. carinii: see Table 13, page 125.** IV rx (base on TMP component): **standard 8–10 mg per kg per day divided q6h, q8h, or q12h. For shigellosis: 2.5 mg per kg IV q6h.** Cost: 160/800 po G $1.15. NB $1.31; 160/800 IV $11.21 NB $1.31; 160/800 IV $11.21, double- Peds susp: 200/40 mg: 100 mL $12.63	Adverse reactions in 10%: GI: nausea, vomiting, anorexia. Skin: Rash, urticaria, photosensitivity. More serious (1–10%): Stevens-Johnson syndrome & toxic epidermal necrolysis. Skin reactions may represent toxic metabolites of SMX (rather than allergy) (JAIDS Pharmacotherapy 20:281, 2000). Dally ascorbic acid 0.5–1.0 gm may promote detoxification (JAIDS 26:104). (See Table 10A, page 63 for more S/S; also Ln1d 6:178, 2006) TMP competes with creatinine for tubular secretion, serum creatinine can ↑. TMP also blocks distal tubule secretion of K⁺, serum K⁺ in 21% of pts (NEJM 124:316, 1996). TMP one etiology of aseptic meningitis (CID 19:431, 1994). TMP-SMX contains sulfites and may trigger asthma in sulfite-sensitive pts. Frequent drug cause of thrombocytopenia (AnIM 129:886, 1998). No cross allergenicity with other sulfonamide non-antibiotic drugs (NEJM 349:1628, 2003). **Rapid Oral TMP-SMX Desensitization:**

Hour	Dose TMP/SMX (mg)
0	0.004/0.02
1	0.04/0.2
2	0.4/2

Hour	Dose TMP/SMX (mg)
3	4/20
4	40/200
5	160/800

Comment: Perform in hospital or clinic. Use oral suspension (40 mg TMP/ 200 mg SMX per 5 mL [tsp]). Take 6 oz water after each dose. Corticosteroids, anti-histamines NOT used. Refs.: CID 20:849, 1995; AIDS 5:311, 1997 |
Topical Antimicrobial Agents		
Bacitracin (Baciguent)	20% skin & bacitracin zinc ointment, apply 3.5 gm Cost $5-10	Active vs. staph, strep & clostridium. Contact dermatitis incidence 9.2% (IDC No Amer 18:717, 2004).
Fusidic acid¹ ointment	2% ointment, apply bid	CID 42:394, 2006. Available in Canada and Europe (Leo Laboratories)
Mupirocin (Bactroban)	Skin cream or ointment 2%: Apply tid times 10 days. 1% ointment 2%: Nasal ointment 2%: apply bid times 5 days. 22 gm NB $60, G $41	Skin cream: itch, burning, stinging 1–1.5%. Nasal: headache 9%, rhinitis 6%, respiratory congestion 5%. Not active vs. enterococci or gm-neg bacteria.
Polymyxin B–Bacitracin (Polysporin)	5000 units/gm; 400 units/gm Cost $25	Apply 1–3 times/day. Polymyxin active vs. gm-neg bacteria but not Proteus sp., Serratia sp. or gm-pos bacteria. See Bacitracin comment above.
Polymyxin B – Bacitracin– Neomycin (Triple antibiotic ointment (TAO))¹ (Neosporin)	5000 units/gm; 400 units/gm; 3.5 mg/gm 3.5 gm $2-8	Apply 1–3 times/day. Neomycin active vs. Staph aureus & gm-neg bacteria and polymyxin B comments above. Neomycin active vs. gm-neg bacteria and polymyxin active vs. streptococci. See Bacitracin comment above. Contact dermatitis incidence 1%, risk of nephro- & oto-toxicity if absorbed.
Retapamulin (Altabax)	1% ointment; apply bid. 5, 10 & 15 gm tubes. 15 gm: $68	TAO spectrum broader than mupirocin and active mupirocin-resistant strains (DMID 54:63, 2006). Microbiologic success in 90% S. aureus infections and 97% of S. pyogenes infections (J Am Acad Derm 55:1003, 2006).

¹ NOTE: all dosage recommendations are for adults (unless otherwise indicated) & assume normal renal function.
† Cost = average wholesale price from 2007 RED Book, Thomson Healthcare, Inc.
(See page 2 for abbreviations)

TABLE 10D – AMINOGLYCOSIDE ONCE-DAILY AND MULTIPLE DAILY DOSING REGIMENS
(See Table 17, page 178, If estimated creatinine clearance <90 mL per min.)

General: Dosage given as both once-daily (OD) and multiple daily dose (MDD) regimens.
Pertinent formulae:

(1) **Estimated creatinine clearance** (CrCl): (140–age)(ideal body weight in kg) ÷ CrCl for men in mL per min; multiply answer times 0.85 for CrCl of women

$$\frac{(140-age)(\text{ideal body weight in kg})}{(72)(serum\ creatinine)}$$ Alternative method to calculate CrCl: see NEJM 354:2473, 2006

(2) **Ideal body weight** (IBW)—Females: 45.5 kg + 2.3 kg per inch over 5' = weight in kg
Males: 50 kg + 2.3 kg per inch over 5' = weight in kg

(3) **Obesity adjustment**: use if actual body weight (ABW) is ≥30% above IBW. To calculate adj dosing weight in kg: IBW + 0.4(ABW–IBW) = adjusted weight
(Pharmacotherapy 27:1081, 2007; CID 25:112, 1997)

DRUG	MDD AND OD IV REGIMENS; TARGETED PEAK (P) AND TROUGH (T) SERUM LEVELS	COST† Name Brand (NB), Generic (G)	COMMENTS For more data on once-daily dosing, see AJM 105:182, 1998, and Table 17, page 178
Gentamicin (Garamycin), **Tobramycin** (Nebcin)	MDD: 2 mg per kg load, then 1.7 mg per kg q8h - - - - P 4–10 mcg/mL, T 1–2 mcg per mL- - - - OD: 5.1 (7 if critically ill) mg per kg q24h - - - - P 16–24 mcg per mL, T <1 mcg per mL	Gentamicin: 80 mg $5.30 Tobramycin: 80 mg NB $7.28, G $4.20	All aminoglycosides have potential to cause tubular necrosis and renal failure, deafness due to cochlear toxicity, vertigo due to damage to vestibular organs, and rarely neuromuscular blockade. Risk minimal with oral or topical application due to small % absorption unless tissues altered by disease.
Kanamycin (Kantrex), **Amikacin** (Amikin), Streptomycin	MDD: 7.5 mg per kg q12h - - - - P 15–30 mcg per mL, T 5–10 mcg per mL- - - OD: 15 mg per kg q24h - - - - P 56–64 mcg per mL, T <1 mcg per mL	Kanamycin: 1 gm $13.12 Amikacin: 500 mg NB $34.26, G $7.80 Streptomycin: 1 gm $9.10	Risk of nephrotoxicity ↑ with concomitant administration of cyclosporine, vancomycin, ampho B, radiocontrast. Risk of nephrotoxicity ↓ by concomitant AP Pen and perhaps by once-daily dosing method (especially if baseline renal function normal).
Netilmicin[NUS]	MDD: 2 mg per kg q8h - - - - P 4–10 mcg per mL, T 1–2 mcg per mL- - - OD: 6.5 mg per kg q24h - - - - P 22–30 mcg per mL, T <1 mcg per mL		In general, same factors influence risk of ototoxicity. **NOTE: There is no known method to eliminate risk of aminoglycoside nephro/ototoxicity. Proper rx attempts to ↓ the % risk.** The clinical trial data of OD aminoglycosides have been reviewed extensively by meta-analysis (CID 24:816, 1997).
Isepamicin[NUS]	Only OD: Severe infections 15 mg per kg q24h, less severe 8 mg per kg q24h	2 gm NB $34.06	**Serum levels:** Collect serum peak level (PSL) exactly 1 hr after the start of the infusion of the 3rd dose. In critically ill pts, it is reasonable to measure the PSL after the 1st dose as well as later doses as volume of distribution and renal function may change rapidly.
Spectinomycin (Trobicin)[NUS]	2 gm IM times 1-gonococcal infections	500 mg G $1.24	For dosing methods and references: For once-daily 7 mg per kg per day of gentamicin—Hartford Hospital method, see AAC 39:650, 1995.
Neomycin—oral	Prophylaxis (GI surgery: 1 gm po times 3 with erythro, see Table 15B, page 168 For hepatic coma: 4–12 gm per day po		

Tobramycin—inhaled (Tobi): See Cystic fibrosis, Table 1, page 39. Adverse effects few: transient voice alteration (13%) and transient tinnitus (3%). Cost: 300 mg $72.00

Paromomycin—oral: See Entamoeba and Cryptosporidia, Table 13, page 123. Cost 250 mg $2.72

† Estimated CrCl invalid if serum creatinine <0.6 mg per dL. Consultation suggested.
§ Cost = average wholesale price from 2007 RED BOOK, Thomson Healthcare, Inc.

TABLE 11A – TREATMENT OF FUNGAL, ACTINOMYCOTIC, AND NOCARDIAL INFECTIONS—ANTIMICROBIAL AGENTS OF CHOICE*
(See Table 11B for Amphotericin B Preparations and Adverse Effects)

TYPE OF INFECTION/ORGANISM/ SITE OF INFECTION	ANTIMICROBIAL AGENTS OF CHOICE		COMMENTS
	PRIMARY	ALTERNATIVE	
Actinomycosis (A. israelii most common, also A. naeslundii, A. viscosus, A. odontolyticus, A. meyeri, A. gerencseriae) Cervicofacial, pulmonary, abdominal, cerebral, & rarely pericarditis (IDCP 12:233, 2004) Classically abdominal actino presents as intraabdominal or pubic mass abscess, fistula tract (Dis Colon Rectum 48:575, 2005) yrs after surgery, may mimic cancer (World J Gastro 11:1722, 2005). Fine needle aspirate of cervicofacial actino estab dx in 15 pts in Spain (Med Oral Patol Oral Cir Bucal 9:467, 2004).	**Ampicillin** 50 mg/kg per day IV times 4-6wks, then 0.5gm **amoxicillin** po tid **OR Penicillin G** 10-20 mil units/day IV x 4-6 wks, then **penicillin V** 2-4gm/ day po. Duration individualized, may be guided by resolution of measurable disease burden (abscess, mass), so duration 3-6mo usually adequate for thoracic & abdominal 3-6wks for cervicofacial	**Doxycycline** or **ceftriaxone** or **clindamycin** or **erythromycin** or **Chloramphenicol** 12.5–15mg/kg IV/po q6h has been recommended for CNS infection in pen-allergic pts	Tuboovarian abscesses may complicate IUDs. Removal of IUD is primary rx. With abscesses, inflammatory mass or fistulae, surgery often required. Penicillin G and ceftriaxone IV are effective; with home IV therapy, agents given q24h, e.g., ceftriaxone, are more practical. Surgery may be necessary for hemoptysis.
Aspergillosis (A. fumigatus most common, also A. flavus and A. terreus) **Allergic bronchopulmonary aspergillosis (ABPA)** Semin Respir. Crit Care Med. 27:185, 2006. ABPA found in 1–2% of pts with asthma & 1–15% with cystic fibrosis (Chest 130:222, 2006). (CID 37 (Suppl.3):37, 2003). Clinical manifestations: wheezing, pulmonary infiltrates, bronchiectasis & fibrosis, Airway colonization assoc. with ↑ blood eosinophils, ↑ serum IgE, ↑ specific serum antibodies	Rx of ABPA: **Itraconazole** 200mg po q24h times 16wks or longer	For failures try **Itra** 200 mg po bid times 12 mos (CID 41:1289, 2003; CID 37 (Suppl.3):S225, 2003). Flucon nasal spray benefited 12/16 pts (ENT J 83: 692, 2004).	In 2 PRCTs[2] Itra ↓ number of exacerbations requiring corticosteroids (p < 0.03), improved immunological markers (eosinophils in sputum & ↓ serum IgE levels), & in 1 study improved lung function & exercise tolerance (Cochrane Database Syst Rev 3:CD001108, 2004).
Allergic fungal sinusitis: relapsing chronic sinusitis; nasal polyps without bony invasion; asthma, eczema or allergic rhinitis; ↑ IgE levels and isolation of Aspergillus, or other dematiaceous sp. (Alternaria, Cladosporium, etc.)	Rx controversial: systemic corticosteroids + surgical debridement. (Allergy 59:231, 2004)		In 1 report, fungal elements identified by histopathology in up to 93% of cases of "chronic sinusitis." In a DBRCT in 24 pts, intranasal ampho was assoc. with a ↓ in mucosal thickening of 8.8% by CT scan vs ↑ of 2.5% in placebo (LnID 4:257, 2004). In another 116 patients in a PBPCT, no benefit from nasal ampho B irrigation (J Allergy Clin Immunol 118:1149, 2006). Controversial area.
Aspergilloma (fungus ball) (J Resp Dis 23:300, 2002)	Efficacy of antimicrobial agents not proven. **Itraconazole** (po) benefit reported anecdotally.		Aspergillus may complicate pulmonary sequestration (Eur J Cardio Thor Surg 27:28, 2005). Paranasal fungus balls respond to surgery, 172 of 175 cases (Med Mycol 44:61, 2006).
Invasive, pulmonary (IPA) or extrapulmonary: (See CID 108:314, 2005; Am J Respir Crit Care Med 173:707, 2006). Good website:doctorfungus.org Posaconazole an option for post-chemotherapy in neutropenic pts (PMN <500 per mm³) but may also present with neutrophil recovery (Mycopathologia 159:181, 2005). Most common pneumonia in (continued on next page)	**Voriconazole** 6mg/kg IV q12h x 2 (or 200mg q12h for body weight ≤40kg, 100mg po q12h for body weight <40kg) then either (4mg/kg IV q12h) or 200mg po q12h. **Lipid-based ampho B** (ABLC/LAB) may be as effective and less nephrotoxic than standard ampho B **but much more expensive** (see footnote[a] for dosages). 50% response with LAB (CID 44:1284 & 1298, 2007)		**Vori** more effective than ampho B in randomized trial of 277 immuno-suppressed pts with IPA. 53% responded vs 32% (x with ampho B. Overall survival (71 vs 58%) (NEJM 347:408, 2002). Vori advantageous in cerebral aspergillosis (CID 39:603, 2004. Blood 106:2641, 2005) & as salvage therapy for refractory infect (Eur J Haematol 73:50, 2004). 40% of 31 pts survived with vori alone. Satisfactory response in 11/20 pts with bone involvement (18 for salvage). (continued on next page)

---

¹ **Oral solution preferred to tablets because of ↑ absorption** (see Table 11B, page 105).

² **PRCTs** = Prospective randomized controlled trials

³ **Dosages: ABLC** 5mg/kg per day IV over 2 hrs; **liposomal Ampho B** 3–5mg/kg per day IV given over 1–2hrs.

See page 2 for abbreviations. All dosage recommendations are for adults (unless otherwise indicated) and assume normal renal function

TABLE 11A (2)

TYPE OF INFECTION/ORGANISM/ SITE OF INFECTION	ANTIMICROBIAL AGENTS OF CHOICE		COMMENTS
	PRIMARY	ALTERNATIVE	
Aspergillosis (continued)			
(continued from previous page)
transplant recipients. Usually a late (≥100 days) complication in allogeneic bone marrow & liver transplantation: 45% survival at 90 days (CID 44:531, 2007). May complicate COPD when corticosteroids used (Clin Micro Inf 11:427, 2005).

Typical x-ray/CT lung lesions (halo sign, cavitation, or mycotic lung sequestration) have 90% positive predictive value for invasive pulmonary aspergillosis in pts with neutropenia (CID 31:859, 2000).

An immunoassay test that detects circulating **galactomannan** is available for dx of invasive aspergillosis (Lancet ID 4:349, 2005). For strengths & weaknesses of the test see CID 42:1417, 2006).

False-pos. tests occur with serum from pts receiving PIP-TZ & AM-CL (Clin Micro 43:2548, 2005). Other causes of false positive galactomannan serum antigen assay: food (pasta, rice, canned vegetables), Geotrichum sp. & Bifidobacterium sp. & electrolyte solution containing sodium gluconate [prodcudialysate fluid, plasmalyte] & used for pronchoalveolar lavage [BAL] & concomitant antifungal rx may also ↓ sensitivity (CID 40:1762, 2005). (MiraVista, 1-866-647-2847). Mucositis of GI tract also associated with positives without evidence of infection. | (continued from previous page)
OR
Some clinicians start with Voriconazole. If it fails to respond clinically in 7-10 days then switch to Lipid-based Ampho B
OR
Combination rx: Vori (in above dosage) + **caspofungin 70 mg iv** on day 1, then 50 mg iv (q24h (35 mg with moderate hepatic insufficiency) are currently used as initial treatment in many bone marrow transplant units, esp. in pts receiving high doses of corticosteroids (Abstracts in Herne & Onc 8:11, 2005).

Micafungin or anidulafungin probably equivalent to **caspofungin** but are not FDA approved for this indication.

Alternative: Caspofungin at doses given above. (Approved for salvage therapy of Aspergillosis)

For all regimens: If response good may switch to oral **vori** after 2-3wks (See on page 94) | (continued from previous page)
CID 40:1141, 2005 & with Subacute IPA & chronic pulmonary Aspergillosis: modest response (Am J Med 119:527, 2006). 15% of patients have subtherapeutic levels at recommended doses (Cancer 109:1532, 2007); check levels & if low, increase vori dose treatment failures or life-threatening infections.

Caspofungin monotherapy (as initial rx): salvage rx in pts who failed to respond to prior antifungal rx (CID 40:S392, 2005). **Ampho B overall success rate 34–42%** (CID 32:358, 2001) in pulmonary aspergillosis in pts rx ≥14 days. Success depended on under-lying disease: 83% in heart/kidney transplants, 54% neutropenic leukemia, 33% bone marrow trans. 20% liver trans (CID 23:608, 1996). **A. terreus infec esp resist to ampho B: 83 cases, 73.4% mortality ampho B rx vs 55.8% vori rx <0.01** (CID 39:192, 2004). **Use vori!**

Caspo: Among 83 pts with IPA, 37 (45%) had favorable response following salvage rx with caspo monotherapy. In pts receiving >7 days of caspo monotherapy, 56% (37/66) responded favorably (J Inf 50:196, 2004). Response in compassionate use program: 44% (J Inf 50:196, 2005). Minimal toxicity reported (Transpl Int Dis 1:25, 2002).

Micafungin: 57% clinical response in an open-label study of "deep-seated" infections, 60% response in IPA (Scand J Int Dis 36:372, 2004).

Posaconazole showed 42% success in 107 pts vs 26% in 86 historical controls in "refractory IA" (Clin Infect Dis 44:2, 2007).

Combo therapy: No controlled trials; they are needed (CID 39:803, 2004). No antag. between triazoles (vori & itra, posa), echinocandins (caspo, mica), & ampho B. Synergy demonstrated vs aspergillus in vitro &/or animal models between triazoles & caspo. In retrospective study of bone marrow transplant pts with IPA who failed ampho B, vori + caspo superior to vori alone (CID 39:797, 2004). In 40 solid organ transplant pts treated with caspo and compared to historical controls given Lipid-based Ampho B, no overall survival benefit found but subset analysis showed ↑ success with combo in A. fumigatus infections and in those with renal failure (Transplantation 81:320, 2006). Need clinical data: posa + (either ampho B: AAC 48:3715, 2004 or vori: AAC 52:2587, 2006). **Is any combo rx better than Vori alone? Don't know yet!** |
| **Blastomycosis** (CID 30:679, 2000)
(Patients initially treated for 2wks; dermatitis, pulmonary or extrapulmonary. For blood/urine antigen, call 1-866-647-2847 | **Itraconazole**¹ oral solution 200-400mg/day po for 6mo. **OR Ampho B**¹ 0.7-1mg/kg/day to total dose of 1.5gm for very sick pts | **Fluconazole** 400-800 mg per day for at least 6 mos. 85%- effective for non-life-threatening disease (CID 25:200, 1997) | |

---

¹ Oral solution preferred to tablets because of ↑ absorption (see Table 11B, page 105).

See page 2 for abbreviations. All dosage recommendations are for adults (unless otherwise indicated) and assume normal renal function.

TABLE 11A (3)

TYPE OF INFECTION/ORGANISM/ SITE OF INFECTION	ANTIMICROBIAL AGENTS OF CHOICE		COMMENTS
	PRIMARY	ALTERNATIVE	

Candidiasis. Candidemia in US is 4th most common nosocomial blood stream infection with up to 30% mortality, 10-21 day increase in length of stay and $40K - $92K increased expense (CID 41:1232, 2005 and CID 39:309,2005) A change in C. albicans & increase in C. albicans & increase in non-albicans species continues. The latter show ↓ susceptibility to antifungal agents (esp. fluconazole). These changes predominantly in immunocompromised pts wherein antifungal prophylaxis (esp. fluconazole) is widely used (JCM 43:2729, 2005; COID 18:490, 2005). Pts who develop disseminated candidiasis while receiving fluconazole are likely to be infected with an azole-resistant C. glabrata or C. krusei (CID 42:244, 2006). In vitro susceptibility profiles help select empiric antifungal rx.

Bloodstream: clinically stable with or without venous catheter — if C. glabrata or C. krusei unlikely (no flu with in 30 days) (IDSA Guidelines: CID 38:161, 2004, CID 42:244, 2006).	**Fluconazole** ≥6 mg/kg per day or for flu with in 30 days) then po for 14 days after last + blood culture	Echinocandin (see **caspofungin, anidulafungin & micafungin** below)	Fluconazole still preferred here because of clinical response studies, favorable safety profile and low cost (JAC 57:384,2006)
All positive blood cultures require therapy!			
• Remove & replace venous catheter ("not over a wire") (J Clin Micro 43:1829, 2005), esp. in non-neutropenic: mortality 21% vs 4% if catheter not removed.			
• Treat for 2wk after last pos. blood culture & resolution of signs & symptoms of infection.			

Bloodstream: unstable	**Caspofungin** 70mg IV on day 1 followed by 50mg IV q24h (reduce to 35mg IV q24h with moderate hepatic insufficiency). **OR** **Micafungin** 100 mg IV q24h **OR** **Anidulafungin** 200 mg IV times 1, then 100 mg IV q24h (no dosage adjustments for renal or hepatic insufficiency)	**Ampho B** 0.7 mg/kg IV q24h, (>0.7mg/kg) IV for C. glabrata, 1mg/kg IV for C. krusei **OR** **ABLC 5 mg/kg/d or LAB 3-5 mg/kg/d** **OR** **Voriconazole**: 6 mg per kg IV q12h times 2 doses, then maintenance doses of 3 mg per kg IV q12h (if >40 kg), or 200 mg q12h, after at least 3 days of IV therapy **OR** **Combination of fluconazole** (flu) 800 mg per day + **ampho B** 0.7 mg per kg per day for first 5-6 days, then switch to flu 400 mg per day po	The echinocandins appear to have similar safety & efficacy, vs candida including candidemia; decisions on use made on the basis of cost. A randomized study (277 pts, 10% were neutropenic) found **caspofungin** equivalent to **ampho B** (0.6-1 mg per kg per day) for invasive candidiasis. For candidemia 71.7% rx with caspo vs 62.8% with ampho B had successful outcomes but caspo had significantly less toxicity (NEJM 347:2020, 2002). Caspo had 70% favorable response vs 56% for ampho B in 58 cancer pts with candidemia (Cancer 101:2866, 2005). **Micafungin**: non-inferior to caspofungin in DBPCT (CID 45:883, 2007). Data from a randomized double-blind study (n=245) (NEJM 356:2472, 2007) show **anidulafungin** was at least equivalent and possibly superior to flu for invasive candidemia/candidiasis: success rate of 75.6% with anidula vs 60.2% with flu. Tolerability was comparable. **Voriconazole** non-inferior to ampho B followed by flu in non-neutropenic candidemia (Lancet 366:1435, 2005). However cross resistance between vori and flu reported in 9 of 28 candida isolates (J Clin Micro 44:529,2006) especially with C. glabrata; vori still active vs. C. krusei (J Clin Micro 44:1740, 2006). Would not recommend as initial rx in those with extensive azole exposure. MICs of candins are higher for C. parapsilosis than for other candida species and clinical response rates may be less.
Failure to respond to fluconazole or deteriorating status (Critical to remove intravenous catheter)			
• Hemodynamic instability (sepsis)			
• C. glabrata or C. krusei likely			
• Neutropenia (immunosuppressed/flu prophylaxis)			
Neutropenic pts and B are similarly effective in neutropenic pts (IDSA Guidelines, 2003).			
Mortality rates inc with delay in initiation of therapy: 15% day 0, 24% day 1, 37% day 2 & 41% >day 4- p >.0009 (CID 43:25, 2006)			

See page 2 for abbreviations. All dosage recommendations are for adults (unless otherwise indicated) and assume normal renal function

TABLE 11A (4)

TYPE OF INFECTION/ORGANISM/ SITE OF INFECTION	ANTIMICROBIAL AGENTS OF CHOICE		COMMENTS
	PRIMARY	ALTERNATIVE	
Candidiasis/Bloodstream: clinically stable with or without venous catheter (continued)			
Cutaneous (including paronychia, Table 1, page 24)	Apply topical **ampho B, clotrimazole, econazole, miconazole,** or **nystatin** 3–4 x daily for 7–14 days or **ketoconazole** 400 mg po once daily x 14 days.	Ciclopirox olamine 1% cream/lotion. Apply topically bid x 7–14 days.*	*Cost (30 gm tube cream): Clo $5–8, Eco $30, Mic $3.20, Nys $3
Endocarditis Causes: C. albicans 24%, non-albicans Candida sp. 24%, Aspergillus sp. 24%, others 27% (CID 32:50, 2001). Surgery may not always be required (Scand J Inf Dis 37:320, 2005).	**(Ampho B** 0.6mg/kg per day IV for 7 days, then 0.8mg/kg IV every other day or **lipid-based ampho B** 3–5mg/kg per day) + **flucytosine** 25–37.5mg/kg per day qid) + surgical resection	**Fluconazole** 200–400 mg po per day for chronic infection when valve cannot be replaced (Chest 122:302, 2002) + Surgical resection	Ciclopirox lotion, 30 mL; $48; cream 30 gm; $51 * *Adjust flucyt dose and interval to produce serum levels; peak 70–80 mg per L, trough 30–40 mg per L. Caspofungin cidal vs candida; several reports of cure (CID 39:1489-e70-3, 2004; CID 40:e-72, 2005).
Endophthalmitis (IDSA Guidelines. CID 38:161, 2004). Occurs in 10% of candidemia (PIDJ 23:635, 2004), thus ophthalmologic consult for all pts. Diagnosis: typical white exudates on retinal exam and/or subjective vision loss.	**[Ampho B** or **lipid-based ampho B** (ABLC 5mg/kg per day)] OR **fluconazole** 400mg/day IV or po either as initial rx or follow-up after ampho B. Role of intravitreal ampho B not well defined but commonly used in pts with substantial vision loss (CID 27:1130, 1998). Treat 6–12 wk.		Treatment results mixed in small series. Fluconazole (CID 20:657, 1995), ABLC (IJ Inf 40:92, 2000), and vitrectomy (CID 27:1130, 1998). Not successful alone or with caspo (Am J Ophthal 139:135, 2005). No clinical trials available.
Oral (thrush)—not AIDS patient (See below for vaginitis)	**Fluconazole** 200 mg single dose **Nystatin** pastilles (200,000 units) or 100 mg/day po x 14 days or clotrimazole 5/day x 14 days	**Nystatin** pastilles (200,000 units) 4–5x/day, or 2 (500,000 units) (swish & swallow) qid or 2 (500,000 units) tabs tid for 14 days **OR** **Clotrimazole** 1 troche (10 mg) 5x/day x 14 days.	Maintenance not required in non-AIDS pts. Usually improves in 3–4 days, longer rx ± relapse. Fluconazole-resistant C. krusei fungemia reported in flucon-rx pts (NEJM 325:1315, 1991).
AIDS patient			
Stomatitis, esophagitis Oral colonization with candida correlates with HIV RNA levels in plasma & with CD4 counts (JID 180:534, 1999). HAART has resulted in dramatic ↓ in prevalence of oropharyngeal & esophageal candidiasis & ↓ in refractory disease. See MMWR 53(RR-15):97, 2004.	**Oropharyngeal**, initial episodes (7–14d rx): • **Fluconazole** 100 mg po q24h; OR • **Itraconazole** oral solution 200 mg po q24h; OR + **nystatin** suspension OR + **nystatin** suspension 4–6 mL q6h or 1–2 flavored pastilles 4–5x/day **Esophageal** (14–21d): • **Flucon** 100mg (up to 400mg) po or IV q24h; OR • **Itra** oral solution 200mg po q24h; OR **Caspofungin** 50mg IV q24h; OR **ampho B** 0.3 mg/kg IV q24h or **ampho liposomal** 3–5 mg/kg IV q24h, or **anidulafungin** 100 mg IV day 1 followed by 50 mg per day.	**Fluconazole-refractory oropharyngeal:** • **Itra** oral solution ≥200 mg po q24h; or • **ampho B** suspension 100mg/mL, 1 mL po q6h; or • **ampho B** 0.3 mg/kg IV q24h **Fluconazole-refractory esophageal:** • **Caspofungin** 50 mg IV q24h; or • **vori** 200 mg po or IV q12h; or • **ampho B** 0.3–0.7 mg/kg IV q24h; or **anidulafungin** 100 mg/d or 150 mg IV q24h or **ABLC** 5 mg/kg IV q24h	**Fluconazole-refractory** disease uncommon (4% in ACTG 816) & is seen in pts with low CD4 counts (<50/mm³). **Flu** superior to oral suspension of **nystatin** (CID 24:1204, 1997). **Itra** 100mg po q12h x14d achieved clinical response in 41/74 (55%) pts unresponsive to flu (AIDS Res Hum Retrovir 15:1413, 1999). **Ampho B oral suspension** gave 42.6% response rate in 54 pts refractory to flu, but 70% of those relapsed (AIDS 14:845, 2000). For esophagitis, **caspofungin** as effective as **fluconazole** (CID 33:1447, 2001). **Micafungin** 100 mg or 150 mg IV per day equal to flu 200 mg per day; relapse rates similar: 15 vs 11% (CID 39:842, 2004). **Anidulafungin** 100 mg IV day to flu 100 mg per day in 494 pts: cure rate 97% vs 98.8% (CID 39:770, 2004) but relapse rate higher (53% vs 19%) with anidulafungin.

*Cost = average wholesale price from 2007 RED BOOK, Thomson Healthcare, Inc.

*See page 2 for abbreviations. All dosage recommendations are for adults (unless otherwise indicated) and assume normal renal function

TABLE 11A (5)

TYPE OF INFECTION/ORGANISM/ SITE OF INFECTION	ANTIMICROBIAL AGENTS OF CHOICE		COMMENTS
	PRIMARY	ALTERNATIVE	
Candidiasis/AIDS patient *(continued)*			
Vulvovaginitis Common among healthy young females & unrelated to HIV status.	• **Topical azoles** (clotrimazole, buto, mico, tico, or terconi x3-7d; or • topical **nystatin** 100,000units/day as vaginal tablet x14d; or • oral **itra** 200 mg q12h x1d or 200 mg q24h x3d; or • oral **fluconan** 150 mg x1 dose		
Peritonitis (Chronic Ambulatory Peritoneal Dialysis) *See Table 19, page 185*	**Fluconazole** 400 mg po q24h x 2–3wks; or **caspofungin** 70mg IV on day 1 followed by 50 mg IV q24h for 14 days.	**Ampho B**, continuous IP dosing at 1.5mg/L of dialysis fluid times 4-6wk	Remove cath immediately or if no clinical improvement in 4-7 days. In 1 study, all 8 pts with candida peritonitis who received caspo responded favorably (as compared to 7/8 pts on ampho B) *(NEJM 347:2020, 2002).*
Urinary: Candiduria • Usually colonization of urinary catheter, a benign event • Rarely may be source of dissemination if it has obstructive uropathy or if undergoing urologic manipulation. Then: **fluconazole** Persistent candiduria in immunocompromised pt warrants ultrasound or CT of kidneys	**Remove urinary catheter or stent**. 40% will clear but only 20% if replaced *(CID 30:14, 2000).* Antifungal rx not indicated unless pt has symptoms of UTI, neutropenic, low birth-weight infant, has renal allograft or is undergoing urologic manipulation. Then: **fluconazole** 200 mg per day po or IV times 7–14 days OR **ampho B** 0.5 mg per day IV times 1–14 days.		**Fluconazole** in placebo-controlled trial, candiduria cleared more rapidly in pts treated with flucon 200mg/day x 14 days; 2wk after completion, clearance not different than placebo group *(CID 30:15, 2000).* **Bladder washout** with ampho B not recommended; will not treat upper tract infection. 5FC may be of value in non-albicans UTI but resistance develops rapidly. **Caspofungin** effective in clearing candiduria in 12 pts (most with candidemia) but urine levels low. **NOTE: Void** not in urine in active form.
Vaginitis—Non-AIDS patients. *Review article: MMWR 51 (RR-6), 2002.* (Candida vaginitis in AIDS patients: see Stomatitis, vaginitis above). (See Table 1, page 23)			
Sporadic/infrequent	**Intravaginal**: Multiple **imidazoles**. See footnote¹ **Oral: Fluconazole** 150 mg po x1 OR **itraconazole** 200 mg po bid x 1 day.** For over-the-counter preparations, see footnote¹		**In general, oral & vaginal rx are similarly effective.** Rx aided by avoiding tight clothing, e.g., pantyhose. Oral drugs + rectal candida & may ↓ relapses. **Ampho B** vaginal 50mg suppository effective in non-albicans candida infec when other rx failed *(Am J Ob Gyn 192:2009 & 2012, 2005).*
Chronic recurrent (5–8%) 24 episodes/yr. Ref.: *NEJM 351:876, 2004*	**Fluconazole** 150 mg po q12h times 3 & then 150 mg po q wk	**Itraconazole** 100 mg po q24h times 18 months (or until following 2-day rx with itra)	After 6 mos. > 90% of 170 women free of disease vs 36% of 173 receiving placebo. By 6 mos. rx. 42.9% free of disease vs 21.9% who received placebo (p <0.001). NEJM 351:2554, 2004. Only 76.9% cured 1 mo. following 3-day rx with itra *(Mycoses 48:165, 2005).*
Chromoblastomycosis (*Cladosporium* or *Fonsecaea*); Cutaneous (usually feet, legs): raised scaly lesions, most common in tropical areas	If lesions small & few, **surgical excision or cryosurgery with liquid nitrogen** *(J Am Acad Derm 42:408, 2003).* If lesions chronic, extensive, burrowing: **itraconazole**	**Itraconazole** 200 mg po q24h *(Int J Dermatol 42:408, 2003).* **Fluconazole** experience disappointing	**13/13 patients rx itra responded** *(CID 15:553, 1992).* **Terbinafine**[HDix] impressive in 35 pts rx for 12 mos. (800 mg per day)—86% mycologic cures *(J Derm Treat 9:29, 1998).* In 4 pts resistance to itra developed on rx with 2 clinical failures *(Mycosis 47:216, 2004).* 5/6 responded to **posaconazole** *(Drugs 65:1560, 2005; Rev Inst Med Trop São Paulo 47:339, 2005).*
Coccidioidomycosis (Coccidioidis imnitis) (San Joaquin or Valley Fever); **Pts low risk persistence/complication**	**Antifungal rx not generally recommended.** Treat if fever, wt loss and/or fatigue do not resolve wks to 2 mo (see below)		Uncomplicated pulmonary most common in endemic areas *[Emerg Infect Dis 12:958, 2006]* Influenza-like illness of 1–2wk duration.

See page 2 for abbreviations. All dosage recommendations are for adults (unless otherwise indicated) and assume normal renal function

---

¹ Intravaginal products for candidiasis: **Butoconazole** 2% cream (5gm) q24h at bedtime x 3 days (2 at bedtime x 3 days) or 1% cream (5gm) at bedtime times 7 days (14 days may ↑ cure rate) or 100mg vaginal tab x 7 days; or **miconazole** 200mg vaginal suppos. (1 at bedtime x 3 days)** or 100mg vaginal suppos. q24h x 7 days or 2% cream (5gm) at bedtime x 7 days; or **terconazole** 80mg vaginal tab. (1 at bedtime x 3 days) or 0.4% cream (5gm) or 0.8% cream 5gm intravaginal q24h x 3 days; or **tioconazole** 6.5% vag. ointment x 1 dose**

** = over-the-counter product

See page 2 for abbreviations. All dosage recommendations are for adults (unless otherwise indicated) and assume normal renal function

TABLE 11A (6)

TYPE OF INFECTION/ORGANISM/ SITE OF INFECTION	ANTIMICROBIAL AGENTS OF CHOICE		COMMENTS
	PRIMARY	ALTERNATIVE	
Coccidioidomycosis (continued)			
Primary pulmonary in pts with ↑ risk for complications or dissemination. Rx indicated: • Immunosuppressive disease: AIDS (CID 41:1174, 2005), post-transplantation (Am J Transpl 6:340,2006), hematological malignancies (AJM 165:113, 2005), or therapies (steroids, TNF-α antagonists) (Arth Rheum 50:1959, 2004) • Pregnancy in 3° trimester • Diabetes • Serum CF antibody titer >1:16 • Pulmonary infiltrates • Dissemination (identification of spherules or culture of organism from ulcer, joint effusion, pus from subcutaneous abscess or bone biopsy, etc.)	**Mild to moderate severity:** Itraconazole solution 200 mg po or IV bid OR Fluconazole 400 mg po q24h for 3–12 mo **Locally severe or disseminated disease** Ampho B 0.6–1mg/kg per day x 7 days then 0.8mg/kg every other day or **liposomal ampho B** 3-5 mg/kg/d IV or **ABLC** 5 mg/kg/d IV, until clinical improvement (usually several wks or longer in disseminated disease), followed by **Itra** or **flu** for at least 1 year. Some use combination of Ampho B & Flu for progressive severe disease; controlled series lacking (Mycosis 46:42, 2003). **Consultation with specialist recommended:** surgery may be required.	**Ampho B** IV as for pulmonary (above) + 0.1–0.3 mg daily intra-thecal (intraventricular) via reservoir device. **OR** itra 400–800 mg po q24h **OR voriconazole** (see Comment)	Ampho B cure rate 50–70%. Responses to azoles are similar. Itra may have slight advantage esp. in soft tissue infection. Relapse rates after rx 49%. Relapse rate ↑↑ if CF titer ≥1:256 (RIH = 4.7) (CID 25:1205, 1997). Following CF titers after completion of rx important; rising titers warrant readministration of rx (CID 25: 1271, 1997). In an RDBS of 198 pts with progressive non-meningeal cocci, 57% responded to flu, 72% to itra (p=0.05). (AnIM 133:676, 2000). **Vori** effective in 1 case of widely disseminated cocci (CID 39:e74, 2004). **Caspofungin** successful in a renal transplant pt (CID 39:879, 2004). **Posaconazole** successful in 5/6 pts with refractory non-meningeal cocci (CID 40:1770, 2005) & in 11/16 cases successful reported overall (Drugs 65:1553, 2005).
Meningitis occurs in 1/3 to 1/2 of pts with disseminated coccidioidomycosis			
Adult (CID 42:103, 2006)	Fluconazole 400–1,000 mg po q24h indefinitely	**Ampho B** (po) indefinitely. Dose not established. Itra 400–800 mg po q24h (see Comment)	80% relapse rate, continue flucon indefinitely. Voriconazole successful in high doses (6 mg/kg IV q12h) followed by oral suppression (400 mg po q12h) (CID 36:1619, 2003; AAC 48: 2341, 2004). Caspofungin also used (JAC 54:292, 2004) & failed in another case (CID 39:879, 2004).
Child	Fluconazole (po) indefinitely, 6 mg/kg per day po (Pediatric dose not established)		
Cryptococcosis (IDSA Guideline, CID 30:710, 2000). Excellent review. Brit Med Bull 72:99, 2005 **Non-meningitis (non-AIDS)** Risk 57% in organ transplant (Transpl Inf Dis 4:183, 2002 & 7:26, 2005) & those receiving other forms of immunosuppressive agents (alemtuzumab—Transplant Proc 37:934, 2005 & adalimumab: EID 13:953, 2007).	**Fluconazole** 200–400 mg solution q24h for 6–12 mo OR **Itraconazole** (po) 200 mg q24h for 8 wk to 6 mo **For more severe disease:** **Ampho B** 0.5–0.8mg/kg per day IV or IV until course then change to **Fluconazole** 400 mg po q24h for 8–10 wk course	**Itraconazole** 200 mg po q24h for 6–12 mo OR **Ampho B** 0.3 mg/kg per day IV + flucytosine 37.5 mg/kg po qid times 6 wk	**Flucon alone 90% effective for meningeal and non-meningeal forms.** Fluconazole as effective as ampho B (CID 32:E145, 2001). Addition of **interferon**-γ (IFN-γ-1b 50 mcg per M² subcut. 3x per wk x 9wk) to liposomal ampho B assoc. with response in pt failing antifungal rx (CID 38: 910, 2004). Posaconazole 400-800 mg also effective in a small series of patients (CID 45:562, 2007; Chest 132:952, 2007).
Meningitis (non-AIDS)	**Ampho B** 0.5–0.8 mg/kg per day IV + **flucytosine** 37.5 mg/kg² po q6h until pt afebrile & cultures neg (~6 wk) (NEJM 301:126, 1979) then stop ampho B/flucyt, start **fluconazole** 200 mg po q24h (NEJM 113:183, 1990) **OR** **Fluconazole** 400 mg po q24h x 8–10wk (less severely ill pt). Some recommend flu for 2 yr to reduce chance of relapse.		CSF opening pressure >250mm H₂O: repeat LPs to drain fluid to control pressure. Outbreaks of C. gattii meningitis have been reported in the Pacific Northwest (Emerg Infect Dis. 13:42, 2007); severity of disease and prognosis appear to be worse than with C. neoformans; initial therapy with ampho B + flucytosine recommended

---

¹ Some experts would reduce to 25 mg per kg q6h

See page 2 for abbreviations. All dosage recommendations are for adults (unless otherwise indicated) and assume normal renal function

TABLE 11A (7)

TYPE OF INFECTION/ORGANISM/ SITE OF INFECTION	ANTIMICROBIAL AGENTS OF CHOICE		COMMENTS
	PRIMARY	ALTERNATIVE	
Cryptococcosis (continued)			
HIV/AIDS: Cryptococcemia and/or Meningitis			
Treatment (see CID 30:710, 2000 & Table 11) Cryptococcus in blood may be manifest by positive blood culture or positive test in serum for cryptococcal antigen (CRAG, >95% sens.), no help in monitoring therapy. With HAART, symptoms of acute meningitis may return: Immune reconstitution Syndrome (see Table 14D). † CSF pressure (>25cm H₂O) associated with high mortality, lower with CSF removal (CID 30:47, 2000). If frequent LPs not possible, ventriculostomy or shunts an option (Surg Neurol 63:529 & 531, 2005).	**[Ampho B 0.7 mg/kg IV q24h + flucytosine 25 mg/kg po q6h]×2 wks** or **Liposomal amphotericin B** 6 mg/kg IV q24h + flucytosine 25 mg/kg po q6h ×2 wks See Comment. **Then** **Consolidation therapy: Fluconazole** 400 mg po q24h to complete a 10-wk course or until CSF culture sterile, then suppression (see below). Start Highly Active Antiretroviral Therapy (HAART) if possible.	**[Fluconazole 400–800 mg/day po or IV for less severe disease** or **Fluconazole 400–800 mg/day po or IV + flucytosine 25 mg/kg po q6h ×4–6 wks** **Itraconazole** 200mg q12h po [If CD4 count rises to >100/mm³ with effective antiretroviral rx some authorities recommend dc suppressive rx. See www.hivatis.org. Authors would only dc if CSF culture negative.]	Early fungicidal activity in CSF greater with Ampho B than fluconazole (Ln 363:1764, 2004). Ampho B + 5FC treatment: 29/236 pts died within 1st 2 wks & 62 (26%) by 10wks; only 129 (55%) were alive & culture-neg. at 10wks (CID 28:82, 1999). In 64 pts, ampho + 5FC↓ crypto CFUs more rapidly than ampho + flu or combination of 3 drugs (p <0.001) (Ln 363:1764, 2004). Monitor 5-FC levels: peak 70–80 mg/L, trough 30–40 mg/L. Higher levels assoc. with bone marrow toxicity. Increased toxicity with concomitant LAB. If normal mental status, >20 cells/mm³ CSF, & CSF crypto antigen <1:1024, flucon alone is reasonable (CID 22:322, 1996). Successful outcomes were observed in 14/29 (48%) subjects with cryptococcal meningitis treated with posaconazole (CID 56:745, 2005). Voriconazole effective in 7 of 18 but relapsed disease in 10 more (SJID 36:1122, 2004). Itraconazole not as effective as fluconazole, 13/51 (25%) pts relapsed vs 2/51 (4%) receiving fluconazole (p = 0.006) (CID 28:291, 1999); at doses of 600 mg/day = flu as consolidation rx in 35 pts in Thai (J Med Assoc Thai 86:293, 2003). No recurrences of crypto meningitis in 22 pts who dc flu suppression with >100 CD4 & undetectable VL ×3 mos. (CID 36:1329, 2003) & 1.53 relapses/100 person-years (CID 38:565, 2004).
Suppression (chronic maintenance Therapy) Discontinuation of antifungal rx can be considered in patients who remain asymptomatic, with CD4 >100–200/mm³ for ≥6 months. Some recommend a lumbar puncture before discontinuation of maintenance rx. Reappearance of pos. serum CRAG may predict relapse.	**Fluconazole** 200 mg po q24h or **Itraconazole** 200 mg po bid	**Itraconazole** 200mg q12h po if flu intolerant or failure	
Dermatophytosis (See Superficial fungal infections, CID 38:1173, 2004)			**Toenail Rx Options:** **Terbinafine** 250 mg po q24h [children <20kg, 67.5 mg/day, 20–40 kg, 125 mg/day; >40 kg 250 mg/day] × 12 wks (76% effective) OR **Itraconazole** 200 mg po q24h ×3 mo. (59% effective) OR **Fluconazole** 150–300 mg po q wk × 6–12 mo (48% effective)[NEJSAJ [Data reflect cure rates from meta-analysis of all randomized controlled trials (Brit J Derm 150:537, 2004)] All agents with similar cure rates (60–100%) in clinical studies (Ped Derm 17:304, 2000). Addition of topical ketoconazole or selenium sulfate shampoo reduces transmissibility of T. tonsurans (J Dermatol 39:261, 2000).
Onychomycosis (Tinea unguium) (Derm Ther 17:517, 2004; Cutis 74:5,6, 2004) Topical nail lacquer (ciclopirox) approved but cure in only 5–9% after 48 wks (Med Lett 42:51, 2000) but † to 50% cure in another study (Cutis 73:81, 2004). May enhance oral rx (Cutis 74:55, 2004). Terbinafine appears to be the most cost-effective rx (Manag Care Interface 18:55, 2005). Overall cure rate from 18 randomized control trials, 76% (J DrugsDerm 4:302, 2005)	**Fingernail Rx Options:** **Terbinafine** 250 mg po q24h [children <20 kg, 67.5 mg/day, 20–40 kg, 125 mg/day, >40 kg 250 mg/day] × 6 wk (79% effective) OR **Itraconazole** 200 mg po q24h × 3 mo [NEJSAJ, or **Itraconazole** 200 mg po bid × 1 wk/mo × 2 mo. **Fluconazole** 150–300 mg po q wk × 3–6 mo. [NEJSAJ **NOTE:** For side-effects, see footnotes; see drug analysis in AJM 120:791, 2007: risk of stopping therapy due to adverse event varied between 2–6% with specific drug & drug regimen.		
Tinea capitis ("ringworm") (Trichophyton tonsurans; Microsporum canis; N. America; other sp. elsewhere) (PIDJ 18:191, 1999)	**Terbinafine** 250 mg po q24h × [for children <20 kg 62.5 mg] 4 wk for T. tonsurans, 4–8 wk for 30 days[NEJSAJ Children 125 mg, or 6–12mg/kg per day (up to 800 mg) (COID 17:97, 2004; Exp Opin Pharm Ther 5:219, 2004).	**Itraconazole** 3–5 mg/kg per day for 30 days[NEJSAJ **Fluconazole** 8 mg/kg q wk × 8–12 wks. Cap at 150 mg q wk **Griseofulvin**: adults 500 mg q24h × 4 wks, children 10–20 mg/ kg per day until hair regrows 6–8 wk.	

¹ Flucytosine = 5-FC

² **Serious but rare cases of hepatic failure** have been reported in pts receiving terbinafine & should not be used in those with chronic or active liver disease.

³ Use of itraconazole tabs has been associated with myocardial depression and with onset of congestive heart failure (see Ln 357:1766, 2001).

See page 2 for abbreviations. All dosage recommendations are for adults (unless otherwise indicated) and assume normal renal function

TABLE 11A (8)

TYPE OF INFECTION/ORGANISM/ SITE OF INFECTION	ANTIMICROBIAL AGENTS OF CHOICE		COMMENTS
	PRIMARY	ALTERNATIVE	
Dermatophytosis (continued)			
Tinea corporis, cruris, or pedis (Trichophyton rubrum, T. mentagrophytes, Epidermophyton floccosum) "Athlete's foot, jock itch," and ringworm	**Topical rx:** Generally applied 2x/day. Available as creams, ointments, sprays, by prescription & over the counter.¹ Apply 2x/day for 2–3wks. **See footnote¹ for names & prices.** Recommend: Lotrimin Ultra or (with AT; contain butenafine and terbinafine—both are fungicidal	**Terbinafine** 250 mg po q24h x 2 wks^NF/OL OR **ketoconazole** 200 mg po q24h x 4 wks OR **fluconazole** 200 mg po once/wk. for 2–4 wks^NF/OL. **Griseofulvin** adults 500 mg q24h times 4–6 wks, children 10–20 mg/kg per day. Duration: 2–4 wks for corporis, 4–8 wks for pedis.	**Keto** po often effective in severe recalcitrant infection. Follow for hepatotoxicity; many drug-drug interactions. **Terbinafine** 87% achieved mycological cure in double-blind study (32 pts) (J Med Assn Thai 76:388, 1993; Brit J Derm 130(543):22, 1994) and fluconazole 78% (J Am Acad Derm 40:S31, 1999).
Tinea versicolor (Malassezia furfur or Pityrosporum orbiculare) Rule out erythrasma—see Table 1, page 49	**Ketoconazole** (400 mg single dose)^NF/OL or (200 mg q24h x 7 days) or (2% cream 1x q24h x 2wks)	**Fluconazole** 400 mg po single dose or **itraconazole** 400 mg po q24h x 3–7 days	**Keto** (po) times 1 dose was 97% effective in 1 study. Another alternative: **Selenium sulfide** (Selsun). 2.5% lotion, apply as lather, leave on 10min then wash off, 1/day x 7 day or 3–5/wk times 2–4wks
Fusariosis Infections in eye, skin, sinus & disseminated diseases—especially in bone marrow transplant pts.	**Voriconazole** 6 mg/kg IV q12h on day 1, then either (4 mg/kg IV q12h) or (200 mg po q12h for body weight ≥40 kg, 100 mg po q12h for body weight <40 kg)	**Ampho B** 1–1.2 mg/kg or **ABLC** 5 mg/kg/d IV or **LAB** 3–5 mg/kg/d IV or **Posa** 400 mg po bid with meals (if not taking meals, 200 mg po qid).	Voriconazole successful in 50% (CID 36:1122, 2003). Posaconazole 800 mg/d in divided doses was effective in 50% in 20 pts who failed Ampho B and 67% that recovered from myelosuppression (CID 42:1398, 2006)
Histoplasmosis (Histoplasma capsulatum): See IDSA Guideline: CID 45:807, 2007 Best diagnostic test is urinary, serum, or CSF histoplasma antigen, MiraVista Diagnostics (1-866-647-2847).			
Acute pulmonary histoplasmosis	**Mild to moderate disease, symptoms <4 wk:** No rx. If symptoms last over one month: **Itraconazole** 200 mg po tid for 3 days then once or twice daily for 6–12 wk. **Moderately severe or severe: Liposomal ampho B**, 3–5 mg/kg/d or **ABLC** 5 mg/kg/d IV or ampho B 0.7–1.0 mg/kg/d for 1–2 wk, then Itra 200 mg tid for 3 days, then bid for 12 wk + **methylprednisolone** 0.5–1.0 mg/kg/d for 1–2 wk.		Ampho B for patients at low risk of nephrotoxicity first.
Chronic cavitary pulmonary histoplasmosis	**Itra** 200 mg tid for 3 days then once or twice daily for at least 12 mo (some prefer 18–24 mo)		Document therapeutic itraconazole blood levels at 2 wk.¹ Relapses occur in 9–15% of patients.
Mediastinal lymphadenitis, mediastinal granuloma, pericarditis; and rheumatologic syndromes	If no response to non-steroidals, **Prednisone** 0.5–1.0 mg/kg/d tapered over 1–2 weeks for 1) pericarditis with hemodynamic compromise, 2) lymphadenitis with obstruction or compression syndromes, or 3) severe rheumatologic syndromes. **Mild cases:** Antifungal therapy not indicated. Nonsteroidal anti-inflammatory drug for pericarditis or rheumatologic syndromes. **Itra** 200 mg po once or twice daily for 6–12 wk for moderately severe to severe cases, or if prednisone is administered.		Check itra blood levels to document therapeutic concentrations.

---

¹ Drug name (trade name) & wholesale price for 15 gm. All are applied to affected area bid. **Prescription drugs:** butenafine (Mentax) $42, ciclopirox (Loprox) $46, clotrimazole (Lotrimin $19, Mycelex $13), econazole (Spectazole) $26, ketoconazole (Nizoral) $20, miconazole (Monistat-Derm) $17, naftifine (Naftin) $31, oxiconazole (Oxistat) $32, terconazole (Terazol) $50, sertaconazole (Ertaczo) $30. **Non-prescription (over-the-counter):** Tolnaftate (Tinactin $6), Ting or Tolnate $2), undecylenic acid (Cruex $5, Desenex $5), Lotrimin AF 1% 12 gm $6.80, Lamisil AF 1% 12 gm $8.15.

See page 2 for abbreviations. All dosage recommendations are for adults (unless otherwise indicated) and assume normal renal function

TABLE 11A (9)

TYPE OF INFECTION/ORGANISM/ SITE OF INFECTION	ANTIMICROBIAL AGENTS OF CHOICE		COMMENTS
	PRIMARY	ALTERNATIVE	
Histoplasmosis (Histoplasma capsulatum) *(continued)*			
Progressive disseminated histoplasmosis	**Mild to moderate disease:** Itra 200 mg po bid for 3 days then bid for at least 12 mo		**Ampho B** 0.7-1.0 mg/kg/d may be used for patients at low risk of nephrotoxicity. Confirm therapeutic Itra blood levels. Azoles are teratogenic; Itra should be avoided in pregnancy; use a lipid ampho formulation. Urinary antigen levels useful for monitoring response to therapy and relapse
	Moderately severe disease: Liposomal ampho B, 3 mg/kg/d or ABLC 5 mg/kg/d for 1-2 weeks then **Itra** 200 mg bid for 3 days, then bid for at least 12 mo. **Liposomal ampho B,** 5 mg/kg/d, for a total of 175 mg/kg over 4-6 wk, then **Itra** 200 mg 2-3x a day for at least 12 mo		
CNS histoplasmosis	**Itra** 200 mg daily		Monitor CNS histo antigen, monitor Itra blood levels.
Prophylaxis	**Itra** 200 mg po daily		Consider primary **prophylaxis in HIV-infected** patients with < 150 CD4 cells/mm³ in high prevalence areas. Secondary prophylaxis (i.e. suppressive therapy) indicated in HIV-infected patients with < 150 CD4 cells/mm³ and other immunosuppression cannot be reversed
Madura foot *(See Nocardia & Scedosporium, below)*			
Mucormycosis & other Zygomycosis—Rhizopus, Rhizomucor, Absidia, (CID 41:521, 2005) Rhinocerebral, pulmonary, cutaneous, disseminated (CID 41:634, 2005; J Clin Microbiol Infect Dis 25:215, 2006 Key to successful rx: early dx with symptoms suggestive of sinusitis (or lateral facial pain or numbness): think mucor with palatal ulcers, &/or black eschars, onset unilateral blindness in immunocompromised or diabetic pt (J Otolaryn 34:166, 2005). Rapidly fatal without rx. Dx by culture of tissue or stain: wide ribbon-like, non-septated with variation in diameter & right angle branching (Comform Infect 12:7, 2005).	**Lipid-based Ampho B OR Ampho B:** Increase rapidly to 0.8-1.5 mg/kg per day IV; when improving, then every other day. Total dose usually 2.5-3 gm.	Posaconazole 400 mg po bid with meals (if not taking meals, 200 mg qid)	Cure dependent on: (1) surgical debridement, (2) rx of hyperglycemia, correction of neutropenia, or reduction in immunosuppression. (3) antifungal rx: liposomal amphotericin (J Clin Micro 43:2012, 2005) longterm rx **posaconazole**—striking improvement reported, 54-70% overall success in refractory zygomycosis vs 25% or less with amphotericin or lipid-based ampho B (Drugs 65:1553, 2005) and 19 of 24 successful, 11 with rhinocerebral (AAC 50:126, 2006). Prolonged use of Voriconazole predisposes to zygomycetes infections, all resistant to vori. (Lancet ID 5:594, 2005)
Nocardiosis (N. asteroides & N brasiliensis) Culture & sensitivity cases: Reference Labs, R.J. Wallace (903) 877-7680 or CDC (404) 639-3158 (IDCP 8:27, 1999)			
Cutaneous and lymphocutaneous (sporotrichoid)	**TMP-SMX** 5-10 mg/kg per day of TMP & 25-50 mg/kg per day of SMX in 2-4 div. doses/day, po or IV	**Sulfisoxazole** 2 gm po qid or **minocycline** 100-200 mg po bid	Survival improved when sulfa-containing regimen used (Medicine 68:38, 1999). **Prosthetic valve endocarditis** with N. asteroides cured with IMP + amikacin times 2mo followed by TMP-SMX times 4 mos. (AJM 115:330, 2003)
Pulmonary, disseminated, brain abscess Duration of rx generally 3mo for immunocompetent host (38%) & 6mos for immunocompromised (62% organ transplant, malignancy, chronic lung disease, diabetes, ETOH use, steroid rx), AIDS, & infliximab rx (Canad Med J 171:1063, 2004)	**TMP-SMX** Initially 15 mg/kg per day of TMP & 75 mg/kg per day of SMX IV q 6h, div. in 2-4 doses. After 3-4 wk, ↓ dose to 10 mg/kg per day TMP in 2-4 doses po. Do serum level *(see Comment)*	**IMP** 500 mg IV q6h) + (**amikacin** 7.5mg/kg IV q12h) times 3-4wk & then po regimen	Measure sulfonamide blood levels: Peak of 100-150mcg/mL 2hrs post-po dose. Increasing sulfa resistance; recommend sensitivity testing (Eur J Clin Micro Inf Dis 24:142, 2005; AAC 48:832, 2004). Linezolid 600mg po bid appears also to be effective (Ann Pharmacother 41:1694, 2007)

See page 2 for abbreviations. All dosage recommendations are for adults (unless otherwise indicated) and assume normal renal function

TABLE 11A (10)

TYPE OF INFECTION/ORGANISM/ SITE OF INFECTION	ANTIMICROBIAL AGENTS OF CHOICE		COMMENTS
	PRIMARY	ALTERNATIVE	
Nocardiosis (N. asteroides & N. brasiliensis) (continued)			
Paracoccidioidomycosis (South American blastomycosis)/ P. brasiliensis	**Itraconazole** 200 mg/day po x 6 mo or **Ketoconazole** 400 mg/day po for 6–18 mo	**Ampho B** 0.4–0.5mg/kg per day IV to total dose of 1.5–2.5gm or **sulfonamides** (dose: see Comment)	Improvement in >90% pts on itra or keto.[MCM4] **Sulfa** 4–6gm/day for > 6 wk, then 500mg/day for 3–5yr also used (CID 14 (Suppl.):S-68, 1992). Low-dose itra (50–100mg/day), keto (200-400mg/day) & sulfadiazine (up to 6g/day) showed similar clinical responses in 4–6mo in a randomized study (Med Mycol 40: 411, 2002). HIV+: TMP-SMX suppressive rx indefinitely (CID 21:1275, 1995).
Lobomycosis (keloidal blastomycosis)/ P. loboi	**Surgical excision**. clofazimine or ampho B		
Penicilliosis (Penicillium marneffei). Common disseminated fungal infection in AIDS pts in SE Asia (esp. Thailand & Vietnam).	**Ampho B** 0.5–1 mg/kg per day times 2 wks followed by **itraconazole** 400 mg/day for 10 wks followed by 200 mg/day po **indefinitely for HIV-infected pts** (CID 26:1107, 1998). See Comment	For less sick patients **itra** 200 mg po bid x 3 days, then 200 mg po bid x 12 wks, then 200 mg po q24-h. (IV if unable to take po)	3rd most common OI in AIDS pts in SE Asia following TBc and cryptococcal meningitis. Prolonged fever, lymphadenopathy, hepatomegaly. Skin nodules are umbilicated (mimic cryptococcal infection or molluscum contagiosum). In AIDS pts, suppression with itra effective in **preventing relapses** (NEJM 339:1739, 1998). Preliminary data suggests vori effective. CID 43:1060, 2006.
Phaeohyphomycosis, Black molds, Dematiaceous fungi (See CID 41:521, 2005, CID 43:S3, 2006) Sinuses, skin, bone & joint, brain abscess, endocarditis, emerging especially in HSCT pts with disseminated disease.	**Surgery + itraconazole** 400 mg/day po, duration not defined, probably IV.[MCM4]	Case report of success with **voriconazole + terbinafine** (Scand J Infect Dis 39:87, 2007). OR **Itraconazole + terbinafine** synergistic against S. prolificans (AAC 44:470, 2000). No clinical data & combination could show ↑ toxicity (see Table 11B, page 105)	**Posaconazole** successful in case of brain abscess (CID 34:1648, 2002). Accounted for 10% of mycelial infections post-transplant (CID 37:221, 2003).
Scedosporium prolificans: Bipolaris, Wangiella, Curvularia, Exophiala, Phialemonium, Scytalidium, Alternaria			**Notoriously resistant to antifungal rx including amphotericin & azoles (CID 34:909, 2002). Mortality >80%.**
Scedosporium apiospermum (Pseudallescheria boydii) (not considered a true dematiaceous mold) (Medicine 81:333, 2002). Skin, subcut (Madura foot), brain abscess, recurrent meningitis. May appear after near-drowning incidents. Also emerging especially in hematopoietic stem cell transplant (HSCT) pts with disseminated disease	**Voriconazole** 6 mg/kg IV q12h on day 1, then either (4 mg/kg IV q12h or 200 mg po q12h for body weight ≥40 kg, but 100 mg po q12h for body weight <40 kg) (PIDJ 21:240, 2002)	Surgery + **itraconazole** 200 mg po bid until clinically well.[MCM4][MCM3] (Many have no resistant or refractory to itra) OR **Posa** 400 mg po bid with meals (if not taking meals, 200 mg po qid)	**Resistant to many antifungal drugs including amphotericin.** In vitro voriconazole more active than itra (J Clin Micro 39: 954, 2001). Case reports of successful rx of disseminated and CNS disease with voriconazole (Clin Micro Inf 9:750, 2003; EJCMID 22:408, 2003) but only 3 of 10 successful in one study (CID 36:1122, 2006). Posaconazole active in vitro and successful in several case reports.

1 **Oral solution preferred to tablets because of ↑ absorption** (see Table 11B, page 105).

See page 2 for abbreviations. All dosage recommendations are for adults (unless otherwise indicated) and assume normal renal function

104

TABLE 11A (11)

TYPE OF INFECTION/ORGANISM/ SITE OF INFECTION	ANTIMICROBIAL AGENTS OF CHOICE		COMMENTS
	PRIMARY	ALTERNATIVE	
Sporotrichosis *IDSA Guideline: CID 45:1255, 2007*			
Cutaneous/Lymphocutaneous	Itraconazole po 200 mg/day for 2-4 wks after all lesions resolved, usually 3-6 mos.	If no response, **itra** 200 mg po bid or **terbinafine** 500 mg po bid or **SSKI** 5 drops (eye drops) tid & increase to 40-50 drops tid	Fluconazole 400-800 mg daily only if no response to primary or alternative suggestions. *Pregnancy or nursing:* local hyperthermia (see below).
Osteoarticular	**itra** 200 mg po bid x 12 mos.	**Liposomal ampho B** 3-5 mg/kg/d IV or **ABLC** 5 mg/kg/d IV or **ampho B deoxycholate** 0.7-1 mg/kg/d IV daily, if response, change to **itra** 200 mg po bid x total 12 mos.	After 2 wks of therapy, document adequate serum levels of itraconazole.
Pulmonary	If severe, **lipid ampho B** 3-5 mg/kg IV or **standard ampho B** 0.7-1 mg/kg IV once daily until response, then **itra** 200 mg po bid. Total of 12 mos.	Less severe: **itraconazole** 200 mg po bid x 12 mos.	After 2 weeks of therapy document adequate serum levels of itra. Surgical resection plus ampho B for localized pulmonary disease.
Meningeal or Disseminated	**Lipid ampho B** 5 mg/kg IV once daily x 4-6 wks, then—if better—**itra** 200 mg po bid for total of 12 mos.	AIDS/Other immunosuppressed pts: chronic therapy with **itra** 200 mg po once daily.	After 2 weeks, document adequate serum levels of itra.
Pregnancy and children	**Pregnancy:** Cutaneous—local hyperthermia. Severe: **lipid ampho B** 3-5 mg/kg IV once daily. **Avoid itraconazole**.	**Children:** Cutaneous: **itra** 6-10 mg/kg (max of 400 mg) daily. Alternative is **SSKI** 1 drop tid increasing to max of 1 drop/kg or 40-50 drops tid/day, whichever is lowest.	For children with disseminated sporotrichosis: Standard ampho B 0.7 mg/kg IV once daily & after response, itra 6-10 mg/kg (max 400 mg) once daily.

See page 2 for abbreviations. All dosage recommendations are for adults (unless otherwise indicated) and assume normal renal function

TABLE 11B – ANTIFUNGAL DRUGS: ADVERSE EFFECTS, COMMENTS, COST

DRUG NAME, GENERIC (TRADE/USUAL DOSAGE/COST)*	ADVERSE EFFECTS/COMMENTS
Non-lipid amphotericin B deoxycholate¹: 0.3–1mg/kg per day as single infusion 50mg $11.64 Mixing ampho B with lipid emulsion results in precipitation and is discouraged (Am J Hlth Pharm 52:1463, 1995)	**Admin:** Ampho B is a colloidal suspension that must be prepared in electrolyte-free D5W at 0.1mg/mL to avoid precipitation. No need to protect suspensions from light. Infusions cause chills/fever, myalgia, anorexia, nausea, rarely hemodynamic collapse/hypotension. Postulated that to proinflammatory cytokines, doesn't appear to be histamine release (Pharmacol 23:966, 2003). Manufacturer recommends test dose of 1mg, but often not done (1ˢᵗ few mL of 1ˢᵗ dose is test). Infusion duration usu. 4+ hrs. No difference found in 1 vs 4 hr infus. (AAC 34:1402, 1992) except chills/fever occurred sooner with 1hr infus. Febrile reactions ↓ with repeat doses. Rare pulmonary reactions (severe dyspnea & focal infiltrates suggest pulmonary edema) assoc with rapid infus (CID 33:75, 2001). Many side effects (see below) can be ameliorated with: **pre-treatment:** diphenhydramine, hydrocortisone (25–50mg) and heparin (1000 units) had no influence on rigors/fever (CID 70:755, 1995). Cytokine postulated in e.g. NSAIDs, cannabinoids may prove efficacious but have risk. **Toxicity:** Major concern is nephrotoxicity (15% of 102 pts surveyed, CID 26:334, 1998). Manifest initially by kaliuresis and hypokalemia, then fall in serum bicarbonate (may proceed to renal tubular acidosis),↓ in renal erythropoietin and anemia, and rising BUN/serum creatinine. Hypomagnesemia may occur. Can reduce risk of renal injury by **(a) pre- & post-infusion hydration with 500mL saline (if clinical status allows salt load). (b)** avoidance of other nephrotoxins, eg, radiocontrast, aminoglycosides, cis-platinum, (c) Use of lipid prep of amphotericin B. Use of low-dose dopamine did not significantly ↓ renal toxicity (AAC 42:1103, 1998). In single randomized controlled trial of 80 neutropenic pts with refractory fever & suspected or proven invasive fungal infection, 0.97mg/kg per day ampho **continuously infused over 24hr period** compared to classic **rapid infusion** of 0.95mg/kg/day, **infused over 4hr**. Continuous infusion produced less nephrotoxicity (28% vs 15% respectively). ↓ in fever, chills & vomiting (p <0.02–0.0003) & appeared as effective as rapid infusion but in very few proven fungal infections (BMJ 322:1, 2001). Continuous infusion allows a dramatic: ↑ in administered dosage without sig. toxicity (CID 36:943, 2003). It is disturbing that these exciting observations have not led to controlled trials examining efficacy in rx of life-threatening fungal infections (CID 36:1213, 2003). Await trials of efficacy in larger number of proven fungal infections!
Lipid-based ampho B products¹: Amphotericin B lipid complex (ABLC) (Abelcet): 5 mg/kg per day as single infusion 100 mg $240	**Admin:** Consists of ampho B complexed w/2 lipid bilayer ribbons. Compared to standard ampho B, larger volume of distribution, rapid blood clearance and high tissue concentrations (liver, spleen, lung). Dosage: **5mg/kg once daily.** infuse at 2.5mg/kg per hr; adult and ped. dose the same. Do NOT use an in-line filter. Do not dilute with saline or mix with other drugs or electrolytes.³ **Toxicity:** Fever and chills in 18%, nausea 9%, vomiting 8%, serum creatinine ↑ in 11%, renal failure 5%, anemia 4%, ↓ K 5%; rash 4%. A fatal case of fat embolism reported following ABLC infusion (Exp Mol Path 177:246, 2004).
Liposomal amphotericin B (LAB, AmBisome): 1–5 mg/kg per day as single infusion. 50 mg $188	**Admin:** Consists of vesicular bilayer liposome with ampho B intercalated within the membrane. Dosage: **3–5mg/kg per day** iv as single dose infused over a period of approx. 120min. If well tolerated, infusion time can be reduced to 60min. (see footnote 2, page 105). Tolerated well in elderly pts (J Inf 50:277, 2005). **Toxicity:** Gen less than ampho B. Nephrotoxic 18.7% vs 33.7% for ampho B, chills 47% vs 75%, nausea 39.7% vs 38.7%, vomiting 31.8% vs 43.9%, rash 24% for both, ↓ Ca 18.4% vs 20.9%, ↓ K 20.4% vs 25.6%, ↓ Mg 20.4% vs 25.6%. Acute infusion-related reactions common with liposomal ampho B, 20–40%. 86% occur within 5min of infusion, incl chest pain, dyspnea, hypoxia or severe abdom, flank or leg pain; 14% dev flushing & urticaria near end of 4hr infusion. All responded to diphenhydramine (1mg/kg) & interruption of infusion. Reactions may be due to complement activation by liposome (CID 36:1213, 2003).

¹ Published data from trials of pts intolerant of or refractory to conventional ampho B deoxycholate (Amp B.d). **None of the lipid ampho B preps has shown superior efficacy compared to ampho B in prospective trials (except liposomal ampho B was more effective vs ampho B in rx of disseminated histoplasmosis)** (AnIM 137:105, 2002; CID 37:415, 2003). **Dosage equivalency has not been established** (CID 36:1500, 2003). Nephrotoxicity ↓ with all lipid ampho B preps (NEJM 340:764, 1999).

² Decreased differences between Abelcet and Ambisome: toxicity (rigors) & febrile episodes with Abelcet (70% vs 36%) but higher frequency of mild hepatic toxicity with AmBisome (59% vs 38%, p=0.05). Mild elevations in serum creatinine were observed in 1/3 of both (BJ Hemat 103:198, 1998; Focus on Fungal Int #9, 1999; Bone Marrow Tx 20:39, 1997; CID 26:1383, 1998)

* From 2007 Red Book, Thomson Healthcare, Inc. Price is **average wholesale price (AWP)**.
See page 2 for abbreviations. All dosage recommendations are for adults (unless otherwise indicated) and assume normal renal function

TABLE 11B (2)

DRUG NAME, GENERIC (TRADE)/USUAL DOSAGE/COST*	ADVERSE EFFECTS/COMMENTS
Amphotericin B cholesteryl complex (amphotericin B colloidal dispersion, ABCD, Amphotec): 3–4mg/kg per day as single infusion 100 mg $93	**Admin:** Consists of ampho B deoxycholate stabilized with cholesteryl sulfate resulting in a disc-shaped colloidal complex. Compared to standard ampho B, larger volume of distribution, rapid blood clearance, high tissue concentrations. Dosage: Initial dose for adults & children: **3–4mg/kg per day.** If necessary, can ↑ to 6mg/kg day. Infuse in D5W & infuse at 1mg/kg per hr. Do NOT use in-line filter. **Toxicity:** Fever 33%, chills 50%, fever 33%, serum creatinine 12–20% & ↓K 17%. Hepatotoxicity more common (incidence 1.5) than other continuing rx ampho B (inc. 0.78/100 pt days) *(CID 41:1301, 2005)* & ↑ with continuing rx.
Caspofungin (Cancidas) 70 mg IV on day 1 followed by 50 mg IV q24hr (reduce to 35 mg IV q24hr with moderate hepatic insufficiency) 70 mg $395; 50 mg $395	An echinocandin which inhibits synthesis of β-(1,3)-D-glucan. Fungicidal against candida (MIC <2mcg/mL), including those resistant to other antifungals & active against aspergillus (MIC 0.4-2.7mcg/mL). In some preclinical studies may have high drug concentrations found less effective *(AAC 48:3407, 2004)*, but has not been demonstrated clinically. Approved indications for caspo incl: empirical rx for febrile, neutropenic pts; rx of candidemia, candida intraabdominal abscesses, peritonitis, & pleural space infections; esophageal candidiasis, & invasive aspergillosis in pts refractory to or intolerant of other therapies. Serum conc. not affected by rifampin. Approved as 1st-line rx for candidemia *(NEJM 347:2020, 2002; NEJM Dial Transplant, July 5, 2005)*. Only 2% of 263 pts in double-blind trial dc drug due to drug-related adverse event *(transpl Inf Dis 7:25, 2002)*. 14% had ↑ transaminases (similar to triazoles). Most common adverse effect: pruritus at infusion site & headache, fever, chills, vomiting, & diarrhea assoc with ampho B rx *(CID Oct. 12, 2005, online)*. For caspo vs 21% short-course ampho B in 422 pts with candidemia ↑ serum creatinine in 8% on caspo vs 21%. Most common adverse effect: pruritus at infusion site. Drug metab in liver & dosage ↓ to 35mg in moderate to severe hepatic failure. Class C for preg (embryotoxic in rats & rabbits). See Table 22, page 198 for drug-drug interactions, esp. cyclosporine (hepatic toxicity) & tacrolimus (drug level monitoring recommended). Reversible thrombocytopenia reported *(Pharmacother 24:1408, 2004)*.
Micafungin (Mycamine) 50 mg/day for prophylaxis post-bone marrow stem cell trans., 100 mg candidemia, 150 mg candida esophagitis: 50 mg $112	The 2nd echinocandin approved by FDA *(Mar 2005)* for rx of esophageal candidiasis & prophylaxis against candida infections in HSCT recipients *(CID 39:1407, 2004)*. Active against most strains of candida sp. & aspergillus sp. incl those resist to fluconazole such as C. glabrata & C. krusei. No antagonism seen when combo with other antifungal drugs & occ. synergism with ampho B *(AAC 49:2994, 2005)*. No dosage adjust for severe renal failure or moderate hepatic impairment. Watch for drug-drug interactions with sirolimus or nifedipine. Most common adverse events incl nausea 2.8%, vomiting 2.4%, & headache 2.4%. Transient ↑ LFTs, BUN, creatinine reported: rare cases of significant hepatitis & renal insufficiency. See *CID 42:1171, 2006*
Anidulafungin (Eraxis) For Candidemia, 200 mg IV on day 1 followed by 100 mg/day (slow IV); Rx forEC: 100 mg IV x 1, then 50 mg/day IV (slow IV) 50 mg/vial NB $112	An echinocandin with antifungal activity (cidal) against candida sp. & aspergillus sp. including ampho B & triazole-resistant strains. FDA approved for treatment of esophageal candidiasis (EC), candidemia, and other complicated Candida infections. Effective in clinical trials of esophageal candidiasis & in 1 trial was superior to fluconazole in rx of invasive candidemia/candidemia in 245 pts (75.6% vs 60.2%) *(ICAAC 2005)*. Few drug-drug interactions (see Table 22) Like other echinocandins, remarkably non-toxic; most common side-effects: nausea, vomiting, ↓ Mg, ↓ K & headache in 11–13% of pts. No dose adjustments for renal or hepatic insufficiency. Few drug-drug interactions (see Table 22) See *CID 43:215, 2006*
Fluconazole (Diflucan) 100 mg tabs NB $33.37, G $2 150 mg tabs NB $16, G $7 200 mg tabs NB $17, G $8 400 mg IV NB $179, G $88 Oral suspension: 50 mg per 5 mL: $42/35 mL bottle—NB	IV—oral dose because of excellent bioavailability. **Pharmacology:** absorbed po, water solubility enables IV. For peak serum levels *(see Table 9, page 77)*. T½ 30hr (range 20–50hr). 12% protein bound. **CSF levels 50–90% of serum in normals.** 1 in meningitis. No effect on mammalian steroid metabolism. **Drug-drug interactions, see Table 22.** Side-effects overall 16% (more common in HIV+ pts [21%]). Nausea 3.7%, headache 1.9%, skin rash 1.8%, abdominal pain 1.7%, vomiting 1.7%, diarrhea 1.5%; SGOT 20%. Alopecia (rare, pubic crest) in 12–20% pts on ≥400mg q24h after median of 3mo (reversible in approx. 6mo) *(AnIM 123:354, 1995)*. Rare: severe hepatotoxicity *(CID 41:301, 2005)*, exfoliative dermatitis. Anaphylaxis *(BMJ 302:1341, 1991)*. Ref: *NEJM 330:263, 1994*
Flucytosine (Ancobon) 500 mg cap $10.50	AEs: Overall 30%. GI 6% (diarrhea, anorexia, nausea, vomiting); hematologic 22% [leukopenia, thrombocytopenia, when serum level >100mcg/mL, esp. in azotemic pts)]; hepatotoxicity (asymptomatic ↑ SGOT, reversible); skin rash 7% (sulfide reversible). False ↑ on serum creatinine on EKTACHEM analyzer.
Griseofulvin (Fulvicin, Grifulvin, Grisactin) 500 mg G $3, susp 125 mg/mL: 120 mL $52	Photosensitivity, urticaria, GI upset, fatigue, headache (rare). Interferes with warfarin drugs. Increases blood and urine porphyrins, should not be used in patients with porphyria. Minor disulfiram-like reactions. Exacerbation of systemic lupus erythematosus. *(JAC 26:171, 2000)*

---

¹ HSCT = hematopoietic stem cell transplant

* From 2007 Red Book, Thomson Healthcare, Inc. **Price is average wholesale price (AWP).**
See page 2 for abbreviations. All dosage recommendations are for adults (unless otherwise indicated) and assume normal renal function

TABLE 11B (3)

DRUG NAME, GENERIC (TRADE)/USUAL DOSAGE/COST*	ADVERSE EFFECTS/COMMENTS
Imidazoles, topical For vaginal and/or skin use	Not recommended in 1st trimester of pregnancy. Local reactions: 0.5-1.5%: dyspareunia, mild vaginal or vulvar erythema, burning, pruritus, urticaria, rash. Rarely similar symptoms in sexual partner.
Itraconazole (Sporanox) 100 mg cap $10 10mg/mL oral solution (fasting state) (150 mL - $158) AAC 42:1862, 1998 IV usual dose 200 mg bid x 4 doses followed by 200 mg q24h for a max of 14 days ($239/250 mg)	**Itraconazole tablet & solution forms not interchangeable, solution preferred.** Many authorities recommend measuring drug serum concentration after 2wk to ensure satisfactory absorption. To obtain highest plasma concentration, tablet is given with food & acidic drinks (e.g., cola) while solution is taken in fasted state; under these conditions, the peak conc. of capsule is approx. 3mcg/mL & of solution 5.4mcg/mL. Peak levels reached faster (2.2 vs 5hrs) with solution. **Peak plasma concentrations after IV injection (200mg) compared to oral capsule (200mg): 2.8mcg/mL (on day 7 of rx) vs 2mcg/mL (on day 36 of rx).** Protein-binding for both preparations is over 99%, which explains virtual absence of penetration into CSF. **(do not use to treat meningitis)**. Most common adverse effects are dose-related nausea and vomiting, diarrhea 8%, vomiting 6%, & abdominal discomfort 6.7%. Allergic rash 8.6%, edema 3.5%, & malaise 27% reported. Doses may produce hypokalemia 8% & ↑ blood pressure 3.2%. Delirium & peripheral neuropathy reported (Psychosomatics 44:260, 2003; Diabetes Care 28:225, 2005). **Reported to produce impairment in cardiac function.** Severe liver failure req transplant in pts receiving pulse rx for onychomycosis; FDA reports 24 cases with 11 deaths out of 50mil people who received the drug prior to 2001 (Eur Acad Derm & Venereol 19:205, 2005). Other concern, as with fluconazole and itraconazole is **drug-drug interactions; see Table 22** Some can be life-threatening.
Ketoconazole (Nizoral) 200 mg tab $5	Gastric acid required for absorption—cimetidine, omeprazole, antacids block absorption. In achlorhydria, dissolve tablet in 4 mL 0.2N HCl, drink with a straw. Coca-Cola® decreased absorption by 65%. CSF levels "none." **Drug-drug interactions important, see Table 22** **Some interactions can be life-threatening. Dose-dependent nausea and vomiting.** Liver toxicity of hepatocellular type reported in about 1:10,000 exposed pts—usually after several days to weeks of exposure. At doses of ≥800 mg per day ↓ serum testosterone and plasma cortisol levels fall. With high doses, adrenal (Addisonian) crisis reported.
Miconazole (Monistat IV) 200 mg—not available in U.S.	IV miconazole indicated in patient critically ill with Scedosporium (Pseudallescheria boydii) infection. Very toxic due to vehicle needed to get into solution.
Nystatin (Mycostatin) 30gm cream NB $30, G $4 500,000 units oral tab $0.70	Topical: virtually no adverse effects. Less effective than imidazoles and triazoles. PO: large doses give occasional GI distress and diarrhea.
Posaconazole (Noxafil) 400 mg po bid with meals (if not taking meals, 200 mg qid) 200 mg po TID (with food) for prophylaxis. 40 mg/mL suspension—105 mL, $576.	An oral triazole with activity against a wide range of fungi refractory to other antifungal rx including: aspergillosis, zygomycosis, fusariosis, Scedosporium (Pseudallescheria), phaeohyphomycosis, histoplasmosis, refractory candidiasis, refractory coccidioidomycosis, refractory cryptococcosis, & refractory chromoblastomycosis as other triazoles. Approved for prophylaxis. Clinical response in 75% of 176 AIDS pts with azole-refractory oral/esophageal candidiasis. Posaconazole has similar toxicities as other triazoles: nausea 9%, vomiting 6%, abd. pain 5%, headache 5%, diarrhea, ↑ ALT, AST, & rash (3% each). In pts rx for >6 mos, serious side-effects have included adrenal insufficiency, nephrotoxicity, & QTc interval prolongation. Significant drug-drug interactions; inhibits CYP3A4 (see Table 22.) (See Drugs 65:1552, 2005)
Terbinafine (Lamisil) 250 mg tab $12	In pts given terbinafine for onychomycosis, rare cases [8] of idiosyncratic & symptomatic hepatic injury & more rarely liver failure leading to death or liver transplant. The drug is **not recommended** for pts with **chronic or active liver disease;** hepatotoxicity may occur in pts with or without pre-existing disease. Pretreatment serum transaminases (ALT & AST) advised & alternate rx used for those with abnormal levels. Pts started on terbinafine should be warned about symptoms suggesting liver dysfunction (persistent nausea, anorexia, fatigue, vomiting, RUQ pain, jaundice, dark urine or pale stools). If symptoms develop, drug should be discontinued & liver function immediately evaluated. In controlled trials, changes in ocular lens and retina reported—clinical significance unknown. Major drug-drug interaction (see Table 22). Adverse effects in 10% of pts: headache usually 2.8% (rx 1.1%, placebo), diarrhea 5.6% rx 2.9, rash 5.6 rx 2.2; taste abnormality 2.8 vs 0.7. Inhibits CYP2D6 enzymes (see Table 22) An acute generalized exanthematous pustulosis has been reported in 13 cases (Brit J Derm 152:780, 2005) & 5 cases of subacute cutaneous lupus erythematosus (Acta Derm Venerol 84:472, 2004).

TABLE 11B (4)

DRUG NAME, GENERIC (TRADE)/USUAL DOSAGE/COST*	ADVERSE EFFECTS/COMMENTS
Voriconazole (Vfend) IV: Loading dose 6 mg per kg q12h times 1 day, then 4 mg per kg q12h IV for invasive aspergillus & serious mold infections; **3 mg per kg IV q12h** for serious candida infections. 200mg IV = $121 **Oral: >40 kg body weight:** 400 mg po q12h times 1 day, then 200 mg po q12h. 200mg po = $39 **<40 kg body weight:** 200 mg po q12h times 1 day, then 100 mg po q12h. **Take oral dose 1 hour before or 1 hour after eating.** Oral suspension (40 mg per mL) $47/200 mg dose. Oral suspension dosing: Same as for oral tabs. Reduce to ½ maintenance dose for moderate hepatic insufficiency	A triazole with activity against Aspergillus sp., **including Ampho resistant strains of A. terreus** (*J Clin Micro* 37:2343, 1999). Active vs Candida sp. (including krusei), Fusarium sp. & various molds. Steady state serum levels reach 2.5–4 mcg per mL. Up to 20% of patients with subtherapeutic levels with oral administration; check levels for suspected treatment failure, life threatening infections. Toxicity similar to other azoles/triazoles including uncommon serious hepatic toxicity (hepatitis, cholestasis & fulminant hepatic failure. Liver function tests should be monitored during rx & drug dc'd if abnormalities develop. Rash reported in up to 20%, occ. photosensitivity & rare Stevens-Johnson, hallucinations (including musical hallucinations (*Infection* 32:293, 2004)) & anaphylactoid infusion reactions with fever and hypotension (*Clin Exp Dermatol* 26:648, 2001). 1 case of QT prolongation with ventricular tachycardia in a 15 y/o with ALL reported (*CID* 39:684, 2004). **Approx. 21% experience a transient visual disturbance** following IV or po ("altered/enhanced visual perception", blurred or colored visual change or photophobia) within 30–60 minutes. Visual changes resolve within 30–60 min. after administration & are attenuated with repeated doses (**do not drive at night for outpatient rx**). No persistence of effect reported. Cause unknown. In patients with CICr <50 mL per min. the drug should be given orally, not IV, since the intravenous vehicle (SBECD-sulfobutyl/ether-B cyclodextrin) may accumulate. Hallucinations, hypoglycemia, electrolyte disturbance & pneumonitis attributed to ↑ drug concentrations (*CID* 39:1241, 2004). Potential for drug-drug interactions high—see *Table 22* (*CID* 36:630, 1087, 1122, 2003). **NOTE:** Not in urine in active form. **Cost:** 50 mg tab $3; 200 mg tab $35; 200 mg IV $109

Table 11C – SUMMARY OF SUGGESTED ANTIFUNGAL DRUGS AGAINST TREATABLE PATHOGENIC FUNGI

Microorganism	Antifungal[1-4]				
	Fluconazole[5]	Voriconazole	Posaconazole	Echinocandin	Polyenes
Candida albicans	+++	+++	+++	+++	+++
Candida glabrata	±	+	+	+++	++
Candida tropicalis	+++	+++	+++	+++	++
Candida parapsilosis[6]	+++	+++	+++	++ (higher MIC)	+++
Candida krusei	-	++	++	+++	++
Candida guilliermondii	+++	+++	+++	++ (higher MIC)	++
Candida lusitaniae	+++	++	++	++	+
Cryptococcus neoformans	+++	+++	+++	-	+++
Aspergillus fumigatus[7]	-	+++	+++	++	++
Aspergillus flavus[7]	-	+++	+++	++	++ (higher MIC)
Aspergillus terreus	-	+++	+++	++	-
Fusarium sp.	-	++	++	-	++ (lipid formulations)
Scedosporium apiospermum (Pseudallescheria boydii)	-	+++	+++	±	±
Scedosporium prolificans[8]	-	±	±	-	-
Trichosporon spp.	±	++	++	-	±
Zygomycetes (e.g., Absidia, Mucor, Rhizopus)	-	-	++	-	+++ (lipid formulations)
Dematiaceous molds[9] (e.g., Alternaria, Bipolaris, Curvularia, Exophiala)	±	+++	+++	+	+
Dimorphic Fungi[10]					
Blastomyces dermatitidis	++	++	++	-	++
Coccidioides immitis/posadasii	+++	++	+++	-	+++
Histoplasma capsulatum	++	++	++	-	+++
Sporothrix schenckii	+	++	++	-	+++

- = no activity; ± = possibly activity; + = active 3rd line therapy (least active clinically)
++ = Active, 2nd line therapy (less active clinically); +++ = Active, 1st line therapy (usually active clinically)

1. Minimum inhibitory concentration values do not always predict clinical outcome.
2. Echinocandins, voriconazole, posaconazole and polyenes have poor urine penetration.
3. During severe immune suppression, success requires immune reconstitution.
4. **Flucytosine** has activity against *Candida* sp., *Cryptococcus* sp., and dematiaceous molds, but is primarily used in combination therapy.
5. For infections secondary to *Candida* sp., patients with prior triazole therapy have higher likelihood of triazole resistance.
6. Successful treatment of infections from *Candida parapsilosis* requires removal of foreign body or intravascular device.
7. Lipid formulations of amphotericin may have greater activity against *A. fumigatus* and *A. flavus* (+++).
8. *Scedosporium prolificans* is poorly susceptible to single agents and may require combination therapy (e.g., addition of terbinafine).
9. Infections from zygomycetes, some *Aspergillus* spp., and dematiaceous molds often require surgical debridement.
10. For dimorphic fungi, itraconazole is first-line therapy and active clinically (+++).

TABLE 12A – TREATMENT OF MYCOBACTERIAL INFECTIONS*

Tuberculin skin test (TST). Same as PPD [MMWR 52(RR-2):15, 2003]

Criteria for positive TST after 5 tuberculin units (intermediate PPD) read at 48-72 hours:
≥5 mm induration: + HIV, immunosuppressed; ≥15 mg prednisone per day, recent close contact
≥10 mm induration: foreign-born, countries with high prevalence, IVDUsers; low income; NH residents; chronic illness; silicosis
≥15 mm induration: otherwise healthy

Two-stage to detect sluggish positivity: If 1st PPD + but <10 mm, repeat intermediate PPD in 1wk. Response to 2nd PPD can also happen in 1wk. If pt received BCG in childhood.
BCG vaccine as child: If ≥10 mm induration, & from country with TBc, should be attributed to M. tuberculosis. In areas of low TB prevalence, TST reactions of ≥18mm more likely from BCG than TB [CID 40:211, 2005]. Prior BCG may result in sluggish reaction in 2-stage TST [AnM 161:1760, 2001; Clin Micro Inf 10:980, 2005].

Routine anergy testing no longer recommended in HIV+ or HIV-negative patients [JAMA 283:2003, 2000].

Whole blood interferon-gamma release assay [QuantiFERON-TB (QFT)] approved by U.S. FDA as diagnostic test for TB [JAMA 286:1740, 2001; CID 34:1449 & 1457, 2002]. CDC recommends TST for
TB suspects & pts at ↑ risk for progression to active TB & suggests either TST or QFT for individuals at ↑ risk for latent TB (LTBI) & for persons who warrant testing but are deemed at low risk for LTBI
[MMWR 52(RR-2):15, 2003]. IFN-γ assay is better indicator of TBc risk than TST in BCG-vaccinated population [JAMA 293:2756, 2005]. A more sensitive assay based on M. tbc-specific antigens
(QuantiFERON-TB GOLD) was approved by the USFDA 5/2/05 and an enzyme-linked immunospot method (ELISpot) using antigens specific for MTB (do not cross-react with BCG) is under evaluation &
looks promising [Thorax 58:916, 2003; Ln 361:1168, 2003; AnIM 140:709, 2004; LnID 4:761, 2005; CID 40:246, 2005; JAMA 293:2756, 2005; MMWR 54:49, 2005]. However, none of these tests can
distinguish latent from active TB and none is 100% sensitive (ELISpot slightly higher sensitivity than QuantiFeron-TB Gold)[AnIM 146:340, 2007; CID 44:74, 2007].

CAUSATIVE AGENT/DISEASE	MODIFYING CIRCUMSTANCES	INITIAL THERAPY	SUGGESTED REGIMENS
			CONTINUATION PHASE OF THERAPY
I. Mycobacterium tuberculosis exposure but TST negative (household members & other close contacts of potentially infectious cases)	Neonate—Rx essential	INH (10mg/kg/day for 3mo)	Repeat tuberculin skin test (TST) in 3mo. If mother's smear neg & chest x-ray (CXR) normal, stop INH. In UK, BCG is then given [Ln 2:1479, 1990], unless mother HIV+. If infant's repeat TST + &/or CXR abnormal (hilar adenopathy &/or infiltrate), INH + RIF [10-20 mg/kg/day] (or SM). Total rx 6mo. If mother is being rx, separation of infant from mother not indicated.
	Children <5 years of age—Rx indicated	As for neonate for 1-3 mos.	If repeat TST at 3mo is negative, stop. If repeat TST +, continue INH for total of 9mo. If INH not given initially, repeat TST at 3mo.
	Older children & adults—Risk 2-4%/1st yr		If + rx with INH for 9 mos. (see Category II below).
			No rx

(Continued on next page)

See page 2 for abbreviations, page 116 for footnotes   * Dosages are for adults (unless otherwise indicated) and assume normal renal function   ¹ **DOT** = directly observed therapy

TABLE 12A (2)

CAUSATIVE AGENT/DISEASE	MODIFYING CIRCUMSTANCES	SUGGESTED REGIMENS — INITIAL THERAPY	SUGGESTED REGIMENS — ALTERNATIVE
II. Treatment of latent infection with M. tuberculosis (formerly known as "prophylaxis) (NEJM 347:1860, 2002; NEJM 350:2060, 2004; JAMA 293:2776, 2005) **A. INH indicated due to high-risk** Assumes INH susceptibility. INH 54–88% effective in preventing active TB for ≥2yr.	(1) + tuberculin reactor & HIV+ risk of active disease 10% per yr, AIDS 170 times (/mo.) (NEJM 9: 113 times 1). Development of active TBc in HIV+ pts after INH usually due to reinfection, not reactivation (NEJM 341:1174) (2) Newly infected persons (TST conversion in past 2 yrs—risk 3.3%, 1ˢᵗ yr) (3) Past tuberculosis, not rx with adequate chemotherapy (INH, RIF, or alternatives) (4) + tuberculin reactors with CXR consistent with non-progressive tuberculous disease (risk 0.5–5.0% per yr) (5) + tuberculin reactors with specific predisposing conditions: illicit IV drug use (MMWR 38:236, 1989), silicosis, diabetes mellitus, prolonged adrenocorticoid rx (>15mg prednisone/day), immunosuppressive rx, hematologic diseases (Hodgkin's), endstage renal disease, clinical condition with rapid substantial weight loss or chronic under-nutrition, previous gastrectomy (ARRD 134: 355, 1986). (6) + tuberculin reactors due to start anti-TNF-(alpha) therapy. For management algorithm see Thorax 60:800, 2005. **NOTE: For HIV, see Sanford Guide to HIV/AIDS Therapy &/or JID 196:S35, 2007**	**INH** (5mg/kg/day, max 300mg/ day for adults; 10mg/kg/day for children). May be used/w/with DOT w/ DOT (MMWR 52:735, 2003). Optimal duration 9 mos. (includes children, HIV–, HIV+, and fibrotic lesions on chest x-ray). In some cases, 6 mos. may be given for cost-effectiveness (AJRCCM 161:S221, 2000). Not all agree with CDC recommendation and HIV+ persons <18yr. or those with fibrotic lesions on chest film (NEJM 345:189, 2001).	If compliance problem: **INH** by DOT† 15mg/kg 2x/wk times 9mo. due **RIF + PZA** regimen effective in HIV– and HIV+ pts (AJRCCM 161:S221, 2000; JAMA 283:1445, 2000). **However, there are descriptions of severe & fatal hepatitis in immunocompetent pts on RIF + PZA** (MMWR 50:289, 2001). Monitoring for cofactors did not seem to allow prediction of fatalities (CID 42:346, 2006). Therefore, regimen is no longer recommended for LTBI treatment (AJRCCM 52:735, 2003; CID 39:484, 2004). Not all agree with CDC recommendation and recent study suggests short course therapy is safe with monitoring and more likely to be completed than longer therapy (CID 43:271, 2006). **RIF** 600mg/kg po for 4mo. (HIV– and HIV+). Meta-analysis suggests 3mo of INH + RIF may be equiv to "standard" (6–12mo) INH therapy (CID 40:670, 2005).
B. TST positive (organisms likely to be [INH-susceptible)	Age no longer considered a modifying factor (see Comments)	**INH** (5 mg/kg per day for adults; 10 mg/kg per day not to exceed 300 mg/day for children). Results with 6 mos. rx not quite as effective as 12 mos. (65% vs 75% reduction in disease). 9 mos. is current recommendation. See IIA above for details and alternate rx.	Reanalysis of earlier studies favors **INH** prophylaxis (if INH related, hepatitis case fatality rate <1% and TB case fatality 26.7%, which appears to be the case) (AnIM 152:2517, 1990). Recent data suggest INH prophylaxis has positive risk-benefit ratio in pts ≥35 if monitored for hepatotoxicity (AnIM 127:1051, 1997). Overall risk of hepatotoxicity 0.1–0.15% (JAMA 281:1014.)
	Pregnancy—Any risk factors (II.A above)	Treat with **INH** as above. For women at risk for progression of latent to active disease, esp. those who are HIV+ or who have been recently infected, rx should not be delayed even during the first trimester.	Risk of INH hepatitis may be ↑ (Ln 346:199, 1995).
	Pregnancy—No risk factors	No initial rx (see Comment)	Delay rx until after delivery (AJRCCM 149:1359, 1994).
C. TST positive & drug resistance likely (For data on worldwide prevalence of drug resistance see NEJM 344:1294, 2001; JID 185:1197, 2002; JID 194:479, 2006; EID 13:380, 2007)	INH-resistant (or adverse reaction to INH), RIF-sensitive organisms likely	**RIF** 600 mg/day po for 4 mos. (HIV+ or HIV–)	IDSA guideline lists rifabutin in 600 mg/day dose as another alternative; however, current recommended max. dose of rifabutin is 300 mg per day. Estimate RIF alone has protective effect of 56%, 26% of pts reported adverse effects (only 2) (157 did not complete 6 mos. rx) (AJRCCM 155:1735, 1997).
	INH- and RIF-resistant organisms likely	Efficacy of all regimens unproven. **PZA** 25–30 mg per day for 4 mos. (HIV+ or HIV–).	**PZA** + ofloxacin has been associated with asymptomatic hepatitis (CID 261:1264, 1997).
		Efficacy of all regimens unproven. **PZA** 25–30 mg per day to max. of 2 gm per day + **ETB** 15–25 mg per kg per day to max. of 2 gm per day times 6–12 mos.	
		PZA 25 mg per kg per day to max. of 2 gm per day) + **levo** 500 mg per day (max 400 mg/day), all po. times 6–12 mos.	

See page 2 for abbreviations, page 116 for footnotes.   * Dosages are for adults (unless otherwise indicated) and assume normal renal function   † **DOT** = directly observed therapy

TABLE 12A (3)

CAUSATIVE AGENT/DISEASE	MODIFYING CIRCUMSTANCES	SUGGESTED REGIMENS						
		INITIAL PHASE[1] DIRECTLY OBSERVED THERAPY (DOT) REGIMENS			CONTINUATION PHASE OF THERAPY[1,2] (In vitro susceptibility known)			
		Regimen: in order of preference	Drugs	Interval/Doses[1] (min. duration)	Regimen	Drugs	Interval/Doses[1,2] (min. duration)	Range of Total Doses (min. duration)
III Mycobacterium tuberculosis A. Pulmonary TB [General reference on rx in adults & children: Ln 362:887, 2003; MMMR 52(RR-11):1, 2003; CID 40(Suppl 1): S1, 2005] Isolation essential Pts with active TB should be isolated in single rooms, not cohorted (MMWR 54(RR-17), 2005). Older observations on infectivity of suscepti-ble & resistant M. tbc before and after rx (ARPD 85:511, 1962) may not be applicable to MDR M. tbc or to the HIV-+ individual. Extended isolation may be appropriate. See footnotes, page 113 USE DOT REGIMENS IF POSSIBLE (continued on next page)	Rate of INH resistance known to be <4% (drug-susceptible organisms) [Modified from MMMR 52:(RR-11):1, 2003]	1 (See Figure 1, page 115)	INH RIF PZA ETB	7 days per wk times 56 doses (8 wk) or 5 days per wk times 40 doses (8 wk)	1a	INH/RIF	7 days per wk times 126 doses (18 wk) or 5 days per wk times 90 doses (18 wk)	182-130 (26 wk)
					1b	INH/RIF	2 times per wk times 36 doses (18 wk)	92-76 (26 wk)[4]
					1c[3]	INH/RFP	1 time per wk times 18 doses (18 wk)	74-58 (26 wk)[4]
		2 (See Figure 1, page 115)	INH RIF PZA ETB	7 days per wk times 14 doses (2 wk), then 2 times per wk times 12 doses (6 wk) or 5 days per wk times 10 doses (2 wk), then 2 times per wk times 12 doses (6 wk)	2a	INH/RIF	2 times per wk times 36 doses (18 wk)	62-58 (26 wk)[4]
					2b[3]	INH/RFP	1 time per wk times 18 doses (18 wk)	44-40 (26 wk)
		3 (See Figure 1, page 115)	INH RIF PZA ETB	3 times per wk times 24 doses (8 wk)	3a	INH/RIF	3 times per wk times 54 doses (18 wk)	78 (26 wk)
		4 (See Figure 1, page 115)	INH RIF ETB	7 days per wk times 56 doses (8 wk) or 5 days per wk times 40 doses (8 wk)	4a	INH/RIF	7 days per wk times 217 doses (31 wk) or 5 days per wk times 155 doses (31 wk)	273-195 (39 wk)
					4b	INH/RIF[3]	2 times per wk times 62 doses (31 wk)	118-102 (39 wk)

COMMENTS

Dose in mg per kg (max. q24h dose)

Regimen* Q24h:	INH	RIF	PZA	ETB	SM	RFB
Child	10-20 (300)	10-20 (600)	15-30 (2000)	15-25	20-40 (1000)	10-20 (300)
Adult	5 (300)	10 (600)	15-30 (2000)	15-25	15- (1000)	5 (300)
2 times per wk (DOT):						
Child	20-40 (900)	10-20 (600)	50-70 (4000)	50	25-30 (1500)	NA
Adult	15 (900)	10 (600)	50-70 (4000)	50	25-30 (1500)	NA
3 times per wk (DOT):						
Child	20-40 (900)	10-20 (600)	50-70 (3000)	25-30	25-30 (1500)	NA
Adult	15 (900)	10 (600)	50-70 (3000)	25-30	25-30 (1500)	NA

Second-line anti-TB agents can be dosed as follows to facilitate DOT: Cycloserine 500-750 mg po q24h (5 times per wk) Ethionamide 500-750 mg po q24h (5 times per wk) Kanamycin or capreomycin 15 mg per kg IM/IV q24h (3-5 times per wk) Ciprofloxacin 750 mg po q24h (5 times per wk) Ofloxacin 600-800 mg po q24h (5 times per wk) Levofloxacin 750 mg po q24h (5 times per wk) (CID 21:1245, 1995)

Risk factors for drug-resistant TB: Recent immigration from Latin America or Asia or living in area of high rate of resistance (>4%), or previous rx without RIF exposure to known MDR TB. Incidence of MDR TB in U.S. appears to have stabilized and may be slightly decreasing in early 1990s (JAMA 278:833, 1997). Incidence of primary drug resistance high (>25%) in parts of China, Thailand, Russia, Estonia & Latvia (NEJM 344:1294, 2001; NEJM 347:1850, 2002). (continued on next page)

See page 2 for abbreviations, page 116 for footnotes   * Dosages are for adults (unless otherwise indicated) and assume normal renal function   [1] DOT = directly observed therapy

TABLE 12A (4)

CAUSATIVE AGENT/DISEASE	MODIFYING CIRCUM-STANCES	SUGGESTED REGIMEN[a]	DURATION OF TREATMENT (mo.)[c]	SPECIFIC COMMENTS[a]	COMMENTS
III **Mycobacterium tuberculosis** **A. Pulmonary TB** *(continued from previous page)* REFERENCES: CID 22:683, 1996; CID 31:633, 2000; Med Lett 5/15; 19.658, 2006; Med Lett 5/15, 2007	INH (± SM) resistance	RIF **PZA** ETB (an **FQ** may strengthen the regimen for pts with extensive disease). Emergence of FQ resistance a concern (JAC 3:432, 2003; AAC 49:3178, 2005)	6	*(continued from previous page)* In British Medical Research Council trials, 6-mo. regimens have yielded ≥95% success rates despite resistance to INH if 4 drugs were used in the initial phase & RIF + ETB or SM was used throughout (ARRD 133: 423, 1986). Additional studies suggested that results were best if PZA was also used throughout the 6 mos (ARRD 136:1339, 1987). FQs were not employed in BMRC studies, but may strengthen the regimen for pts with extensive disease. INH should be stopped in cases of INH resistance [see MMWR 52(RR-11):1, 2003 for additional discussion].	*(continued from previous page)* For MDR TB, consider rifabutin (~30% RIF-resistant strains are rifabutin-susceptible). Note that CIP not as effective as PZA + ETB in multidrug regimen for susceptible TB (CID 22:287, 1996). Moxifloxacin and levofloxacin have enhanced activity compared with CIP against M. tuberculosis (AAC 46: 1022, 2002; AAC 47:2442, 2003; AAC 47:3117, 2003; JAC 53:441, 2004; AAC 48:780, 2004). FQ resistance may be seen in pts previously treated with FQ (CID 37:1448, 2003). Linezolid has excellent in vitro activity, including MDR strains (AAC 47: 416, 2003). Mortality reviewed: CI 349:71, 1997. Rapid (24-hr) diagnostic tests for M. tuberculosis: (1) the Amplified Mycobacterium tuberculosis Direct Test amplifies and detects M. tuberculosis ribosomal RNA; (2) the AMPLICOR Mycobacterium tuberculosis Test amplifies and detects M. tuberculosis DNA. Both tests have sensitivities & specificities >95% in sputum samples that are AFS-positive. In negative smears, specificity remains >95% but sensitivity is 40–77% (ARRD 155:1497, 1997). Note that MTB may grow out on standard blood agar plates in 1–2 wks (J Clin Micro 41: 1710,2003).
Multidrug-Resistant Tuberculosis (MDR TB): Defined as resistant to at least 2 drugs including INH & RIF. In pts clusters with high mortality (ANM 118:17, 1994; E JCMID 23: 174, 2004; MMWR 55:305, 2006; JID 194:1194, 2006)	Resistance to INH & RIF (± SM)	**FQ PZA ETB** ± alternative agent[7]	18–24	In such cases, extended rx is needed to ↓ the risk of relapse. In cases with extensive disease, the use of an additional agent (alternative agents) may be prudent to ↓ the risk of failure & additional acquired drug resistance. Resectional surgery may be appropriate.	
	Resistance to INH, RIF (± SM) & ETB or PZA	**FQ [ETB** or **PZA** if active), **IA** & 2 alternative agents[7]	24	Use the first-line agents to which there is susceptibility. Add 2 or more alternative agents in case of extensive disease. Surgery should be considered. Survival ↑ in pts receiving active FQ & surgical intervention (AJRCCM 169:1103, 2004).	
	Resistance to RIF	**INH ETB FQ**, supplemented with **PZA** for the first 2 mo (an IA may be included for the first 2 mos. for pts with extensive disease)	12–18	Q24h & 3 times per wk regimens of INH, PZA & SM given for 9 mos. were effective in a BMRC trial (ARRD 115:727, 1977). However, extended use of an IA may not be feasible. In pts receiving a shorter, all-oral regimen times 12–18 mos. duration (e.g., to 12 mos.), an IA may be added in the initial 2 mos. of rx.	
Extensively Drug-Resistant Tuberculosis (XDR-TB): Defined as resistant to INH & RIF plus any FQ and at least 1 of the 3 second-line drugs: capreomycin, kanamycin, or amikacin (MMWR 56:250, 2007). **See footnotes, page 113** Reviews of therapy for MDR TB: JAC 54:593, 2004; Med Lett 2:83, 2004. For XDR-TB see MMWR 56:250, 2007.	XDR-TB	See Comments	18–24	Therapy requires multiple second-line drugs to which infecting organism is susceptible, including multiple second-line drugs (MMWR 56:250, 2007). Increased mortality seen primarily in HIV+ patients	

See page 2 for abbreviations, page 116 for footnotes.

Dosages are for adults (unless otherwise indicated) and assume normal renal function   † DOT = directly observed therapy

TABLE 12A (5)

CAUSATIVE AGENT/DISEASE; MODIFYING CIRCUMSTANCES	SUGGESTED REGIMENS		COMMENTS
	INITIAL THERAPY	CONTINUATION PHASE OF THERAPY (In vitro susceptibility known)	
B. Extrapulmonary TB	**INH + RIF** (or **RFB**) + **PZA** q24h times 2 months ... Authors add **pyridoxine** 25–50 mg po q24h to regimens that include INH.	**INH + RIF** (or **RFB**)	6mo regimens probably effective. Most experience with 9–12mo regimens. Am Acad Ped (1994) recommends 6mo rx for isolated cervical adenitis, renal and 12mo for meningitis, miliary, bone/joint. DOT useful here as well as for pulmonary tuberculosis. IDSA recommends 6mo for lymph node, pleural, pericarditis, disseminated disease, genitourinary & peritoneal TBc; 6–8mo for bone & joint; 9–12mo for CNS (including meningeal) TBc. Corticosteroids "strongly rec" only for pericarditis & meningeal TBc. [MMWR 52(RR-11):1, 2003]
C. Tuberculous meningitis *For critical appraisal of adjunctive steroids: CID 25:872, 1997*	**INH + RIF + ETB + PZA**	May omit ETB when susceptibility to **INH** and **RIF** established. See Table 9, page 78, for CSF drug penetration. Initial reg of INH + RIF + SM + PZA also effective, even in patients with INH resistant organisms (JID 192:79, 2005).	3 drugs often rec for initial rx. May sub ethionamide for ETB. Infection with MDR TB ↑ mortality & morbidity (CID 38:851, 2004; JID 192:79, 2005). Dexamethasone (for 1st mo) has been shown to ↓ complications (Pediatrics 99:226, 1997) & ↑ survival in pts >14yr old (NEJM 351:1741, 2004). PCR of CSF markedly ↑ diagnostic sensitivity and provides rapid dx (Neurol 45:2228, 1995; Arkeuo 53:771, 1996) but considerable variability in sensitivity depending on method used (LnID 3:633, 2003). ↓survival in HIV pts (JID 192:2134, 2005)

See page 2 for abbreviations, page 116 for footnotes   * Dosages are for adults (unless otherwise indicated) and assume normal renal function   † **DOT** = directly observed therapy

TABLE 12A (6)
FIGURE 1: TREATMENT ALGORITHM FOR TUBERCULOSIS [Modified from MMWR 52(RR-11):1, 2003]

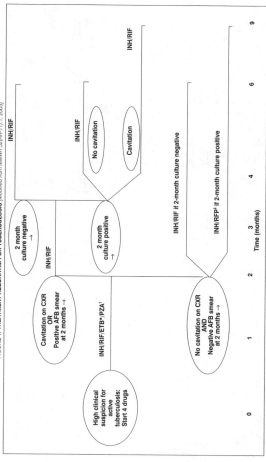

If the pt has HIV infection & the CD4 cell count is <100 per mcL, the continuation phase should consist of q24h or 3 times per wk INH & RIF for 4-7 months.
* ETB may be discontinued in <2 months if drug susceptibility testing indicate no drug resistance. † PZA may be discontinued after 2 months (56 doses).
‡ RFP should not be used in HIV patients with tuberculosis or in patients with extrapulmonary tuberculosis.

See page 2 for abbreviations

TABLE 12A (7)

CAUSATIVE AGENT/DISEASE; MODIFYING CIRCUMSTANCES	SUGGESTED REGIMENS		COMMENTS
	INITIAL THERAPY	CONTINUATION PHASE OF THERAPY (in vitro susceptibility known)	
III. Mycobacterium tuberculosis (continued)			
D. Tuberculosis during pregnancy	**INH + RIF + ETB** for 9mo		PZA not recommended: teratogenicity data inadequate. Because of potential ototoxicity to fetus throughout gestation (16%), SM should not be used unless other drugs contraindicated. Add pyridoxine 25 mg per day for pregnant women on INH. Breast-feeding should not be discouraged in pts on first-line drugs (MMWR 52(RR-11):1, 2003).
E. Treatment failure or relapse: Usually due to poor compliance or resistant organisms (AJM 102/164, 1997).	Directly observed therapy (DOT). Check susceptibilities. (See section III.A, page 112 & above)		Pts whose sputum has not converted after 5–6 mos. = treatment failures. Failures may be due to non-compliance or resistant organisms. Check susceptibilities of original isolates. Non-compliance common. Reinstitute DOT. If isolates show resistance, modify regimen to include at least 2 effective agents, preferably ones which pt has not received. Surgery may be necessary for "failure." In HIV+ patients, reinfection is a possible explanation for "failure." NB, patients with MDR-TB usually convert sputum within 12 weeks of successful therapy (AnIM 144:650, 2006).

CAUSATIVE AGENT/DISEASE	MODIFYING CIRCUMSTANCES	SUGGESTED REGIMENS		COMMENTS
		PRIMARY	ALTERNATIVE	
F. HIV infection or AIDS pulmonary or extrapulmonary (NOTE: 60–70% of HIV+ pts with TB have extra-pulmonary disease)	**INH + RIF (or RFB) + PZA** q24h times 2 months. (Authors use **pyridoxine** 25–50 mg q24h in regimens that include INH.)	**INH + RIF** (or RFB) q24h times 4 months (total 6 mos.). May treat q24h (or min 3x/wk) depending on delayed response.	**Alternative regimen:** **INH + SM + PZA +** **ETB** times 2 (7), then **INH + SM + PZA** 2–3 x per wk for 7 mo. May be used with a PI regimen. May be prolonged up to 12 mo in pts with delayed response.	1. Because of possibility of developing resistance to RIF in pts with low CD4 cell counts who receive wkly or every (2x/wk) doses of RFB, it is recom. that such pts receive q24h (or min 3x/wk) doses of RFB for initiation & continuation phase of rx (MMWR 51:214, 2002). 2. Clinical & microbiologic response same as in HIV-neg patient although there is considerable variability in outcomes among currently available studies (CID 32:623, 2001). 3. Post-treatment suppression not necessary for drug-susceptible strains. 4. Rate of INH resistance known to be <4% (for † rates of resistance, see Section III.A). 5. More info, see MMWR 47(RR-20):1, 1998; CID 28:139, 1999; MMWR 52(RR-11):1, 2003 6. May use early intermittent therapy: 1 dose per day for 2 weeks followed by 2–3 doses per wk for 24wk (MMWR 47(RR-20), 1998). 7. Adjunctive prednisolone of NO benefit in HIV+ patients with TBc pleurisy (JID 190:869, 2004). (JID 195:856, 2005) or in patients with TBc pericarditis.
Concomitant protease inhibitor (PI) therapy (Modified from MMWR 49:185, 2000; AJRCCM 162:7, 2001).	**Initial & cont. therapy:** **INH** 300 mg + **RFB** (see below for dose) + **PZA** 25 mg per kg + **ETB** 15 mg per kg q24h times 2 mos., then **INH + RFB** times 4 mos. (up to 7 mos.)			**Comments:** Rifamycins induce cytochrome CYP450 enzymes (RIF > RFB > RPT) & reduce serum levels of concomitantly administered Pis. Conversely, Pis (ritonavir > amprenavir > indinavir > nelfinavir > saquinavir) inhibit CYP450 & ↑ serum levels of RFB & RFB. If dose of RFB is not reduced, toxicity ↑. RFB/PI combinations are therapeutically effective (CID 30:779, 2000). RFB has no effect on nelfinavir levels at dose of 1250 mg bid (Can JID 10:21B, 1999). **Although RFB is preferred, rifampin can be used for rx of active TB in pts on regimens containing efavirenz or ritonavir. RIF should not be administered to pts on ritonavir + saquinavir because drug-induced hepatitis with marked transaminase elevations has been seen in healthy volunteers receiving this regimen** (www.fda.gov).
	PI Regimen	RFB Dose		
	Nelfinavir 1200mg q12h or indinavir 1000mg q8h or amprenavir 1200mg q12h	150 mg q24h or 300 mg intermittently		
	Lopinavir/ritonavir—standard doses	150 mg 3x per wk		

FOOTNOTES: [1] When DOT is used, drug may be given 5 days/wk & necessary number of doses compare 5 with 7 q24h doses, indicates this would be an effective practice. [2] Patients with cavitation on initial chest x-ray & positive cultures at completion of 2mo of rx should receive a 7mo (31 wk; either 217 doses [q24h] or 62 doses [2x/wk] continuation phase. [3] 5day/wk admin is always given by DOT. [4] Not recommended for HIV-infected pts with CD4 cell counts <100 cells/mL. [5] Options 1c & 2b should be used only in HIV-neg. pts who have neg. sputum smears at the time of completion of 2mo rx & do not have cavitation on initial chest x-ray. For pts started on this regimen who have + culture from 2mo specimen, rx should be extended extra 3mo. [6] Options 4a & 4b should be considered under options 1–3 cannot be given. Alternative agents – ethionamide, cycloserine, p-aminosalicylic acid, clarithromycin, AM-CL, linezolid. [7] Modified from MMWR 52(RR-11):1, 2003. See also IDCP 11:329, 2002. [8] Continuation regimen with INH/RIF classed thus INH/RIF (Lancet 364:1244, 2004).

See page 2 for abbreviations, page 116 for footnotes   * Dosages are for adults (unless otherwise indicated) and assume normal renal function   † DOT = directly observed therapy

TABLE 12A (8)

CAUSATIVE AGENT/DISEASE	MODIFYING CIRCUMSTANCES	SUGGESTED REGIMENS		COMMENTS
		PRIMARY	ALTERNATIVE	
IV. Other Mycobacterial Disease ("Atypical") (See ATS Consensus: AJRCCM 152:51, 1997; IDC No. Amer. March 2002; CMR 15:716, 2002; CID 42:1756, 2006)				
A. M. bovis		**INH + RIF + ETB**		The M. tuberculosis complex includes M. bovis. All isolates resistant to PZA. 9–12 months of rx if drug susceptibility authorities. Isolation not required.
B. Bacillus Calmette-Guerin (BCG) (derived from M. bovis)	Only fever (>38.5°C) for 12–24 hrs.	INH 300 mg q24h time 3 months		Intravesical BCG effective in superficial bladder tumors and carcinoma in situ. Adverse effects: fever 2.9%, granulomatous prostatitis, pneumonitis, hepatitis 0.7%, sepsis 0.4% (J Urol 147:596, 1992).
	Systemic illness or sepsis	INH 300 mg + RiF 600 mg + **ETB** 1200 mg po q24h times 6 mos.		With sepsis, consider initial adjunctive prednisone. Resistant to PZA. BCG may cause regional adenitis or pulmonary disease in HIV-infected children (CID 37:1226, 2003)
C. M. avium-intracellulare complex (MAC, MAI, or Battey bacillus) *Clin Chest Med 23:633, 2002; ATS/IDSA Consensus Statement: AJRCCM 175:367, 2007; alternative ref: CID 42:1756, 2006*	**Immunocompetent patients**			See AJRCCM 175:367, 2007 for details of dosing and duration of therapy. Intermittent (tiw) therapy not recommended for patients with cavitary disease, patients who have been previously treated or patients with moderate of severe disease. The primary microbiologic goal of therapy is 12 months of negative sputum cultures on therapy.
	Nodular/Bronchiectatic disease	**[Clarithro** 1000 mg tiw or **azithro** 500–600 mg tiw] + **ETB** 25 mg/kg tiw + **RIF** 600 mg tiw		**'Classic' pulmonary MAC:** Men 50–75, smokers, COPD. May be associated with hot tub use (Clin Chest Med 23:675, 2002).
	Cavitary disease	**[Clarithro** 500–1000mg/day (lower dose for wt <50 kg) or **azithro** 250–300 mg/day] + **ETB** 15 mg/kg/day + **RIF** 450-600 mg/day] + **streptomycin** or **amikacin**		**'New' pulmonary MAC:** Women 50–70, scoliosis, mitral valve prolapse, (bronchiectasis), pectus excavatum ('Lady Windermere syndrome'). May also be associated with interferon gamma deficiency (AJM 113:756, 2002).
	Advanced (severe) or previously treated disease	**Clarithro** 500–1000mg/day (lower dose for wt <50 kg) or **azithro** 250-300 mg/day] + **ETB** 15 mg/kg/day ± **streptomycin** or **amikacin**		For cervicofacial lymphadenitis (localized) in immunocompetent children, surgical excision is as effective as chemotherapy (CID 44:1057, 2007).
	Immunocompromised pts: Primary prophylaxis—Pt's CD4 count <50–100 per mm³	**Azithro** 1200 mg po weekly OR **Clarithro** 500 mg po bid	**RFB** 300 mg po q24h OR **Azithro** 1200 mg po weekly + **RIF** 300 mg po q24h	RFB reduces MAC infection rate by 55% by 69% (30% survival benefit); azithro by 59% (68% survival benefit) (CID 26:611, 1998). Azithro + RFB more effective than either alone but not as well tolerated (NEJM 335:392, 1996). **Many drug-drug interactions,** see Table 22, pages 200, 201. Drug-resistant MAC disease seen in 29–58% of pts in whom disease develops while taking clarithro prophylaxis & in 11% of those on azithro but has not been observed with RFB prophylaxis (J Inf 38:6, 1999). Clarithro resistance more likely in pts with extremely low CD4 counts at initiation (CID 27:807, 1998).
	Discontinue when CD4 count >100 per mm³ in response to HAART (NEJM 342:1085, 2000; CID 34:662, 2002). Guideline: AnIM 137:435, 2002.			Need to be sure no active M. tbc; RFB used for prophylaxis may promote selection of rifampin-resistant M. tbc (NEJM 335:384 & 428, 1996)
	Treatment Either presumptive dx or after + culture of blood, bone marrow, or usually, sterile body fluids, eg liver	**Clarithro** 500 mg* po bid + **ETB** 15 mg/kg/day + **RFB** 15 mg/kg po/day	**Azithro** 500 mg po/day + **ETB** 15 mg/kg/day + **RFB** 300-450 mg po/day	Median time to neg. blood culture: clarithro + ETB 4.4 wks vs azithro + ETB 3 wks. At 16 wks, clearance of bacteremia seen in 37.5% of azithro- & 85.7% of clarithro-treated pts (CID 27:1278, 1998). More recent study suggests similar clearance rates for azithro (46%) vs clarithro (56%) at 24 wks when combined with ETB (CID 31:1245, 2000). Azithro 250 mg po q24h not effective, but azithro 600 mg po q24h yields fewer adverse effects (AAC 43:2869, 1999)
		Higher doses of clari (1000 mg bid) may be associated with ↑ mortality (CID 29:125, 1999)		*(continued on next page)*

See page 2 for abbreviations.   * Dosages are for adults (unless otherwise indicated) and assume normal renal function   ¹ **DOT** = directly observed therapy

TABLE 12A (9)

CAUSATIVE AGENT/DISEASE	MODIFYING CIRCUMSTANCES	SUGGESTED REGIMENS		COMMENTS
		PRIMARY	ALTERNATIVE	
IV. Other Mycobacterial Disease ("Atypical") (continued)				
C. M. avium-intracellulare complex (continued)				*(continued from previous page)* Addition of RFB to clarithro ↓ ETB ↓ relapse rate & ↑ emergence of resistance to clari, ↓ survival (CID 37:1234, 2003). Data on clofazimine difficult to assess. Earlier study improves survival (CID 21:1234, 2003). Data on clofazimine difficult to assess. Earlier study suggested adding CLO of no value (CID 25:621, 1997). More recent study suggests it may be as effective as RFB in 3 drug regimens containing clari & ETB (CID 29:125, 1999) although it may not be as effective as RFB at preventing clari resistance (CID 28:136, 1999). Thus, pending more data, we still do not recommend CLO for MAI in HIV+ pts. Drug toxicity: With clarithro, 23% pts had to stop drug 2° to dose-limiting adverse reaction (AnIM 121:905, 1994). Combination of clarithro, ETB and RFB led to uveitis and pseudojaundice (NE-JM 330:438, 1994); result is reduction in max dose of RFB to 300 mg. Treatment failure rate is high. Reasons: drug toxicity, development of drug resistance, & inadequate serum levels of clarithro ↓ in pts also given RIF or RFB (JID 171:747, 1995). If pt not responding to initial regimen after 2–4 weeks, add one or more drugs. Several anecdotal reports of pts not responding to usual primary regimen who gained weight and became afebrile with dexamethasone 2–4 mg per day po (AAC 38:2215, 1994; CID 26:682, 1998).
	Chronic post-treatment suppression—secondary prophylaxis	**Always necessary.** (Clarithro or azithro) + ETB (15mg/kg/day (dosage above))	**Clarithro or azithro or RFB** (dosage above)	Recurrences almost universal without chronic suppression However, in patients on HAART with robust CD4 cell responses, it is possible to discontinue chronic suppression (JID 178:1446, 1998; NEJM 340:1301, 1999).
D. Mycobacterium celatum	Treatment, optimal regimen not defined		**Clarithro, FQ** (CIP or above)	Isolated from pulmonary lesions and blood in AIDS patients (CID 24:144, 1997). Easily confused with M. xenopi (and MAC). Susceptibilities similar to MAC. Clarithro-resistant strains now described (J CID 24:140, 1997).
E. Mycobacterium chelonae ssp. abscessus	Treatment, optimal regimen not defined; Surgical excision may facilitate clarithro rx in subcutaneous abscess and is important adjunct to rx (CID 24:1147, 1997)	**Clarithro FQ** (CIP above) May be susceptible to clarithro (Am Micro Inf 3:5482, 1997). Suggest rx "like MAI" but often resistant to RIF (JInf 38:157, 1999). Most reported cases received 3 or 4 drugs. usually clarithro + ETB ± CIP ± RFB (EID 9:399, 2003)		M. abscessus susceptible to AMK (70%), clarithro (95%), cefoxitin (70%), CLO, cotrimazole, IMP, azithro, cipro, doxy, mino, tigecycline (CID 42:1756, 2006). Single isolates of M. abscessus often not associated with disease. Clarithro-resistant strains now described (J Clin Micro Rev 39: 2745, 2001). M. chelonae susceptible to AMK (80%), clarithro, azithro, tobramycin (100%), IMP (60%), moxifloxacin (AAC 46:3283, 2002), cipro, mino, doxy, linezolid (CID 42:1756, 2006). Resistant to cefoxitin, FQ (CID 24:1147, 1997; AJRCCM 156:S1, 1997).
Mycobacterium chelonae ssp. chelonae				
F. Mycobacterium fortuitum	Treatment, optimal regimen not defined. Surgical excision of infected areas.	**AMK + cefoxitin + probenecid** 2–6wk, then po **TMP- SMX, or doxy** 2–6 mo. Usually responds to 6–12mo of oral rx with 2 drugs to which it is susceptible (AAC 46: 3283, 2002; Clin Micro Rev 15:716, 2002). Nail salon-acquired infections respond to 4–6 mo of minocycline, doxy, or CIP (CID 38:38, 2004).	**Resistant to all standard anti-Tbc drugs.** Sensitive in vitro to doxycycline, minocycline, cefoxitin, IMP, AMK, TMP-SMX, CIP, oflox, azithro, clarithro, linezolid (Clin Micro Rev 15:716, 2002). May be resistant to azithromycin, rifabutin (AAC 36:S16, 1997). For fortuitum pulmonary disease treat with at least 2 agents active in vitro until sputum cultures negative for 12 months (AJRCCM 175:367, 2007).	

See page 2 for abbreviations.

* Dosages are for adults (unless otherwise indicated) and assume normal renal function † **DOT** = directly observed therapy

TABLE 12A (10)

CAUSATIVE AGENT/DISEASE; MODIFYING CIRCUMSTANCES	SUGGESTED REGIMENS		COMMENTS
	PRIMARY	ALTERNATIVE	
IV. Other Mycobacterial Disease ("Atypical") (continued)			
G. Mycobacterium haemophilum	Regimen(s) not defined. In animal model, **clarithro** effective (AAC 39:2316, 1995). In clinical experience limited (Clin Micro Rev 9:435, 1996). Surgical debridement may be necessary.	**CIP + RIF + clarithro**	Clinical: Ulcerating skin lesions, synovitis, osteomyelitis, cervicofacial lymphadenitis in children (CID 41:1569, 1994). Lab: Requires supplemented media to isolate. Fastidious, in vitro tx. Over ½ resistant to: INH, RIF, ETB, PZA (AnIM 120:118, 1994). For localized cervicofacial lymphadenitis in immunocompetent children, surgical excision as effective as chemotherapy (CID 44:1057, 2007).
H. Mycobacterium genavense	Regimens used include ≥2 drugs: **ETB, RIF, RFB, CLO, clarithro** & **ETB** shown effective in reducing bacterial counts; CIP not effective in animal model (AAC 42:483, 1998).		Clinical: CD4 <50. Symptoms of fever, weight loss, diarrhea. Lab: Growth in BACTEC vials slow (mean 42 days). Subcultures grow only on Middlebrook 7H11 agar containing 2 mcg per mL mycobactin J—growth still insufficient for in vitro sensitivity testing (LnID 3:340, 2008; JCM 42:3630, 2004; AnIM 117:586, 1992). Survival ↑ from 81 to 263 days in pts rx for at least 1 month with ≥2 drugs (AIDS 155:400, 1995).
I. Mycobacterium gordonae	Regimen(s) not defined, but consider **RIF + ETB + KM** or **CIP** (J Inf 38:157, 1999) or **linezolid** (AJRCCM 175:367, 2007)		In vitro, sensitive to ETB, RIF, AMK, CIP, clarithro, linezolid (AAC 47:1736, 2003). Resistant to INH (CID 14:1229, 1992).
J. Mycobacterium kansasii	Q24h po: **INH** (300 mg) + **RIF** (600 mg) + **ETB** (25 mg per kg times 2 mos., then 15 mg per kg). Rx for 18 mos. (until culture-neg. sputum times 15 mos.) (See Comment)	If RIF-resistant, po q24h: **INH** (900 mg) + **ETB** (50 mg) + **pyridoxine** (50 mg) + **sulfamethoxazole** (1.0 gm tid). Rx until all 12 neg. times 15 mos. (See Comment) **Clari + ETB + RIF** also effective in small study (AJRCCM 156:51, 1997; Eur J Clin Microbiol ID 25:609, 2006). Surgical excision.	All isolates are resistant to PZA. Rifapentine, azithro, ETB effective alone or in combination in athymic mice (JAC 47:417, 2001). Highly susceptible to linezolid in vitro (AAC 47:1736, 2003) and to clarithro and moxifloxacin (JAC 55:950, 2005). If HIV+ pt taking protease inhibitor, substitute either clarithro (500 mg bid) or RFB (150 mg per day) for RIF (AJRCCM 156:51, 1997). Because of variable susceptibility to INH, some substitute clarithro 500–750 mg q24h for INH. Resistance to clarithro reported (DMID 31:369, 1998), but most strains susceptible to clarithro as well as moxifloxacin (AAC 48:4562, 2004). Prognosis related to level of immunosuppression (CID 37:584, 2003).
K. Mycobacterium marinum	**Clarithro** 500 mg bid) or (**minocycline** 100–200 mg q24h) or (**doxycycline** 100–200 mg q24h) or **TMP-SMX** 160/800 mg po bid), or (**RIF + ETB**) for 3 mos. (AJRCCM 156:51, 1997; Eur J Clin Microbiol ID 25:609, 2006). Surgical excision.		Resistant to INH & PZA (AJRCCM 156:51, 1997. Also susceptible in vitro to linezolid (AAC 47:1736, 2003). CIP, moxifloxacin also show moderate in vitro activity (AAC 46:1114, 2002).
L. Mycobacterium scrofulaceum	Surgical excision. Chemotherapy seldom indicated. Although regimens not defined, **clarithro + CLO** with or **without ETB**, **INH**, **RIF**, **strep**, **cycloserine** have also been used		In vitro resistant to INH, RIF, ETB, PZA, AMK, CIP (CID 20: 549, 1995). Susceptible to clarithro, strep, erythromycin.
M. Mycobacterium simiae	Regimen(s) not defined. Start 4 drugs as for disseminated MAI.		Most isolates resistant to all 1st-line anti-tbc drugs. Isolates often not clinically significant (CID 26: 625, 1998).
N. Mycobacterium ulcerans (Buruli ulcer)	**RIF + AMK** (7.5 mg per kg IM bid) or (**ETB + TMP-SMX** (160/800 mg po bid) for 4–8 weeks. Surgical excision important. WHO recommends RIF + SM for 8 weeks regardless of whether they not clear (Lancet Infection 6:288, 2006; Lancet 367:1849, 2006; AAC 51:645, 2007).		Susceptible in vitro to RIF, strep, CLO, clarithro, CIP, ofox, amikacin, moxi, linezolid (AAC 42:2070, 1998; JAC 45: 231, 2000; AAC 46:3193, 2002; AAC 52:1921, 2006). Monotherapy with RIF selects resistant mutants in mice (AAC 47:1228, 2003). RIF + strep effective in small study (AAC 49:3182, 2005). Treatment generally disappointing—see review. Ln 354:1013, 1999. RIF + dapsone only slightly better (82% improved) than placebo (75%) in small study (IntJ Inf Dis 6:60, 2002).
O. Mycobacterium xenopi	Regimen(s) not defined (CID 24:226 & 233, 1997). Some recommend a **macrolide** + (**RIF** or **rifabutin**) + **ETB** ± **SM** (AJRCCM 156:51, 1997) or **RIF** + **INH** ± **ETB** (Resp Med 97:439, 2003) but recent study suggests no need to treat in most pts with HIV (CID 37:1250, 2003)		In vitro sensitive to clarithro (AAC 36:2841, 1992) and rifabutin (JAC 39:567, 1997) and many standard antimycobacterial drugs. Clarithro-containing regimens more effective than RIF/INH/ETB regimens in mice (AAC 45:3229, 2001). FQs, linezolid also active in vitro.

See page 2 for abbreviations.

* Dosages are for adults (unless otherwise indicated) and assume normal renal function.   † **DOT** = directly observed therapy

TABLE 12A (11)

CAUSATIVE AGENT/DISEASE	MODIFYING CIRCUMSTANCES	SUGGESTED REGIMENS PRIMARY	ALTERNATIVE	COMMENTS
Mycobacterium leprae (leprosy) Classification: CID 44:1096, 2007.	There are 2 sets of therapeutic recommendations here: one from USA (National Hansen's Disease Programs [NHDP], Baton Rouge, LA) and one from WHO. Both are based on expert recommendations and neither has been subjected to controlled clinical trial (*P. Joyce & D. Scollard, Conn's Current Therapy 2004; MP Joyce, Immigration Medicine, in press 2006; J Am Acad Dermato 51:417, 2004*).			
	Type of Disease	**NHDP Regimen**		COMMENTS
Paucibacillary Forms: (Intermediate, Tuberculoid, Borderline tuberculoid)	Paucibacillary leprosy	Dapsone 100 mg/day + RIF 600 mg po/day for 12 months		Side effects overall 0.4%
Single lesion paucibacillary		Treat as paucibacillary leprosy for 12 months.		
	Type of Disease	**WHO Regimen**		
Paucibacillary Forms: (Intermediate, Tuberculoid, Borderline tuberculoid)		Dapsone 100 mg/day + RIF 600 mg po/day for 6 mo		
Single lesion paucibacillary		Single dose ROM therapy: (RIF 600 mg + Oflox 400 mg + Mino 100 mg) (Ln 353:655, 1999).		
Multibacillary forms: Borderline Borderline-lepromatous Lepromatous See Comment for *erythema nodosum leprosum* Rev. *Lancet 363:1209, 2004*	**NHDP Regimen:** (Dapsone 100 mg/day + CLO 50mg/day + RIF 600mg/day) for 24mo **Alternative regimen:** (Dapsone 100 mg/day + RIF 600 mg/day + Minocycline 100mg/day for 24mo if CLO is refused or unavailable.)	**WHO Regimen** (Dapsone 100 mg/day + CLO 50 mg/day (both unsupervised) + RIF 600 mg + CLO 300 mg once monthly (supervised)). Continue regimen for 12 months.		Side-effects overall 5.1%. For erythema nodosum leprosum: prednisone 60–80mg/day or thalidomide 100–400mg/day (*BMJ 44: 775, 1988; AJM 108:487, 2000*). Thalidomide available in US at 1-800-4-CELGENE. Altho thalidomide effective, WHO no longer rec because of potential toxicity (*UID 193:1743, 2006*) however the majority of leprosy experts feel thalidomide remains drug of choice for ENL under strict supervision. CLO (Clofazimine) (250mg/24hr) or **prothionamide** (375mg q24h) may be subst for CLO. Oflox 400mg po q24h; bactericidal and effective clinically with 4 log₄ ↓ in organisms in small trials (*AAC 38:662, 1994; AAC 38:61, 1994*). Clarithro also rapidly bactericidal (*AAC 38:515, 1994; Ln 345:4, 1995*.) Regimens incorporating clarithro, minocycline, RIF, moxifloxacin, and/or oflox also show promise (*AAC 44:2919, 2000; AAC 50:1568, 2006*). High relapse rate in pts treated with q24h RIF + oflox for 4wk (*Ln 41:1953, 1997*). Resistance to dapsone, RIF & oflox reported (*Ln 349:103, 1997*). Dapsone monotherapy has been abandoned due to emergence of resistance, but older patients previously treated with dapsone monotherapy may remain on lifelong maintenance therapy. Dapsone (or acedapsone⁴⁸) effective for prophylaxis in one study (*JI 41:137, 2000*).

TABLE 12B – DOSAGE, PRICE AND SELECTED ADVERSE EFFECTS OF ANTIMYCOBACTERIAL DRUGS

AGENT (TRADE NAME)[1]	USUAL DOSAGE*	ROUTE[1] / DRUG RESISTANCE (RES) US[3]/COST**	SIDE-EFFECTS, TOXICITY AND PRECAUTIONS	SURVEILLANCE
FIRST LINE DRUGS				
Ethambutol (Myambutol)	25mg/kg/day for 2mo then 15mg/kg/q24h; or as indicated [< 10% resistance] [Bacteriostatic to both extra-cellular & intracellular organisms]	po RES: 0.3% (0–0.7%) 400 mg tab $1.80	**Optic neuritis** with decreased visual acuity, central scotomata, and loss of green and red color vision (esp. high dose), peripheral neuropathy and headache (1.3%), rashes (rare), arthralgia (rare), hyperuricemia (rare). Anaphylactoid reaction (rare). *Primarily used to inhibit resistance.* Disrupts outer cell membrane in M. avium with ↑ activity to other drugs.	Monthly visual acuity & red/green with doses >15mg/kg/day; ≥10% loss considered significant. Usually reversible if drug discontinued.

---

[1] Note: Malabsorption of antimycobacterial drugs may occur in patients with AIDS enteropathy. For review of adverse effects, see *AJRCCM 167:1472, 2003.*

[2] RES = % resistance of M. tuberculosis

[1] DOT = directly observed therapy

** Cost = average wholesale price from 2007 RED BOOK, Thomson Healthcare, Inc.

[2] Dosages are for adults (unless otherwise indicated) and assume normal renal function

See page 2 for abbreviations.

TABLE 12B (2)

AGENT (TRADE NAME)[1]	USUAL DOSAGE*	ROUTE/[1] DRUG RESISTANCE (RES) US$[1]/COST**	SIDE-EFFECTS, TOXICITY AND PRECAUTIONS	SURVEILLANCE
FIRST LINE DRUGS *(continued)*				
Isoniazid (INH) (Nydrazid, Laniazid, Teebaconin)	Q24h dose: 5–10mg/kg/day up to 300mg/day as 1 dose. 2x/wk dose: 15mg/kg (900mg max dose) (< 10% protein binding) [Bactericidal to both intracellular and intracellular organisms] Add pyridoxine in alcoholic, pregnant, or malnourished pts.	po RES: 4.1% (2.6–8.5%) 300 mg tab $0.02 IM (IV route not FDA-approved but has been used, esp. in AIDS) 100 mg per mL in 10 mL vials (IM) $16.64	Overall –1%. Liver: **Hep** (children 10% mild ↑ SGOT; normalizes with continued rx, age ~<20yr (rare), 20–34yr 1.2%, ≥50yr 2.3%) [also ↑ with q24h alcohol & previous exposure to Hep C (usually asymptomatic—*CID* 36:293, 2003)]. May be fatal. With prodromal sx, dark urine, obs LFTs, discontinue. **Peripheral neuropathy** (17% on 6mg/kg per day, less on 300mg, incidence ↑ in slow acetylators); **pyridoxine 10mg q24h will ↓ incidence** of/or neurologic sequelae: convulsions, optic neuritis, toxic encephalopathy, psychosis, muscle twitching, dizziness, coma (all rare). Skin rashes, fever, minor disulfiram-like reaction, flushing after Swiss cheese, blood dyscrasias (rare); + antinuclear (20%). **Drug-drug interactions common, see *Table 22***	Pre-rx liver functions. Repeat if symptoms (fatigue, weakness, malaise, anorexia, nausea or vomiting) >3 days (*AJRCCM* 152:1705, 1995). Some recommend SGOT at 2, 4, 6 mo esp. if age >50yr. Clinical evaluation every mo.
Pyrazinamide	25 mg per kg per day (maximum 2.5 gm per day) q24h as 1 dose [Bactericidal for intracellular organisms]	po RES: 0.2% (0–0.3%) 300 mg cap $2 [IV available, Merrell-Dow. Cost 600 mg ($7.4/M)]	**Arthralgia; hyperuricemia** (with or without symptoms); hepatitis (if recommended dose not exceeded); gastric irritation; photosensitivity (rare).	Pre-rx liver functions. Monthly SGOT, uric acid. Measure serum uric acid if symptomatic gouty attack occurs
Rifamate— combination tablet	2 tablets single dose q24h	po (1 hr before meal) 1 tab $3	1 tablet contains 150 mg INH, 300 mg RIF	As with individual drugs
Rifampin (Rifadin, Rimactane, Rifocin)	10.0 mg per kg per day up to 600 mg (600 mg q24h as 1 dose (60–90% protein binding) [Bactericidal to all populations of organisms]	po (1 hr before meal) 300 mg cap $2 600 mg $3.27	INH-RIF decr'd in ~3% for toxicity; gastrointestinal irritation, antibiotic-associated colitis, drug fever (1%), pruritus with or without skin rash (1%), anaphylactoid reactions in HIV+ pts, mental confusion, thrombocytopenia (1%), leukopenia (1%), headache, bone pain, transient shortness of breath) seen if RIF taken regularly or if q24h dose restarted after an interval of no rx. **Discolors urine, sweat, contact lens an orange-brownish color.** May cause drug-induced lupus erythematosus (*Ln* 349:1521, 1977).	Pre-rx liver function. Repeat if symptoms. **Multiple significant drug-drug interactions, see *Table 22***
Rifater— combination tablet (See *Side-Effects*)	Wt ≥55 kg, 6 tablets single dose q24h	po (1 hr before meal) 1 tab $1.21	1 tablet contains 50 mg INH, 120 mg RIF, 300 mg PZA. Used in 1st 2 months of rx (PZA 25 mg per kg) but ↑ compliance (*AWM* 122: 951, 1995) but cost 1.58 more. Side-effects = individual drugs	As with individual drugs, PZA 25 mg per kg
Streptomycin	15 mg per kg IM q24h, 0.75–1.0 gm per day initially for 60–90 days, then 1.0 gm 2–3 times per week (15 mg per kg per day q24h as 1 dose	IM (or IV) RES: 3.9% (2.7–7.6%) 1.0 gm $9.10	Overall 8%. **Ototoxicity** vestibular dysfunction (vertigo), paresthesias; dizziness & nausea (all less in pts receiving ≤2.3 doses per week); tinnitus and high frequency loss (1%). Discontinuation rates 8%. Available from X-Gen Pharmaceuticals, 607-732-4411, Ref. re: *N—CID* 19:1150, 1994 nephrotoxicity (rare); peripheral neuropathy (rare); allergic skin rashes (4–5%); drug fever. Toxicity similar with q24h vs bid dosing (*CID* 38:1538, 2004).	Monthly audiogram. In older pts, serum creatinine or BUN at start of rx and weekly if pt stable
SECOND LINE DRUGS (more difficult to use and/or less effective than first line drugs)				
Amikacin (Amikin)	7.5–10.0 mg per kg q24h [Bactericidal for extracellular organisms]	IV or IM RES: (est 0.1%) 500 mg $7.80	See *Table 10, pages 80 & 93* Toxicity similar with qd vs bid dosing (*CID* 38:1538, 2004).	Monthly audiogram. Serum creatinine or BUN weekly if pt stable
Capreomycin sulfate (Capastat sulfate)	1 gm per day (15 mg per kg per day) q24h as 1 dose	IM or IV RES: 0.1% (0–0.9%) 1 gm $63.54	Nephrotoxicity (36%), ototoxicity (auditory 11%), eosinophilia, leukopenia, skin rash, fever, hypokalemia, neuromuscular blockade.	Monthly audiogram, biweekly serum creatinine or BUN
Ciprofloxacin (Cipro)	750 mg bid	po 750 mg (po) $7	TB not an FDA-approved indication for CIP. Desired CIP serum levels 4–6 mcg per mL, requires median dose 800 mg (*AJRCCM* 151:2006, 1995). Discontinuation rates 6%. CIP well tolerated (*AJRCCM* 151:2006, 1995). FQ-resistant M. Tb identified in New York (*Ln* 345:1148, 1995). See *Table 10, pages 83 & 90* for adverse effects.	None

See page 2 for abbreviations.   * Dosages are for adults (*unless otherwise indicated*)   [1] DOT = directly observed therapy
** Cost = average wholesale price from 2007 RED BOOK, Thomson Healthcare, Inc.   † Mean (range) (higher in Hispanics, Asians, and patients < 10 years old)

TABLE 12B (3)

AGENT (TRADE NAME)[1]	USUAL DOSAGE*	ROUTE/[1] DRUG RESISTANCE (RES) US[1]/COST**	SIDE-EFFECTS, TOXICITY AND PRECAUTIONS	SURVEILLANCE
SECOND LINE DRUGS (continued)				
Clofazimine (Lamprene)	50 mg per day (unsupervised) + 300 mg 1 time per month supervised or 100 mg per day	po (with meals) 50 mg $0.20	Skin: **pigmentation (pink-brownish black)** 75–100%; dryness 20%; pruritus 5%. GI: abdominal pain 50% (rarely severe leading to exploratory laparoscopy), splenic infarction (VR), bowel obstruction (VR), GI bleeding (VR). Eye: conjunctival irritation, retinal crystal deposits.	None
Cycloserine (Seromycin)	750–1000 mg per day (15 mg per kg per day) 2–4 doses per day $4 [Bacteriostatic for both extra-cellular & intracellular organisms]	po RES: 0.1% (0–0.3%) 250 mg cap $4	Convulsions, **psychoses** (5–10% of those receiving 1.0 gm per day); headache, somnolence; hyperreflexia, increased CSF protein and pressure, **peripheral neuropathy**. 100 mg pyridoxine (or more) q24h should be given concomitantly. Contraindicated in epileptics.	None
Dapsone	100 mg per day	po 100 mg $0.20	Blood: ↓ hemoglobin (1–2 gm) & ↑ retics (2–12%) in most pts. Hemolysis in G6PD deficiency. **Methemoglobinemia.** CNS: peripheral neuropathy (rare). GI: nausea, vomiting. Renal: albuminuria, nephrotic syndrome. Erythema nodosum leprosum in pts rx for leprosy (½–⅓ int'l year).	None
Ethionamide (Trecator-SC)	500–1000 mg per day (15–20 mg per kg per day) 1–3 doses per day [Bacteriostatic for extracellular organisms only]	po RES: 0.8% (0–1.5%) 250 mg tab $3.20	Gastrointestinal irritation (up to 50% on large dose); goiter; peripheral neuropathy (rare); convulsions (rare); changes in affect (rare); difficulty in diabetes control; rashes; hepatitis; purpura; stomatitis, gynecomastia, menstrual irregularity. Give drug with meals or antacids; 50–100 mg pyridoxine per day concomitantly. SGOT monthly. Possibly teratogenic.	None
Ofloxacin (Floxin)	400 mg bid	po, IV 400 mg (po) $6	Not FDA-approved. Overall adverse effects 11%, 4% discontinued due to side-effects. GI: nausea 3%, diarrhea 1%. CNS: insomnia 3%, headache 1%, dizziness 1%.	None
Para-aminosalicylic acid (PAS, Paser) (Na⁺ or K⁺ salt)	4–6 gm bid (200 mg per kg per day) [Bacteriostatic for extracellular organisms only]	po RES: 0.8% (0–1.5%) 450 mg tab $0.08 (see Comment)	Gastrointestinal irritation (10–15%); goitrogenic action (rare); depressed prothrombin activity (rare); G6PD-mediated hemolytic anemia (rare), drug fever; rashes; hepatitis; myalgia; arthralgia. Retards hepatic enzyme induction, may ↑ INH hepatotoxicity. Available from: CDC (404) 639-3670. Jacobus Pharm. Co. (609) 921-7447.	None
Rifabutin (Mycobutin)	300 mg per day (prophylaxis or treatment)	po 150 mg $8	Polymyalgia, polyarthralgia, leukopenia, granulocytopenia. Anterior uveitis when given with concomitant clarithromycin; avoid 600 mg dose (NEJM 330:438, 1994). Uveitis reported with 300 mg per day (AnIM 12:510, 1994). Reddish urine, orange skin (pseudojaundice).	None
Rifapentine (Priftin)	600 mg twice weekly for 1st 2 mos., then 600 mg q4wk	po 150 mg $3.38	Similar to other rifabutins. (See RIF, RFB). Causes red-orange discoloration of body fluids. Note ↑ prevalence of RIF resistance in pts on weekly rx (Ln 353:1843, 1999).	None
Thalidomide (Thalomid)	100–300 mg po q24h (may use up to 400 mg po q24h for severe erythema nodosum leprosum)	po 50 mg $79	Contraindicated in pregnancy. Causes severe life-threatening birth defects. Both male and female patients must use barrier contraceptive methods (Pregnancy Category X). Frequently causes drowsiness or somnolence. May cause peripheral neuropathy (AnIM 108:487, 2000) For review, see Ln 363:1802, 2004	Available only through pharmacists participating in System for Thalidomide Education and Prescribing Safety (S.T.E.P.S.)

See page 2 for abbreviations.   * Dosages are for adults (*unless otherwise indicated*) and assume normal renal function   † **DOT** = directly observed therapy
** Cost= average wholesale price from 2007 RED BOOK, Thomson Healthcare, Inc.   ‡ Mean (range) (higher in Hispanics, Asians, and patients <10 years old)

TABLE 13A – TREATMENT OF PARASITIC INFECTIONS*

Many of the drugs suggested are not licensed in the US. The following are helpful resources available through the Center for Disease Control and Prevention (CDC) in Atlanta. Website is www.cdc.gov.
General advice for parasitic diseases other than malaria: (770) 488-7760 or (770) 488-7775.
For CDC Drug Service* 8:00 a.m. – 4:30 p.m. EST: (404) 639-3670 (or -2888); emergency after hours: (404) 639-2888; fax: (404) 639-3717.
For malaria: Prophylaxis advice (770) 488-7788; treatment (770) 488-7760; website: www.cdc.gov/travel
NOTE: All dosage regimens are for adults with normal renal function unless otherwise stated.
For licensed drugs, suggest checking package inserts to verify dosage and side-effects. Occasionally, post-licensure data may alter dosage as compared to package inserts.
For abbreviations of journal titles, see page's. **Reference with peds dosages: *Medical Letter "Drugs for Parasitic Infections" (Suppl), 2007. General resource: www.gideononline.com**

INFECTING ORGANISM	SUGGESTED REGIMENS		COMMENTS
	PRIMARY	ALTERNATIVE	
PROTOZOA—INTESTINAL (non-pathogenic: E. hartmanni, E. dispar, E. coli, Iodamoeba butschlii, Endolimax nana, Chilomastix mesnili)			
Balantidium coli	Tetracycline 500 mg po tid x 10 days	Metronidazole 750 mg po tid x 5 days	*Another alternative: Iodoquinol 650 mg po tid x 20 days.*
Blastocystis hominis: Role as pathogen controversial	Nitazoxanide: Adults 500mg tabs (children 200mg oral suspension)—both po q12h x 3 days (*AJTMH 68:384, 2003*).	Metronidazole 1.5 gm po as single dose 1x/day x 10 d (placebo-controlled trial in *J Travel Med 10:128, 2003*). Alternatives: Iodoquinol 650 mg po tid x 20 days or **TMP-SMX-DS**, one bid x 7 days	Nitazoxanide: Approved in liquid formulation for rx of children & 500mg tabs for adults. Ref.: *CID 40:1173, 2005.*
Cryptosporidium parvum & hominis Treatment is unsatisfactory Ref. *CID 39:504, 2004*	**Immunocompetent—No Rx:** Nitazoxanide 500 mg po bid x3 days	**HIV with immunodeficiency:** (1) Effective anti-retroviral therapy best therapy; (2) Nitazoxanide 500 mg po bid x 14 days in adults (60% response). No response in HIV+ children.	C. hominis assoc. with [+] in post-infection eye & joint pain, recurrent headache, & dizzy spells (*CID 39:504, 2004*)
Cyclospora cayetanensis	Immunocompetent pts: **TMP-SMX-DS** tab 1 po bid x 7–10 days	AIDS Pts: **TMP-SMX-DS** tab 1 po qid x 10 days; then tab 1 po 3x/wk	If AIDS pts: **CIP** 500mg po bid x7 days & then 1 tab po 3x/wk x 2wk or **Nitazoxanide** 500 mg po q12h x 7 days (*CID 44:466, 2007*).
Dientamoeba fragilis Treat if patient symptomatic	Iodoquinol 650 mg po tid x 20 days	Tetracycline 500 mg po qid x 10 days OR Metronidazole 500–750 mg po tid x 10 days	Other alternatives: doxy 100mg po bid x 10 days; paromomycin 25-35 mg/kg/day po in 3 divided doses x 7 days.
Entamoeba histolytica; amebiasis	Reviews: *Ln 361:1025, 2003; NEJM 348:1563, 2003*		Metronidazole not effective vs cysts.
Asymptomatic cyst passer	Paromomycin (aminosidine in U.K.) 500 mg po tid x 7 days OR Iodoquinol 650 mg po tid x20 days	Diloxanide furoate[NUS] (Furamide) 500 mg po tid x 10 days (Source: Panorama Compound. Pharm., 800-247-9767).	
Patient with diarrhea/dysentery; mild/moderate disease. Oral therapy possible	Metronidazole 500–750 mg po tid x 10 days or tinidazole 2 gm 1x/day x3 days, followed by: Either {paromomycin 25-35 mg/kg/day po divided in 3 doses x7 days} or {iodoquinol 650 mg po tid x 20 days} to clear intestinal cysts. See comment.	Tinidazole[+] 1 gm po q12h x 3 days} or {ornidazole[NUS] 500 mg po q12h x 5 days} followed by:	Colitis can mimic ulcerative colitis; ameboma can mimic adenocarcinoma of colon. Dx: antigen detection & PCR better than O&P. Nitazoxanide 500 mg po bid x 3 days effective in 2 controlled studies (*JID 184:381, 2001 & Tran R Soc Trop Med & Hyg 101:1025, 2007).*
Severe or extraintestinal infection, e.g. hepatic abscess	Metronidazole 750 mg **IV** or **PO** tid x10 days or tinidazole 2 gm 1x/day x 5 days} followed by paromomycin 25-35 mg/kg/day po divided in 3 doses		Serology positive (antibody present) with extraintestinal disease.
Giardia lamblia; giardiasis	{Tinidazole 2 gm po x 1} OR {nitazoxanide 500 mg po bid x3 days}	Metronidazole 250 mg po tid x 5 days (high frequency of GI side-effects). See Comment. Rx if preg: Paromomycin 500 mg 4x /day x7 days	Refractory pts: {metro 750mg po + quinacrine[+] 100 mg po}—both 3x/day x 3wk. Ref. *CID 33:22, 2001.*
Isospora belli	**TMP-SMX-DS** tab 1 po bid x 10 days; if AIDS Pt: **TMP-SMX-DS** qid x 10 days & then bid x 3wk.	Pyrimethamine 75 mg/day po + folinic acid 10mg/day po] x 14 days **CIP** 500 mg po bid x 7 days—87% response (*AnIM 132:885, 2000*).	Chronic suppression in AIDS: either 1 **TMP-SMX-DS** tab 3x/wk OR {pyrimethamine 25mg/day po + folinic acid 5mg/day po}.

[1] Drugs available from CDC Drug Service: 404-639-2888 or -3670 www.cdc.gov/ncidod/srp/drugs/formulary.html; melarsoprol, nifurtimox, stibogluconate (Pentostam), suramin.

[2] Quinacrine available from Panorama Compounding Pharmacy, (800) 247-9767, (818) 988-7979.

* See page's for abbreviations. All dosage recommendations are for adults (unless otherwise indicated) and assume normal renal function.

** Cost = average wholesale price from 2007 RED BOOK, Thomson Healthcare, Inc.

TABLE 13A (2)

INFECTING ORGANISM	SUGGESTED REGIMENS		COMMENTS
	PRIMARY	ALTERNATIVE	
PROTOZOA—INTESTINAL (continued)			
Microsporidiosis			
Ocular: Encephalitozoon hellum or cuniculi, Vittaforma (Nosema) corneae, Nosema ocularum	Albendazole 400 mg po bid x 3wk plus fumagillin eye drops (see Comment)	For HIV pts, antiretroviral therapy key	To obtain fumagillin: 800-292-6773 or www.leiterrx.com. Neutropenia & thrombocytopenia serious adverse events. Dx: Most labs use modified trichrome stain. Need electron micrographs for species identification. FA and PCR methods in development.
Intestinal (diarrhea): Enterocytozoon bieneusi, Encephalitozoon (Septata) intestinalis	Albendazole 400 mg po bid x 3wk; peds dose 15 mg/kg per day into 2 daily doses x 7 days	For V. corneae, may need vitrectomy.	Peds dose ref.: PIDJ 23:915, 2004
Disseminated: E. hellum, cuniculi or intestinalis, Pleistophora sp., others in Comment	Albendazole 400 mg po bid x 3wk	Oral **fumagillin 20 mg po tid** reported effective for **E. bieneusi** (NEJM 346:1963, 2002)—see Comment	For Trachipleistophora sp., try itraconazole + albendazole (NEJM 351:42, 2004).
		No established rx for Pleistophora sp.	Other pathogens: Brachiola vesiculatum & algerae (NEJM 351:42, 2004)
PROTOZOA—EXTRAINTESTINAL			
Amebic meningoencephalitis			
Acanthamoeba sp.— no proven rx Rev. FEMS Immuno/ Med Micro 50:1, 2007.	Success with IV **pentamidine**, topical **chlorhexidine** & 2% **ketoconazole** cream & then po **itra** (NEJM 331:85, 1994). 2 children responded to po rx: **TMP-SMX + rifampin+ keto** (PIDJ 20:623, 2001).		For treatment of keratitis, see Table 1, page 12
Balamuthia mandrillaris	**Pentamidine + clarithro + flucon + sulfadiazine + fluctyosine** (CID 37:1304, 2003; Arch Path Lab Med 128:466, 2004).		
Naegleria fowleri. >95% mortality	A cause of chronic granulomatous meningitis		
	Ampho B 1.5mg/kg per day in 2 div. doses x 3 days, then 1 mg/kg/da x 6 days plus 1.5 mg/da intrathecal 2 days, then 1 mg/da intrathecal qod x 8 days.	**Ampho B + azithro** synergistic in vitro & in mouse model (AAC 51:23, 2007).	
Sappinia diploidea	**Azithro + pentamidine + itra + flucytosine** (JAMA 285:2450, 2001)		
Babesia microti; babesiosis (CID 32:1117, 2001)	**Atovaquone** 750mg bid po x 7-10 days + **azithro** 500 mg po x 1 dose, then 250 mg q24h x 7 days (NEJM 343:1454, 2000)	(**Clindamycin** 600mg po tid) + (**quinine** 650mg po tid) x 7-10 days for adults, can give **clinda** IV as 1.2gm bid.	Can cause overwhelming infection in asplenic patients. Reported in Washington State (EID 10:622, 2004).
Ehrlichiosis—See Table 1, page 51			
Leishmaniasis. Complicated—consultation suggested. Refs: Ln366:1561, 2005 & LnID 6:342, 2006 & LnID 7:581, 2007 & CID 195:1846, 2007			
Cutaneous (C) & Mucocutaneous (MC) disease.	**Always start with antimony for mucocutaneous disease.**		Concern for species that disseminate to mucosa. Method of choice for speciation is PCR - not widely available, so empirically treat for species with potential to disseminate.
New World (Mexico/Cen./S. Amer.):	**(C)** Sodium stibogluconate (**Pentostam**) from CDC drug service (404-639-3670) or **meglumine antimoniate (Glucantime)** from France & Latin America. Dose: 20 mg/kg/d IV x 28 d. Dilute in 120mL of D5W & infuse over 2 hr. Ideally, monitor EKG. Note: only antimony drugs efficacious vs L. braziliensis.	**Amphotericin B** 1 mg/kg IV q.o.d. x 20 doses **or Liposomal Amphotericin B (Ambisome)** 3 mg/kg per day for 6 d for cutaneous & 3 wks for mucocutaneous. **Or miltefosine**[us] effective vs L. panamensis, marginal vs L. mexicana, failed vs L. braziliensis. Obtain from Zentaris, Germany. Impavido @ Zentaris.de. Dose 2.5mg/kg/d x 28 d. Bolivia results: CID 44:350, 2007.	Spontaneous resolution varies by species: L. mexicana: 75% in 3 mo; L. braziliensis: 10% in 3 mo; L. major 90% in 2-4 mo; L. tropica: 90% in 6-15 mo.
L. viannia includes braziliensis (C, MC), guyanensis (C, MC), panamensis (C, MC), peruviana (C) **& L. mexicana** Includes mexicana (C), amazonensis (C), venezuelensis (C), pifanoi (C). **NOTE:** antimony resistance of L. vianna reported JID 193, 1375, 2006)	**(MC):** Rx with antimony as above plus **pentoxifylline** 400 mg po tid x 30 days superior to antimony alone (CID 44:788, 2007).		For antimony AEs, see Table 13 B(1).
			Other therapies for cutaneous leishmaniasis reviewed in LnID 7:581, 2007; all have limitations.
Old World (Europe, Asia, Africa) L. major, L. tropica, L. aethiopica, L. infantum, L. chagas	**Stibogluconate or meglumine antimoniate** as above: 20mg/kg/d x 10 d		

* See page for abbreviations. All dosage recommendations are for adults (unless otherwise indicated) and assume normal renal function.

** Cost = average wholesale price from 2007 RED BOOK, Thomson Healthcare, Inc.

TABLE 13A (3)

INFECTING ORGANISM	SUGGESTED REGIMENS		COMMENTS
	PRIMARY	ALTERNATIVE	

PROTOZOA—EXTRAINTESTINAL (continued)

Visceral leishmaniasis – Kala-Azar –
New World & Old World
L. donovani: India, Africa
L. infantum: Mediterranean
L. chagasi: New World

Liposomal ampho B FDA-approved in immunocompetent hosts: 3 mg/kg once daily days 1–5 & days 14, 21; HIV 4 mg/kg on 2 consecutive days. All IV.	Stibogluconate or meglumine antimoniate (resistance in India & Mediterranean): 20 mg/kg/day IV in single dose x 28 days OR Miltefosine[NFS] 1.5–2.5 mg/kg/day po x 28 days.	Another alternative: standard ampho B 1 mg/kg IV qod daily x 20 days. Ref: liposomal ampho B:CID 43:917, 2006.	

Malaria (Plasmodia species)—NOTE: CDC Malaria info—prophylaxis/treatment (770) 488-7788. After hours: 770-488-7100. Refs: JAMA 297:2251, 2264 & 2285, 2007.

Prophylaxis—Drugs influence personal protection: screens, nets, 30–35% DEET skin repellent (avoid 95% products in children), permethrin spray on clothing and mosquito nets
Websites: www.cdc.gov/malaria; www.who.int/health-topics/malaria.htm.

For areas free of chloroquine (CQ)-resistant P. falciparum: Central America, Haiti, Dom. Republic, Cen America, west & north of the Panama Canal, & parts of Middle East

CQ 500 mg, (300 mg base) as per wk	**CQ Peds dose:** 8.3 mg/kg (5 mg/kg of base) po 1×/wk up to 300 mg (base) max. dose **or AP** by weight (peds tabs): 11–20kg, 1 tab; 21–30 kg, 2 tabs; 31–40 kg, 3 tabs; >40 kg, 1 adult tab per day	CQ safe during pregnancy. **The areas free of CQ-resistant malaria continue to shrink:** Central America west of Panama Canal, Haiti, and parts of Middle East. CQ-resistant falciparum malaria reported from Saudi Arabia, Yemen, Oman, & Iran.	

For areas free of chloroquine begin 1–2 wk before travel, during travel, & 4 wks after travel or **atovaquone-proguanil (AP)** 1 adult tab per day (1 day prior to, during, & 7 days post-travel). Note May exacerbate psoriasis.

For areas with CQ-resistant P. falciparum:
CDC info on prophylaxis (770) 488-7788 or website: www.cdc.gov & LnID 6:139, 2006

Atovaquone-proguanil 100mg (Malarone) comb. tablet, 1 per day with food 1–2 days prior to, during, & 7 days post-travel. Peds dose in footnote* Cost per 2wks: $125. Not in pregnancy. Another option for adults: **primaquine (PQ)** 30 mg (base) po daily in non-pregnant G6PD-neg. travelers 88% protective vs P. falciparum; >92% vs P. vivax (CID 33:1990, 2001).	**Doxycycline** 100 mg po daily for adults & children >8yr of age¹ Take 1–2 days before, during, & for 4 wks after travel. Cost per 2wks: $30 **OR Mefloquine (MQ)** 250 mg (228 mg base) po once per wk. Start 1–2 wks before travel, during, & for 4 wks after travel. (Mk. 1–2 wks before, during, & for 4 wks after travel. Peds dose in footnote¹) [Cost per 2wks: $68].	**Pregnancy: MQ current best option.** Insufficient data with Malarone. **Avoid doxycycline and primaquine.** **Primaquine:** Used only if prolonged exposure to endemic area (e.g., Peace Corps). **Can cause hemolytic anemia if G6PD deficiency present.** **MQ not recommended** for cardiac conduction abnormalities, seizures, or psychiatric disorders; e.g. depression, psychosis. MQ outside U.S. 275 mg tab, contains 250 mg of base.	

Treatment of Malaria

Clinical Severity/ Plasmodia sp.	Region Acquired	Suggested Treatment Regimens (Drug)		Comments
		Primary—Adults	**Alternative & Peds**	
Uncomplicated/ P. falciparum (or species not identified)	Cen. Amer., Dom Rep. of Panama Canal, Haiti, Dom. Republic, & most of Mid East—**CQ-sensitive**	**CQ** 1gm salt (600 mg base) po, then 0.5 gm in 6 hrs, then 0.5gm daily x 2 days. Total 2500 mg salt	**Peds CQ** 10 mg/kg of base po, then 5 mg/kg of base at 6, 24, & 48 hrs. Total 25 mg/kg base	Peds dose should never exceed adult dose.
	CQ-resistant or unknown resistance	**QS** 650 mg po bid) + **(Doxy** 100 mg po bid) or **tetra** 250 mg po qid) or **clinda** 20 mg/kg/d divided tid) x 7 days **OR** **Atovaquone-proguanil** 1gm–400 mg (4 adult tabs) po 1×/day x 3 days w/ food or **mefloquine** 750 mg po x 1 dose, then 500 mg po x 1 dose 6–12hr later.	**MQ** 750 mg po, then 500 mg po in 12 hrs. **OR** **clinda** (QS 10 mg/kg po tid) + **clinda** (20 mg/kg per day tid) – both x 7 days	Can substitute clinda for doxy/tetra. 20 mg/kg per day po div. tid x 7 days. MQ alternative due to neuropsych. reactions. Avoid if malaria acquired in SE Asia due to resistance.
Malaria rapid diagnostic test (Binax NOW) approved MMWR 56:686, 2007				
Uncomplicated / P. malariae	All regions	**CQ** as above: adults & peds		

---

¹ **Peds prophylaxis dosages** (Ref: CID 34:493, 2002): **Mefloquine** weekly dose by **weight** in kg: <15 = 5 mg/kg; 15–19 = ¼ adult dose; 20–30 = ½ adult dose; 31–45 = ¾ adult dose; >45 = adult dose. **Atovaquone/proguanil** by **weight** in kg, single daily dose using peds tab (62.5 mg atovaquone & 25 mg proguanil): <11 kg—do not use; 11–20 kg, 1 tab; 21–30 kg, 2 tabs; 31–40 kg, 3 tabs; ≥41 kg, one adult tab. **Doxycycline** ages >8–12 yrs: 2 mg per kg per day up to 100 mg/day. Continue daily x 4 wks after leaving risk area. Side effects: photosensitivity, nausea, yeast vaginitis.

* See page for abbreviations. All dosage recommendations are for adults (unless otherwise indicated) and assume normal renal function.
** Cost = average wholesale price from 2007 RED BOOK, Thomson Healthcare, Inc.

TABLE 13A (4)

PROTOZOA—EXTRAINTESTINAL/Malaria/Treatment *(continued)*

INFECTING ORGANISM		SUGGESTED REGIMENS		COMMENTS
Clinical Severity/ Plasmodia sp.	Region Acquired	PRIMARY	ALTERNATIVE	Comments
		Primary—Adults	Alternative & Peds (Drug)	
Uncomplicated/ **P. vivax or P. ovale**	All except Papua, New Guinea & Indonesia (CQ-resistant)	**CQ** as above + **PQ** base: 30 mg po once daily x 14 days	**Peds: CQ** as above + **PQ** base 0.5 mg po once daily x 14 days	PQ added to eradicate latent parasites in liver. Screen for G6PD def. before starting PQ. If G6PD positive, dose PQ as 45mg po once weekly x 8wk. Avoid PQ in pregnancy.
Uncomplicated/ **P. vivax**	CQ-sensitive areas; CQ-resistant P. vivax Papua, New Guinea & Indonesia	**QS + (doxy or tetra) + PQ** as above	**MQ + PQ** as above **Peds** (<8yrs old): **QS** alone x 7 days or **MQ** alone. If latter fail, add **doxy** or **tetra**	Doxy or tetra used if benefits outweigh risks. No controlled studies of AP in pregnancy. Possible association of MQ & number of stillbirths. If P. vivax or P. ovale, after pregnancy check for G6PD & give PQ 30 mg daily, times 14 days.
Uncomplicated **Malaria/Alternatives for** **Pregnancy** Ref. LnID 7:118 & 136, 2007	CQ-sensitive areas; CQ-resistant P. falciparum	**CQ** as above **QS + clinda** as above	**CQ** as above If failing or intolerant, **QS + clinda**	
	CQ-resistant P. vivax	**QS** 650mg po bid x 7 days		
Severe malaria (i.e. impaired consciousness, severe anemia, renal failure, pulmonary edema, ARDS, DIC, jaundice, acidosis, seizures, parasitemia >5%. One or more of latter	All regions	**Quinidine gluconate** in normal saline: 10 mg/kg (salt) IV over 1 hr then 0.02 mg/ kg/min by constant infusion OR 24 mg/kg IV over 4 hrs & then 12 mg/kg over 4 hrs q8h. Once parasite density <1% & can take po (QS, QS as above x 7 days (SE Asia) or 3 days elsewhere **PLUS** (**Doxy** 100 mg IV q12h x 7 days) **OR** (**clinda** 10 mg/kg IV load & then 5 mg/kg IV q8h x 7 days)	**Peds: Quinidine gluconate IV—** same mg/kg dose as for adults **PLUS** (**Doxy** (if <45 kg), 4 mg/kg per kg IV q12h; if ≥45 kg dose as for adults) OR **Clinda**, same mg/kg dose as for adults	During quinidine IV: monitor BP; EKG (prolongation of QTc), & blood glucose (hypoglycemia). Consider exchange transfusion if parasitemia >10%. Switch to oral QS, doxy, & clinda when patient able. Steroids not recommended for cerebral malaria. If quinidine not available, or patient intolerant of high level parasitemia, IV artesunate available from CDC Drug Service (770-488-7788 or 770-488-7100) (Ref. CID 44:1067 & 1075, 2007)
Almost invariably P. falciparum				
Malaria—self-initiated treatment: Only for emergency situation where medical care not available		Atovaquone-proguanil (**AP**) 4 adult tabs (1 gm/400 mg) po daily x 3 days	**Peds:** Using adult **AP** tabs for 3 consecutive days: 11–20 kg, 1 tab; 21–30 kg, 2 tabs; 31–40 kg, 3 tabs; >41 kg, 4 tabs.	Do not use for renal insufficiency pts. Do not use if weight <11kg, pregnant, or breast-feeding.
Pneumocystis carinii pneumonia (PCP). New name is **Pneumocystis jiroveci** (yee-row-vek-ee). Refs.: CID 42:1208, 2006; LnID 7:3, 2007.				
Not acutely ill, able to take po meds. PaO₂ >70 mmHg Interest in detection of PCP by serum assay for B-Glucan (AnM 147:70, 2007 & Chest 131:1173, 2007)		(**TMP-SMX-DS**, 2 tabs po q8h x 21 days) OR (**Dapsone** 100 mg po q24h + trimethoprim 5 mg/kg po tid x 21 days) NOTE: Concomitant use of corticosteroids usually reserved for sicker pts with PaO₂ < 70 (see below).	(**Clindamycin** 300–450 mg po q6h + **primaquine** 15 mg base po q24h) x 21 days OR **Atovaquone** suspension 750 mg po bid with food x 21 days.	Mutations in gene of the enzyme target (dihydropteroate synthetase) of sulfamethoxazole identified. Unclear whether mutations result in resist. to TMP-SMX or dapsone + TMP (EID 10:1721, 2004). Dapsone ref.: CID 27:191, 1998. After 21 days, chronic suppression in AIDS pts (see below—post-treatment suppression).
Acutely ill, po or po not possible. PaO₂ <70 mmHg		**Prednisone** (15–30 min. before TMP-SMX) 40 mg po bid times 5 days, then 40 mg po q24h times 5 days, then 20 mg po q24h times 11 days) + **TMP-SMX** (15 mg/ of TMP component per kg per day) IV div. q6-8h times 21 days) Can substitute IV prednisone (reduce dose 25%) for po prednisone	**Prednisone** as in primary PLUS (**Clinda** 600 mg IV q8h) + primaquine 30 mg base po q24h) times 21 days OR **Pentamidine** 4 mg per kg per day IV times 21 days. Caspofungin active in animal models: CID 36:1445, 2003.	After 21 days, chronic suppression in AIDS pts (see below—post-treatment suppression). PCP can occur in absence of HIV infection & steroids (CID 25:215 & 219, 1997). Wait at least 1–8 days before declaring treatment failure & switching to clinda + primaquine or pentamidine. See above regarding gene mutations.

* See page for abbreviations. All dosage recommendations are for adults (unless otherwise indicated) and assume normal renal function.
** Cost = average wholesale price from 2007 RED BOOK, Thomson Healthcare, Inc.

TABLE 13A (5)

INFECTING ORGANISM	SUGGESTED REGIMENS		COMMENTS
	PRIMARY	ALTERNATIVE	
PROTOZOA—EXTRAINTESTINAL/Pneumocystis carinii pneumonia (PCP) *(continued)*			
Primary prophylaxis and post-treatment suppression	**TMP-SMX-DS** or **-SS** 1 tab po q24h or 1 DS 3x/wk) OR **(dapsone** 100 mg po q24h). DC when CD4 >200 x3mo *(NEJM 344:159, 2001).*	**Pentamidine** 300 mg q4wk in 6mL sterile water by aerosol q4 wks) OR **(dapsone** 200 mg po + **pyrimethamine** 75 mg po + **folinic acid** 25 mg po—**all once a week)** or **atovaquone** 1500 mg po q24h with food.	TMP-SMX-DS regimen provides cross-protection vs toxo and other bacterial infections. Dapsone + pyrimethamine protects vs toxo. Atovaquone suspension 1500 mg once daily effective as daily dapsone *(NEJM 339:1889, 1998)* or inhaled pentamidine *(JID 180:369, 1999)*.
Toxoplasma gondii (Reference: *Ln 363:1965, 2004)*			
Immunologically normal patients *(For pediatric doses, see reference)*			
Acute illness w/ lymphadenopathy. Acq. via transfusion (lab accident)	No specific rx unless severe/persistent symptoms or evidence of vital organ damage		
Active chorioretinitis	Treat as for active chorioretinitis.		
Active chorioretinitis: meningitis: lowered resistance due to steroids or cytotoxic drugs	**Pyrimethamine** (pyri) 200 mg po on 1st day, then 50–75 mg q24h) + (**sulfadiazine** (see footnote[1]) 1–1.5gm po qid) + (**leucovorin (folinic acid)** 5–20mg 3x/wk). Treat 1–2wk beyond resolution of signs/symptoms; continue leucovorin 1wk after stopping pyri.		For congenital toxo, toxo meningitis in adults, & chorioretinitis, **add prednisone 1mg/kg/day in 2 div. doses** until CSF protein conc. falls or vision-threatening inflammation subsides. Adjust folinic acid dose by following CBC results.
Acute in pregnant women	**Spiramycin** [From FDA, (301) 827-2335] 1 gm po q8h (w/o food) until term or until fetal infection. NOTE: Use caution interpreting commercial tests for toxoplasma IgM antibody for help. FDA Advisory (301) 594-3060. Toxoplasma Serology Lab, Palo Alto Med. Found. (650) 853-4828.		IgG avidity test of help in 1st trimester *(J Clin Micro 42:941, 2004).*
Fetal/congenital	Mgmt complex. Combo rx with pyrimethamine + sulfadiazine + leucovorin—see Comment.		Details in *Ln 363:1965, 2004.* **Consultation advisable.**
Acquired immunodeficiency syndrome (AIDS)			
Cerebral toxoplasmosis Ref.: *Ln 363:1965, 2004; CID 40(Suppl.3):S131, 2005*	**(Pyrimethamine** (pyri) 200 mg x 1, then 75 mg/day) + (**sulfadiazine** 1–1.5gm po q6h) + **folinic acid** 10–20mg/day for 4–6wks after resolution of signs/symptoms, and then suppressive rx (see below) OR **TMP-SMX** 5mg/kg (TMP component) IV or po q12h x 30 days *(AAC 42:1346, 1998).*	**Pyri** + **folinic acid** (as in primary regimen) + 1 of the following: (1) **Clinda** 600 mg po/IV q6h or (2) **clarithro** 1gm po bid or (3) **azithro** 1.2–1.5 gm po q24h or (4) **atovaquone** 750 mg po q6h. Treat 4–6 wks after resolution of signs/symptoms, then suppression.	Use alternative regimen for pts with severe sulfa allergy. If multiple ring-enhancing brain lesions (CT or MRI), >85% of pts respond to 7–10 days of empiric rx. If no response, suggest brain biopsy. Pyri penetrates brain even if no inflammation; folinic acid prevents pyrimethamine hematologic toxicity.
Primary prophylaxis AIDS pts—lgG Toxo antibody + CD4 count <100 per mcL	**TMP-SMX-DS** 1 tab po q24h or (**TMP-SMX-SS** 1 tab po q24h).	**(Dapsone** 50 mg po q24h) + (**pyri** 50 mg po q wk) + **folinic acid** 25 mg (po q wk)) OR **atovaquone** 1500 mg po q24h	Prophylaxis for pneumocystis also effective vs toxo. Refs.: *MMWR 51(RR-8), 6/14/2002; AnIM 137:435, 2002*
Suppression after rx of cerebral toxo	(**Sulfadiazine** 500–1000 mg po 4x/day) + (**pyri** 25–50 mg po q24h) + (**folinic acid** 10–25 mg po q24h) Dc if CD4 count >200 x 3mo	(**Clinda** 300–450 mg po q6–8h) + **pyri** 25–50 mg po q24h) + (**folinic acid** 10–25mg po q6–12h	(Pyri + sulfa) prevents PCP and toxo; (clinda + pyri) prevents toxo only.
Trichomonas vaginalis	See *Vaginitis, Table 1, page 23*		
Trypanosomiasis. Ref.: *Ln 362:1469, 2003*			
West African sleeping sickness (T. brucei gambiense)			
Early: Blood/lymphatic—CNS OK	**Pentamidine** 4mg/kg IM daily x 10 days	**(Suramin** 100mg IV (test dose), then 1gm IV on days 1, 3, 7, 14, & 21	
Late: Encephalitis	**Melarsoprol** 2.2mg/kg/day IV x 10 days (melarsoprol + nifurtimox superior to melarsoprol alone) *(JID 195:311 & 322, 2007)).*	**Eflornithine** 100mg/kg/day IV x 14 days *(CID 41:748, 2005)*	Combination of IV eflornithine, 400 mg/kg/day divided q12h x 7 days, plus nifurtimox, 15 mg/kg/day po, divided q8h x 10 days more efficacious than standard dose eflornithine *(CID 45:1455 & 1473, 2007).*
Prophylaxis	**Pentamidine** 3mg/kg IM q6 mos.	Not for casual visitor	

[1] Sulfonamides for toxo. Sulfadiazine now commercially available. Sulfisoxazole much less effective.

* See page for abbreviations. All dosage recommendations are for adults (unless otherwise indicated) and assume normal renal function.

** Cost = average wholesale price from 2007 RED BOOK, Thomson Healthcare, Inc.

TABLE 13A (6)

INFECTING ORGANISM	SUGGESTED REGIMENS		COMMENTS
	PRIMARY	ALTERNATIVE	
PROTOZOA—EXTRAINTESTINAL/Trypanosomiasis (continued)			
East African sleeping sickness (T. brucei rhodesiense)			
Early: Blood/lymphatic	**Suramin** 100 mg IV (test dose), then 1gm IV on days 1, 3, 7, 14, & 21	None	
Late: Encephalitis	**Melarsoprol** 2–3.6 mg/kg per day IV × 3 days; repeat after 7 days & for 3rd time 7 days after 2nd course	Prednisone may prevent/attenuate encephalopathy	
T. cruzi—**Chagas disease** or acute American trypanosomiasis Ref.: Ln 357:797, 2001 For chronic disease: see Comment.	**Nifurtimox**[xs] 8–10 mg/kg per day po div. 4x/day after meals x 120 days Ages 11–16yrs: 12.5–15 mg/kg per day div. qid po x 90 days Children <11yrs: 15–20 mg/kg per day div. qid po x 90 days	**Benznidazole**[xs] 5–7 mg/kg per day po div. 2x/day x 30–90 days (AJTMH 63:111, 2000). NOTE: Avoid tetracycline and steroids.	Chronic disease: 1) Immunosuppression for heart transplant can reactivate chronic Chagas disease. 2) Reduced progression with 30 of benznidazole 5 mg/kg per day. AnIM 144:724, 2006
NEMATODES—INTESTINAL (Roundworms). Eosinophilia? Think Strongyloides, Schistosomiasis and filariasis CID 34:407, 2005; 42:1781 & 1655, 2006			
Anisakis simplex **(anisakiasis)** CID 41:1297, 2005; LnID 4:294, 2004	Physical removal: endoscope or surgery (IgE antibody test x 4; samples may help diagnosis	Anecdotal reports of possible treatment benefit from albendazole (Ln 360:54, 2002; CID 41:1825, 2005)	Anisakiasis acquired by eating raw fish: herring, salmon, mackerel, cod, squid. Similar illness due to Pseudoterranova species acquired from cod, halibut, red snapper.
Ascaris lumbricoides **(ascariasis)** Ln 367:1521, 2006	**Albendazole** 400 mg po x 1 dose or **mebendazole** 100 mg po bid x 3 days or 500 mg po x 1 dose	**Ivermectin** 150–200 mcg/kg po x 1 dose or **Nitazoxanide: Adults**—500 mg po bid x 3 days; **children 4–11**—200 mg oral susp. po q12h	Can present with intestinal obstruction.
Capillaria philippinensis **(capillariasis)**	**Mebendazole** 200 mg po bid x 20 days	**Albendazole** 200 mg po bid x 10 days	
Enterobius vermicularis **(pinworm)**	**Albendazole** 400 mg po x 1, repeat in 2wks OR **mebendazole** 100 mg po x 1, repeat in 2wks	**Pyrantel pamoate** 11 mg/kg base (to max. dose of 1gm) po x 1 dose; repeat in 2wks	Side-effects in Table 13B, pages 132, 134
Gongylonemiasis	Surgical removal or **albendazole** 400 mg/day po x 3 days		
NEMATODES—EXTRAINTESTINAL (Roundworm)			
Ancylostoma braziliense & caninum: causes **cutaneous larva migrans** (Dog & cat hookworm)	**Ivermectin** 200 mcg/kg po x 1 dose/day x 1–2 days	**Albendazole** 400 mg po x 3 days	Also called "creeping eruption," dog and cat hookworm. Ivermectin cure rate 77% (1 dose) to 97% (2–3 doses) (CID 31:493, 2000)
Baylisascariasis (Raccoon ascaris)	No drug proven efficacious. Try po **albendazole**.		Some add steroids (CID 39:1484, 2004).
Dracunculus medinensis: **Guinea worm** (CMAJ 170:495, 2004)	Slow extraction of pre-emergent worm	**Metronidazole** 250 mg po tid x 10 days used to ↓ inflammatory response and facilitate removal. Immersion in warm water promotes worm emergence. Mebendazole 400–800mg/day x 6 days may kill worm.	
NEMATODES—INTESTINAL (Roundworms)			
Hookworm (Necator americanus and Ancylostoma duodenale)	**Albendazole** 400 mg po x 1 dose or **mebendazole** 500 mg po x 1 dose	**Pyrantel pamoate** 11 mg/kg po x 1 dose or 1 gm) po daily x 3 days	NOTE: Ivermectin not effective. Eosinophilia may be absent but eggs in stool (NEJM 351:799, 2004).
Strongyloides stercoralis **(strongyloidiasis)** (See Comment)	**Ivermectin** 200 mcg/kg po x 2 days	**Albendazole** 400 mg po bid x 7 days : less effective	For hyperinfections, repeat at 15 days. For hyperinfection: veterinary ivermectin has been given subcutaneously or rectally.
Trichostrongylus orientalis	**Albendazole** 400 mg po x 1 dose	**Pyrantel pamoate** 11mg/kg (max. 1gm) po x 1	**Mebendazole** 100 mg po bid x 3 days
Trichuris trichura **(whipworm)** Ln 367:1521, 2006	**Albendazole** 400 mg po 1x/day x 3 days	**Mebendazole** 100 mg po bid x 3 days or 500 mg po x 1 dose once	**Ivermectin** 200 mcg/kg daily po x 3 days

[1] Available from CDC Drug Service; see footnote 1 page 123
[xs] See page for abbreviations. All dosage recommendations are for adults (unless otherwise indicated) and assume normal renal function.
[**] Cost = average wholesale price from 2007 RED BOOK, Thomson Healthcare, Inc.

TABLE 13A (7)

INFECTING ORGANISM	SUGGESTED REGIMENS		COMMENTS
	PRIMARY	ALTERNATIVE	
NEMATODES—EXTRAINTESTINAL (Roundworms) (continued)			
Filariasis. Wolbachia bacteria needed for filarial development. Rx with dory 100–200 mg/day x 4–6wks ↓ number of wolbachia & ↓ number of microfilaria but no effect on adult worms *(BMJ 326:207, 2003)*			
Filariasis (Elephantiasis): Wuchereria bancrofti or Brugia malayi or B. timori	**Diethylcarbamazine** ² (DEC): po; Day 1, 50 mg; Day 2, 50 mg tid; Day 3, 100 mg tid; Days 4–14, 2 mg/kg q8h for total of 72 mg over 14 days (see comment)	**Albendazole** 200 mg po bid x 21 days	**Diethylcarbamazine** ² (DEC); Day 1, 50 mg; Interest in combining albendazole with DEC; no trials comparing combination vs. DEC alone.
Cutaneous Loiasis: **Loa loa**, eyeworm disease	**Diethylcarbamazine** (DEC); ²,³ Day 1, 50 mg; Day 2, 50 mg tid; Day 3, 100 mg tid; Days 4–21: 8–10 mg/kg/day in 3 divided doses	If **ivermectin** fails, consider **suramin** (from CDC Drug Service)	If concomitant oncho & Loa loa, treat oncho first. If ovrs 5,000 microfilaria/mL of blood, DEC can cause encephalopathy. Might start with albendazole x few days ± steroids, then DEC.
Onchocerca volvulus (onchocerciasis)—river blindness *(Ln 360:203, 2002)*	**ivermectin** 150 mcg/kg po for 6–12 months.	**Albendazole** in high dose x 3 weeks.	Oncho & Loa loa may both be present. Check peripheral smear; if Loa loa microfilaria present, treat oncho first with ivermectin before DEC for Loa loa.
Body cavity Mansonella perstans (dipetalonemiasis)	Nothing works well. Try DEC as for lymphatic filariasis	Chronic pruritic hypopigmented lesions that may be confused with leprosy.	**ivermectin** has no activity. Ref: Trans R Soc Trop Med Hyg 100:458, 2006.
Mansonella streptocerca	**Diethylcarbamazine** ² as above for Wuchereria OR **ivermectin** 150 mcg/kg x 1		
Mansonella ozzardi	**ivermectin** 200 mcg/kg x 1 dose may be effective	Usually asymptomatic. Articular pain, pruritus, lymphadenopathy reported. May have allergic reaction from dying organisms	Can be asymptomatic.
Dirofilariasis: Heartworms D. immitis, dog heartworm D. tenius (raccoon), D. ursi (bear), D. repens (dogs, cats)	No effective drugs; surgical removal only option; No effective drugs	Worms migrate to conjunctivae, subcutaneous tissue, scrotum, breasts, extremities	Can lodge in pulmonary artery → coin lesion. Eosinophilia rare.
Gnathostoma spinigerum: eosinophilic myeloencephalitis	**Albendazole** 400 mg po q24h or bid times 21 days		**ivermectin** 200 mcg per kg per day times 2 days
	Rx directed at relief of symptoms as infection self-limited, e.g., steroids & antihistamines; use of anthelminthics controversial		
Toxocariasis: Clin Micro Rev 16:265, 2003			
Visceral larval migrans	**Albendazole** 400 mg po bid x 5 days	**Mebendazole** 100–200 mg po bid times 5 days	Severe lung, heart or CNS disease may warrant steroids. Differential dx of larval migrans syndromes: Toxocara canis & catis, Ancylostoma spp., Gnathostoma spp., Spirometra spp.
Ocular larval migrans	First 4 wks of illness: (Oral **prednisone** 30–60 mg po q24h + subtenon **triamcinolone** 40 mg/wk) x 2wk		No added benefit of antihelminthic drugs. Rx of little effect after 4wk.
Trichinosis (**trichinosis**)—muscle infection	**Albendazole** 400 mg po bid x 8–14 days	**Mebendazole** 200–400 mg po tid x 3 days, then 400–500 mg po tid x 10 days	Use albendazole/mebendazole with caution during pregnancy.
	Concomitant **prednisone** 40–60 mg po q24h		

¹ Available from CDC Drug Service; see footnote 1 page 123

² May need antihistamine or corticosteroid for allergic reaction from disintegrating organisms

* See page for abbreviations. All dosage recommendations are for adults (unless otherwise indicated) and assume normal renal function.

** Cost = average wholesale price from 2007 RED BOOK, Thomson Healthcare, Inc.

TABLE 13A (8)

INFECTING ORGANISM	SUGGESTED REGIMENS		COMMENTS
	PRIMARY	ALTERNATIVE	
TREMATODES (Flukes)			
Clonorchis sinensis (liver fluke)	**Praziquantel** 25 mg/kg po tid x 2 days or **albendazole** 10 mg/kg per day po x 7 days		Same dose in children
Dicrocoelium dendriticum	**Praziquantel** 25 mg/kg po tid x 1 day		Ingestion of raw or undercooked sheep liver (CID 44:145, 2007)
Fasciola buski (intestinal fluke)	**Praziquantel** 25 mg/kg po tid x 1 day		Same dose in children
Fasciola hepatica (sheep liver fluke)	**Triclabendazole**[NUS] (Egaten; Novartis. Contact Victoria Pharmacy, Zurich: +41-211-24-32) 10 mg/kg po x 1 dose (Ref: Clin Micro Infect 11:859, 2005) or **Nitazoxanide** 500 mg po bid x 7 days.		**Bithionol**[1] Adults and children: 30-50 mg/kg (max. dose 2 gm/day) every other day times 10-15 doses
Heterophyes heterophyes (intestinal fluke); Metagonimus yokogawai (intestinal fluke); Opisthorchis viverrini (liver fluke)	**Praziquantel** 25 mg/kg po tid x 2 days		Same dose in children. Same regimen for **Metorchis conjunctus (North American liver fluke). Nanophyetus salmincola:** Praziquantel 20 mg/kg po td x 1 day
Paragonimus westermani (lung fluke)	**Praziquantel** 25 mg/kg po tid x 2 days or **bithionol**[1] 30-50 mg/kg po x 1 every other day x 10 days		Same dose in children. Alternative: metrifonate 10mg/kg per dose po q2 wks for 3 doses.
Schistosoma haematobium; GU bilharziasis. (NEJM 346:1212, 2002)	**Praziquantel** 20 mg/kg po bid x 1 day (2 doses)		Same dose in children
Schistosoma intercalatum.	**Praziquantel** 20 mg/kg po bid x 1 day (2 doses)		Same dose in children
Schistosoma japonicum; Oriental schisto. (NEJM 346:1212, 2002)	**Praziquantel** 20 mg/kg po **tid x 1 day (3 doses)**		Cures 60-90% pts.
Schistosoma mansoni (intestinal bilharziasis) Possible praziquantel resistance (JID 176:304, 1997) (NEJM 346:1212, 2002). Schisto, (NEJM 346:1212, 2002)	**Praziquantel** 20 mg/kg po bid x 1 day (2 doses)	**Oxamniquine**[NUS] single dose of 15 mg/kg po once; in North and East Africa 30 mg/kg po daily x 3 days. Do not use during pregnancy.	Same dose for children. Cures 60-90% pts. Report of success treating myeloradiculopathy with single po dose of praziquantel, 50 mg/kg, + prednisone for 6 mo (CID 39:1618, 2004)
Toxemic schisto; Katayama fever	**Praziquantel** 20 mg per kg po **tid times 1 day (3 doses)**		Massive infection with either S. japonicum or S. mansoni
CESTODES (Tapeworms)			
Echinococcus granulosus (hydatid disease) (CID 37:1073, 2003; Ln 362:1295, 2003)	**Praziquantel** 20 mg per kg po bid x 3-6 days (LnID 7:218, 2007)		Meta-analysis supports percutaneous aspiration-injection-reaspiration (PAIR) + albendazole. **albendazole** ≥60 kg, 400 mg po bid or <60 kg, 15 mg/kg per day div. bid, with meals. Then: Puncture (P) & needle aspirate (A) cyst content, Instill (I) hypertonic saline (15–30%) or absolute alcohol, wait 20-30 min, then re-aspirate (R) with final irrigation. **Continue albendazole x 28 days** Cure in 96% as comp to 90% pts with surgical resection.
Echinococcus multilocularis (alveolar cyst disease) (CID 16:437, 2003)	**Albendazole** efficacy not clearly demonstrated, can try in dosages used for hydatid disease. Wide surgical resection only reliable rx; technique evolving (AJM 18:195, 2005).		
Intestinal tapeworms			
Diphyllobothrium latum (fish), Dipylidium caninum (dog), Taenia saginata (beef), & T. solium (pork)	**Praziquantel** 5-10 mg/kg po x 1 dose for children and adults. manufacturer is Bayer, Germany		**Alternative was Niclosamide (Yomesan)** 2 gm po x 1; however, drug no longer available.
Hymenolepis diminuta (rats) and H. nana (humans)	**Praziquantel** 25 mg/kg po x 1 dose for children and adults. available; manufacturer is Bayer, Germany		**Alternative was Niclosamide (Yomesan)** 500 mg po q24h x 3 days; however, drug no longer available.
Neurocysticercosis (NCC). Larval form of T. solium Ref: AJTMH 72:3, 2005	**Praziquantel** 5-10 mg/kg po x 1 dose for children & adults.		NOTE: **Treat T. solium (intestinal tapeworms),** if present, with **praziquantel** 5-10 mg/kg po x 1 dose for children and adults.

[1] Available from CDC Drug Service, see footnote 1 page 123
* See page for abbreviations. All dosage recommendations are for adults (unless otherwise indicated) and assume normal renal function.
** Cost = average wholesale price from 2007 RED BOOK, Thomson Healthcare, Inc.

TABLE 13A (9)

INFECTING ORGANISM	SUGGESTED REGIMENS		COMMENTS
	PRIMARY	ALTERNATIVE	

CESTODES (Tapeworms) / Neurocysticercosis (NCC) (continued)

INFECTING ORGANISM	PRIMARY	ALTERNATIVE	COMMENTS
Parenchymal NCC	[Albendazole ≥60 kg 400 mg bid with meals or <60 kg: 15 mg/kg per day in 2 div. doses (max. 800mg/day) **+** Dexamethasone 0.1 mg/kg per day ± Anti-seizure medication] — all x 8-30 days	(Praziquantel 100 mg/kg per day in 3 div. doses x 1 day, then 50 mg/kg/d in 3 doses plus dexamethasone **+** Anti-seizure medication) — all x 29 days. See Comment	Albendazole assoc. with 46% ↓ in seizures (NEJM 350:249, 2004). Praziquantel less cysticidal activity. Steroids decrease serum levels of praziquantel. NIH reports methotrexate at ≤20 mg/wk allows a reduction in steroid use (CID 44:449, 2007).
"Viable" cysts by CT/MRI Meta-analysis: Treatment assoc. with cyst resolution, ↓ seizures, and ↓ seizure recurrence. Ann IM 145:43, 2006.			**Treatment improves prognosis of associated seizures.**
"Degenerating" cysts	Albendazole + dexamethasone as above		
Dead calcified cysts	No treatment indicated		
Subarachnoid NCC	(Albendazole + steroids as above) + shunting for hydrocephalus. Without shunt, 50% died within 9yrs (J Neurosurg 66:686, 1987).		
Intraventricular NCC	Albendazole + dexamethasone + neuroendoscopic removal (if available)		
Sparganosis (Spirometra mansonoides) Larval cysts, dogs—frogs/snakes	Surgical resection or ethanol injection of subcutaneous masses (NEJM 330:1887, 1994).		

ECTOPARASITES Ref. CID 36:1355, 2003; Ln 363:889, 2004. **NOTE: Due to potential neurotoxicity and risk of aplastic anemia, lindane not recommended.**

DISEASE	INFECTING ORGANISM	SUGGESTED REGIMENS		COMMENTS
		PRIMARY	ALTERNATIVE	
Head lice Med Lett 47:68, 2005	Pediculus humanus, var. capitis	Permethrin 1% (generic lotion or cream rinse (Nix): Apply to shampooed dried hair for 10min., repeat in 1wk. **OR** Malathion 0.5% (Ovide): Apply to dry hair for 8-14 hrs, then shampoo. 2 doses 7 days apart.	Ivermectin 200-400mcg/kg po once, 3 doses at 7 day interval reported effective (JID 193:474, 2006).	**Permethrin** success in 78%. Extra combing of no benefit. Resistance increasing. No advantage to 5% permethrin. **Malathion**: Report that 1-2 20-min. applications 98% effective Ped Derm 21:670, 2004). In alcohol—potentially flammable.
Pubic lice (crabs)	Phthirus pubis	Pubic hair: Permethrin OR malathion as for head lice	Eyelids: Petroleum jelly applied qid x 10 days OR yellow oxide of mercury 1% qid x 14 days	Costs: Permethrin 1% lotion/cream $9-9 Malathion 0.5% lotion $119 Ivermectin $20
Body lice	Pediculus humanus, var. corporis	No drugs for pt. treat the clothing. Organism lives in & deposits eggs in seams of clothing. Discard clothing; if not possible, treat clothing with 1% malathion powder or 10% DDT powder. Success with ivermectin 12mg po on days 0, 7, & 14 (JID 193:474, 2006)		
Scabies Refs. LnID 6:769, 2006	Sarcoptes scabiei	**Primary: Permethrin** 5% cream (ELIMITE). Apply entire skin from chin to toes. Leave on 8-14hr. Repeat 1wk. Safe for children >2mo old. **Alternative: Ivermectin** 200mcg/kg po x 1; 2nd dose 14 days later.	**Ivermectin** 200-400mcg/kg po once; 2nd dose 14 days later.	Trim fingernails. Reapply to hands after handwashing. Pruritus may persist times 2wk after mites gone. **Less effective: Crotamiton** 10% cream, apply x 24 hr. rinse off, then reapply x 24 hr. Norwegian scabies in AIDS pts. Extensive, crusted. Can mimic psoriasis. Not pruritic. ELIMITE: 60 gm $18.60. Ivermectin $19.62
	Immunocompromised patients CD4 <150 per mm³ (Norwegian scabies—see Comments)	For Norwegian scabies: Permethrin as above on day 1, then 6% sulfur in petrolatum daily on days 2-7, then repeat times several weeks. Ivermectin 200mcg/kg po x 1 reported effective.		**Highly contagious—isolate!**
Myiasis Due to larvae of flies		Usually cutaneous/subcutaneous nodule with central punctum. Treatment: Occlude punctum to prevent gas exchange with petrolatum, fingernail polish, makeup cream or bacon. When larva migrates, manually remove.		

* See page for abbreviations. All dosage recommendations are for adults (unless otherwise indicated) and assume normal renal function.

** Cost = average wholesale price from 2007 RED BOOK, Thomson Healthcare, Inc.

TABLE 13B – DOSAGE, PRICE, AND SELECTED ADVERSE EFFECTS OF ANTIPARASITIC DRUGS

NOTE: Drugs available from CDC Drug Service indicated by "CDC." Call (404) 639-3670 (or -2888).
Doses vary with indication. For convenience: drugs divided by type of parasite; some drugs used for multiple types of parasites, e.g.: albendazole.
COMMENT: Cost data represent average wholesale le prices as listed in 2007 RED BOOK, Thomson Healthcare, Inc.

CLASS, AGENT, GENERIC NAME (TRADE NAME)	USUAL ADULT DOSAGE (Cost**)	ADVERSE REACTIONS/COMMENTS
Antiprotozoan Drugs		
Intestinal Parasites		
Albendazole (Albenza)	Doses vary with indication, 200–400 mg bid po 200 mg tab $1.58	Teratogenic. Pregnancy, Cat. C; give after negative pregnancy test. Abdominal pain, nausea/vomiting, alopecia, ↑ serum transaminase. Rare leukopenia.
Dehydroemetine (CDC)*	1.5 mg/kg per day to max. of 90 mg IM	Local pain. ECG changes, cardiac arrhythmias, precordial pain, paresthesias, weakness, peripheral neuropathy, GI: nausea/vomiting, diarrhea. Avoid strenuous exercise for 4 wks after rx.
Iodoquinol (Yodoxin) (650 mg $1.20)	Adults: 650 mg po tid; children: 40 mg/kg per day div. tid.	Rarely causes nausea, abdominal cramps, rash, acne. Contraindicated if iodine intolerance.
Metronidazole/Ornidazole[AUS] (Tiberal)	Side-effects similar for all. See *metronidazole in Table 10A, page 83, & Table 10C, page 97.*	
Paromomycin (Humatin) Aminosidine in U.K.	Up to 750 mg qid. 250 mg caps $2.72	Drug is aminoglycoside similar to neomycin; if absorbed due to concomitant inflammatory bowel disease can result in oto/nephrotoxicity. Doses >3 gm assoc. with nausea, abdominal cramps, diarrhea.
Quinacrine[AUS] (Atabrine, Mepacrine)	100 mg tid. No longer available in U.S.; 2 pharmacies will prepare as a service: (1) Connecticut 203-785-6818; (2) California 800-247-9767	Contraindicated for pts with history of psoriasis or psychosis. Yellow staining of skin. Dizziness, headache, vomiting, toxic psychosis (1.5%), hemolytic anemia, leukopenia, thrombocytopenia, urticaria, rash, fever, minor disulfiram-like reactions
Antiprotozoan Drugs: Non-Intestinal Protozoa		
Tinidazole (Tindamax)	500 mg. Doses similar to metronidazole. Cost: 500 mg tab $4-56	Chemical structure similar to metronidazole but better tolerated. Seizures/peripheral neuropathy reported. **Adverse effects:** Metallic taste 4-6%, nausea 3-5%, anorexia 2-3%.
Extraintestinal Parasites		
Antimony compounds[AUS] Stibogluconate sodium (Pentostam) from CDC or Meglumine antimonate (Glucantime—French tradenames	Dilute in 120 mL of D,W and infuse over 2hr. Ideally, monitor EKG.	Fatigue, myalgia, N/V and diarrhea common. ALT/AST ↑s, ↑ amylase and lipase occur. **NOTE: Reversible T wave changes in 30-60%. Risk of QTc prolongation.**
Atovaquone (Mepron) Ref. AAC 46:1163, 2002	Suspension: 1 tsp (750 mg) po bid 750 mg/5 mL. Cost: 210 mL $566.	No. pts stopping rx due to side-effects was 9%: rash 22%, GI 20%, headache 16%, insomnia 10%, fever 14%
Atovaquone and proguanil (Malarone) For prophylaxis of P. falciparum; little data on P. vivax	**Prophylaxis:** 1 tab po (250mg + 100mg) q24h with food **Treatment:** 4 tabs po (1000mg + 400mg) once daily with food x 3 days. *See drug interactions, Table 22B.* Adult tab: 250/100 mg, Peds tab 62.5/25mg. Peds dosage: *footnote 1, page 97* Cost: 250/100 mg tab $5.88	Adverse effects in rx trials: Adults—abd. pain 17%, N/V 12%, headache 10%, dizziness 5%. Rx stopped in 1%. Asymptomatic mild ↑ in ALT/AST. Children—cough, headache, anorexia, vomiting, abd pain 1-2%. Safe in G6PD-deficient pts. Can crush tabs for children and give with milk or other liquid nutrients. Renal insufficiency: contraindicated if CrCl <30 mL per min.
Benznidazole[AUS] (Rochagan, Roche, Brazil)	7.5 mg/kg per day po	Photosensitivity in 50% of pts. GI: abdominal pain, nausea/vomiting/anorexia. CNS: disorientation, insomnia, twitching/seizures, paresthesias, polyneuritis. **Contraindicated in pregnancy**
Chloroquine phosphate (Aralen)	Dose varies—see *Malaria Prophylaxis and rx, pages 125-126.* 500mg tabs $5.50	Minor: anorexia/nausea/vomiting, headache, dizziness, blurred vision, pruritus in dark-skinned pts. Major: protracted rx in rheumatoid arthritis can lead to retinopathy. Can exacerbate psoriasis. Can block response to rabies vaccine. Contraindicated in pts with epilepsy.

* See page for abbreviations. All dosage recommendations are for adults (unless otherwise indicated) and assume normal renal function.

** Cost = average wholesale price from 2007 RED BOOK, Thomson Healthcare, Inc.

TABLE 13B (2)

CLASS, AGENT, GENERIC NAME (TRADE NAME)	USUAL ADULT DOSAGE (Cost**)	ADVERSE REACTIONS/COMMENTS
Antiprotozoan Drugs/Extraintestinal Parasites (continued)		
Dapsone Ref.: CID 27:191, 1998	100 mg po q24h 100 mg tabs $0.20	Usually tolerated by pts with rash after TMP-SMX. Adverse effects: nausea/vomiting, rash, oral lesions (CID 18:630, 1994). Methemoglobinemia (usually asymptomatic); if >10–15%, stop drug. Hemolytic anemia if G6PD deficient. Sulfone syndrome: fever, rash, hemolytic anemia, atypical lymphocytes, and liver injury (West J Med 156:303, 1992).
Eflornithine[AUS] (Ornidyl)	Approved in US for trypanosome infections but not marketed. Aventis product.	Diarrhea in ½ pts, vomiting, abdominal pain, anemia/leukopenia in ½ pts, seizures, alopecia, jaundice, ↓ hearing. Contraindicated in pregnancy
Fumagillin	Eyedrops + po. 20 mg po tid Leiter's: 800-292-6773	Adverse events: Neutropenia & thrombocytopenia
Mefloquine (Lariam)	One 250 mg tab/wk for malaria prophylaxis; for rx, 1250 mg x 1 or 750 mg & then 500 mg in 6-8hrs. 250 mg tab $12.40. In U.S. 250 mg tab = 228 mg base; outside U.S. 275 mg tab = 250 mg base	Side-effects in roughly 3%. Minor: headache, irritability, insomnia, weakness, diarrhea. Toxic psychosis, seizures occur. Teratogenic—do not use in pregnancy. Do not use with quinine, quinidine, or halofantrine. Rare: Prolonged QT interval and toxic epidermal necrolysis (Ln 349:101, 1997). Not used for self-rx due to neuropsychiatric side-effects.
Melarsoprol (CDC) (Mel B, Arsobal) (Manufactured in France)	See Trypanosomiasis for adult dose. Peds dose: 0.36 mg/kg IV, then gradual ↑ to 3.6 mg/kg q1–5 days for total of 9–10 doses	Post-rx encephalopathy (10%) with 50% mortality overall, risk of death 2° to rx 4–8%. Prednisolone 1 mg per kg per day po may ↓ encephalopathy. Other: Heart damage, albuminuria, abdominal pain, vomiting, peripheral neuropathy. Herxheimer-like reaction, pruritus
Miltefosine[AUS] (Zentaris, Impavido) (Expert Rev Anti Infect Ther 4:177, 2006)	100–150 mg (approx. 2.25 mg/kg per day) po x 28 days Cutaneous leishmaniasis 2.25 mg/kg po q24h x 6wk	Contact Zentaris (Frankfurt, Ger): info@zentaris.com **Pregnancy—No**, teratogenic. Side-effects vary: kala-azar pts, vomiting in up to 40%, diarrhea in 17%, "motion sickness", headache & increased creatinine
Nifurtimox (Lampit) (CDC) (Manufactured in Germany by Bayer)	8–10mg/kg per day po div 4 x per day	Side-effects in 40–70% of pts. GI: abdominal pain, nausea/vomiting. CNS: polyneuritis (1/3), disorientation, insomnia, twitching, seizures. Skin rash. Hemolysis in G6PD deficiency
Nitazoxanide (Alinia)	Adults: 500 mg po x 3 days. Children 4-11: 200 mg susp. po q12h Take with food. 500 mg tabs $13.02	Abdominal pain 7.8%, diarrhea 2.1%. Rev.: CID 40:1173, 2005; Expert Opin Pharmacother 7:953, 2006.
Pentamidine (NebuPent)	300 mg via aerosol q month. Also used IM. 300 mg $98.75 + admin. costs	Hypotension, hypoglycemia followed by hyperglycemia, pancreatitis. Neutropenia (15%), thrombocytopenia. Nephrotoxicity. Others: nausea/vomiting, ↑ liver tests, rash
Primaquine phosphate	26.3 mg (= 15 mg base) $1.03	In G6PD def. pts, can cause hemolytic anemia with hemoglobinuria. esp. African, Asian peoples. Methemoglobinemia. Nausea/abdominal pain if pt. fasting. (CID 39:1336, 2004). **Pregnancy: No.**
Pyrimethamine (Daraprim, Malocide) Also combined with sulfadoxine as **Fansidar** (25–500 mg) $4.13	100 mg. then 25 mg/day. 25mg $0.58. Cost of folinic acid (leucovorin) 5mg $2.36	Major problem is hematologic: megaloblastic anemia, ↓ WBC, ↓ platelets. Can give 5 mg folinic acid per day to ↓ bone marrow depression and not interfere with antitoxoplasmosis effect. If high-dose pyrimethamine, ↑ folinic acid to 10-50mg/day. Pyrimethamine + sulfadiazine can cause mental changes due to carnitine deficiency (AJM 95:112, 1993).
Quinacrine[AUS]	For giardiasis: 100 mg po tid x 5 days Peds dose: 2mg/kg po bid (max. 300mg/day) x 5 days	Compounded by Med. Center Pharm., New Haven, CT: (203) 688-6816 or Panorama Compound. Pharm, Van Nuys, CA: (800) 247-9767. Other: Rash, vomiting, diarrhea, xerostomia
Quinidine gluconate Cardiotoxicity ref: LnID 7:549, 2007	Loading dose of 10mg (equiv to 6.2mg of quinidine base) kg IV over 1-2hr, then constant infusion of 0.02mg/of quinidine gluconate / kg per minute.	Adverse reactions of quinidine/quinine similar: (1) IV bolus injection can cause fatal hypotension, (2) hyperinsulinemic hypoglycemia, esp. in pregnancy, (3) ↓ rate of infusion of IV quinidine if QT interval ↑ >25% of baseline, (4) reduce dose 30–50% after day 3 due to ↓ renal clearance and ↓ vol. of distribution
Quinine sulfate (300 mg salt = 250mg base)	324 mg tabs. No IV prep. in US. Oral rx of chloroquine-resistant falciparum malaria: 624 mg po tid x 3 days, then (tetra)q24h 250 mg po qid or doxy 100 mg bid) x 7 days 324 mg $0.16	Cinchonism: tinnitus, headache, nausea, abdominal pain, blurred vision. Rarely: blood dyscrasias, drug fever, asthma, hypoglycemia. Transient blindness in < 1% (AnIM 136:339, 2002). **Contraindicated if prolonged QTc, myasthenia gravis, optic neuritis.**

* See page for abbreviations. All dosage recommendations are for adults (unless otherwise indicated) and assume normal renal function.
** Cost = average wholesale price from 2007 RED BOOK, Thomson Healthcare, Inc.

134

TABLE 13B (3)

CLASS, AGENT, GENERIC NAME (TRADE NAME)	USUAL ADULT DOSAGE (Cost**)	ADVERSE REACTIONS/COMMENTS
Antiprotozoan Drugs/Extraintestinal Parasites *(continued)*		
Spiramycin (Rovamycin) *(JAC 42:572, 1998)*	Up to 3-4 gm/day. Not available in U.S. Can by FDA: (301) 827-2335.	GI and allergic reactions have occurred. Not available in U.S.
Sulfadiazine	1-1.5 gm po q6h. 500 mg 500 $0.34	*See Table 10C, page 92, for sulfonamide side-effects*
Sulfadoxine & pyrimethamine combination (Fansidar)	Contains 500 mg sulfadoxine & 25 mg pyrimethamine. One tab $4.13	Very long mean half-life of both drugs: Sulfadoxine 169hrs, pyrimethamine 111hrs allows weekly dosage. Do not use in pregnancy. Fatalities reported due to Stevens-Johnson syndrome and toxic epidermal necrolysis. Renal excretion—use with caution in pts with renal impairment.
DRUGS USED TO TREAT NEMATODES, TREMATODES, AND CESTODES		
Bithionol *(CDC)*	Adults & children: 30-40 mg/kg (to max. of 2gm/day) po every other day x 10-15 doses	Photosensitivity, skin reactions, urticaria, GI upset.
Diethylcarbamazine (Hetrazan) *(CDC)*	Used to treat filariasis. Licensed (Lederle) but not available in U.S.	Headache, dizziness, nausea, fever. Host may experience inflammatory reaction to death of adult worms: fever, urticaria, asthma, GI upset (Mazzotti reaction). **Pregnancy—No.**
Ivermectin (Stromectol, Mectizan)	Strongyloidiasis dose 200 mcg/kg x 2 doses po. Onchocerciasis: 150mcg/kg x 1 po. Scabies: 200 mcg/kg po x 1. 3 mg tabs $5.40	Mild side-effects: fever, pruritus, rash. In rx of onchocerciasis, can see tender lymphadenopathy, headache, bone/joint pain. Can cause Mazzotti reaction (see above).
Mebendazole (Vermox)	Doses vary with indication. 100mg tab $13.23	Rarely causes abdominal pain, nausea, diarrhea. Contraindicated in pregnancy & children <2 yrs old.
Oxamniquine (Vansil)^AUS	For S. mansoni. Some experts suggest 40-60 mg/kg over 2-3 days in all of Africa.	Rarely: dizziness, drowsiness, neuropsychiatric symptoms, GI upset. EKG/EEG changes. Orange/red urine. **Pregnancy—No.**
Praziquantel (Biltricide)	Doses vary with parasite; see Table 13A. 600 mg $13.16	Mild: dizziness/drowsiness, N/V, rash, fever. Only contraindication is ocular cysticercosis. Metab.-induced by anticonvulsants and steroids; can negate effect with cimetidine 400mg po tid.
Pyrantel pamoate (over-the-counter as Reese's Pinworm Medicine)	Oral suspension. Dose for all ages: 11 mg/kg (to max. of 1gm) x 1 dose	Rare GI upset, headache, dizziness, rash
Suramin (Germanin) *(CDC)*	For early trypanosomiasis. Drug powder mixed to 10% solution with 5 ml water and used within 30 min	Does not cross blood-brain barrier; no effect on CNS infection. Side-effects: vomiting, pruritus, urticaria, fever, paresthesias, albuminuria (discontinue drug if casts appear). Do not use if renal/liver disease present. Deaths from vascular collapse reported.
Thiabendazole (Mintezol)	Take after meals. Dose varies with parasite, see Table 12A. 500 mg $1.25	Nausea/vomiting, headache, dizziness. Rarely: liver damage, ↓ BP, angioneurotic edema, Stevens-Johnson syndrome. May ↓ mental alertness.

TABLE 13C - PARASITES THAT CAUSE EOSINOPHILIA

Frequent and Intense (>5000 ?/mm³)	Moderate to Marked Early Infections	During Larval Migration; Absent or Mild During Chronic Infections	Other
Strongyloides (absent in compromised hosts); Lymphatic Filariasis; Toxocara	Ascaris; Hookworm; Clonorchis; Paragonemis	Opisthorchis	Schistosomiasis; Cysticercosis; Trichuris; Angiostrongylus; Non-lymphatic filariasis; Gnathastoma; Capillaria; Trichostrongylus

---

* See page for abbreviations. All dosage recommendations are for adults (unless otherwise indicated) and assume normal renal/renal function.
** Cost = average wholesale price from 2007 RED BOOK, Thomson Healthcare, Inc.

TABLE 14A – ANTIVIRAL THERAPY (NON-HIV)*

VIRUS/DISEASE	DRUG/DOSAGE	SIDE EFFECTS/COMMENTS
Adenovirus: Cause of RTIs including fatal pneumonia in children & young adults and 60% mortality in transplant pts *(CID 43:331, 2006).* **Findings include:** fever, ↑ liver enzymes, leukopenia, thrombocytopenia, diarrhea, pneumonia, or hemorrhagic cystitis.	In severe cases of pneumonia or post HSCT[1]: **Cidofovir** • 5 mg/kg wk x 2 wks, then q 2 wks + **probenecid** 1.25 gm/M² given 3hrs before cidofovir and 3 & 9 hrs after each infusion • Or 1 mg/kg IV 3x/wk. For adenovirus hemorrhagic cystitis *(CID 40:199, 2005)*. Intravesical **cidofovir** (5 mg/kg in 100 mL saline instilled into bladder)	Successful in 3/8 immunosuppressed children *(CID 38:45, 2004)* & 8 of 10 children *with HSCT (CID 41:1812, 2005).* ↓ in virus load predicted response to cidofovir.
Coronavirus—SARS-CoV (Severe Acute Respiratory Distress Syn.) *(see CID 38:1420, 2004)* A new coronavirus, isolated Spring 2003 *[NEJM 348:1953 & 1967, 2003]* emerged from China & spread from Hong Kong to 32 countries. Effective infection control guidelines controlled the epidemic.	Therapy remains predominantly **supportive care.** Therapy tried or under evaluation (see Comments): **Ribavirin**—ineffective. Interferon alfa ± steroids—small case series. Pegylated IFN-α effective in monkeys. Value of corticosteroids alone unclear. Inhaled nitric oxide improved oxygenation & improved chest x-ray *(CID 39:1531, 2004).*	Other coronaviruses (HCoV-229E, OC43, NL63, etc.) implicated as cause of croup, asthma exacerbations, & other RTIs in children *(CID 40:1721, 2005; JID 191:492, 2005).* May be associated with Kawasaki disease *(JID 191:489, 2005).*
Enterovirus—Meningitis: most common cause of aseptic meningitis. PCR or CSF valuable for early dx *(Scand J Inf Dis 34:359, 2002)* but ↓ sensitivity >2 days of symptoms. PCR on feces pos. in 12/13 specimens, 5–16 days after clinical onset *(CID 40:982, 2005).*	**No rx currently recommended;** however, **pleconaril** (VP 63843) still under investigation.	No clinical benefit demonstrated in double-blind placebo-controlled study in 21 infants with enteroviral aseptic meningitis *(PIDJ 22:335, 2003).*
Hemorrhagic Fever Virus Infections: For excellent reviews, see *Med Lab Observer, May 2005, p. 16, Lancet Infectious Disease Vol 6 No 4.* **Congo-Crimean Hemorrhagic Fever (HF)** *[CID 39:284, 2004]* TicKborne; symptoms include N/V, fever, headache, myalgias, & stupor (1/3). Signs: conjunctival injection, hepatomegaly, petechiae (1/3). Lab: ↓ platelets, ↓ WBC, ↑ ALT, AST, LDH & CPK (100%).	Oral **ribavirin, 30mg/kg** as initial loading dose & (15mg/kg q6h x 4 days then 7.5mg/kg x 6 days (WHO recommendation) (see Comment).	33 healthcare workers in Pakistan had complete recovery *(Ln 346:472, 1995)*, & 61/69 (89%) with confirmed CCHF rx with ribavirin survived in Iran *(CID 36:1613, 2003)*. Shorter time of hospitalization among ribavirin treated pts (7.7 vs. 10.3 days), but no difference in mortality or transfusion needs in study done in Turkey *(J Infection 52: 207-215, 2006)*
Ebola/Marburg HF (Central Africa) Severe outbreak of Ebola in Angola 309 cases with 277 deaths by 5/2/05 *(NEJM 352:2155, 2005; UnID 5:331, 2005)*. Major epidemic of Marburg 1998-2000 in Congo & 2004-5 in Angola *[NEJM355:866, 2006]*	**No effective antiviral rx** *(J Virol 77: 9733, 2003)*.	Can infect gorillas & chimps that come in contact with other dead animal carcasses *(Science 303:387, 2004)*. Marburg reported in African Fruit Bat, *Rousettus aegyptiacus* (PLoS ONE, Aug 22, 2007).
With pulmonary syndrome: Hantavirus pulmonary syndrome, "sin nombre virus"	**No benefit from ribavirin has been demonstrated** *(CID 39:1307, 2004).*	Acute onset of fever, headache, myalgias, non-productive cough, thrombocytopenia and non-cardiogenic pulmonary edema with respiratory insufficiency following exposure to rodents.
With renal syndrome: Lassa, Venezuelan, Korean HF, Sabia, Argentinian HF, Bolivian HF, Junin, Machupo	Oral **ribavirin**, 30 mg/kg as initial loading dose & 15 mg/kg q6h x 4 days & then 7.5 mg/kg x 6 days (WHO recommendation) (see Comment).	Toxicity low, hemolysis reported but recovery when treatment stopped. No significant changes in WBC, platelets, hepatic or renal function. See *CID 36:1254, 2003,* for management of contacts.

[1] HSCT = Hematopoietic stem cell transplant

* See page 2 for abbreviations. NOTE: *All dosage recommendations are for adults (unless otherwise indicated) and assume normal renal function.*

TABLE 14A (2)

VIRUS/DISEASE	DRUG/DOSAGE	SIDE EFFECTS/COMMENTS
Hemorrhagic Fever Virus Infections (continued) **Dengue and dengue hemorrhagic fever (DHF)** http://www.cdc.gov/ncidod/dvbid/dengue/dengue-hcp.htm Think dengue in traveler to tropics or subtropics (incubation period usually 4-7 days) with fever, bleeding, thrombocytopenia, or isolation or serology: serum to CDC (telephone 787-706-2399)	**No data on antiviral rx.** Fluid replacement with careful hemodynamic monitoring critical. Rx of **DHF** with colloids effective: 6% hydroxyethyl starch preferred in 1 study (NEJM 353:9, 2005). Review in Semin Ped Infect Dis 16: 60-65, 2005.	Of 77 cases dx at CDC (2001–2004), recent (2-wk) travel to Caribbean island 30%, Asia 17%, Central America 15%, S. America 15%, (MMWR 54:556, June 10, 2005). 5 pts with severe **DHF** rx with dengue antibody-neg, admiting globulin 500 mg per kg q24h IV for 3-5 days; rapid ↑ in platelet counts (CID 36:1623, 2003)
West Nile virus (see AnIM 104:545, 2004) A flavivirus transmitted by mosquitoes, blood transfusions, transplanted organs (NEJM 348: 2196, 2003; CID 38:1257, 2004), & breast-feeding (MMWR 51:877, 2002). Birds (>200 species) are main host with man & horses incidental hosts. The US epidemic continues.	**No proven rx to date.** 2 clinical trials in progress: (1) Interferon alfa-N3 (CID 40:764, 2005). See www.nyha.org/posting/rahal.html. (2) IVIG from Israel with high titer antibody West Nile (JID 188:5, 2003; Transpl Inf Dis 4:160, 2003). Contact NIH, 301-496-7453; see www.clinicaltrials.gov/show/NCT0036055 Reviewed in Lancet Neurology 6: 171–181, 2007	Usually nonspecific febrile disease but 1/150 cases develops meningoencephalitis, aseptic meningitis or polio-like paralysis (AnIM 104:545, 2004; JCI 113: 1102, 2004). Long-term sequelae (neuromuscular weakness & psychiatric) common (CID 43:723, 2006) Dx by ↑ IgM in serum & CSF or CSF PCR (contact State Health Dept./ CDC). Blood supply now tested in U.S.: ↑ serum lipase in 11/17 cases (NEJM 352-420, 2005)
Yellow fever	**No data on antiviral rx.** Guidelines for use of preventative vaccine (MMWR 51: RR17, 2002)	Reemergence in Africa & S. Amer. due to urbanization of susceptible population (Lancet Inf 5:604, 2005). Vaccination effective. (JAMA 276:1157, 1996)
Chikungunya fever A self limited arbovirus illness spread by Aedes mosquito.	No antiviral therapy	Clinical presentation: high fever, severe myalgias & headache, macular papular rash with occ thrombocytopenia. Rarely hemorrhagic complications. Dx by increase in IgM antibody.
Hepatitis Viral Infections **Hepatitis A** (Ln 351:1643, 1998)	No therapy recommended. If within 2 wks of exposure, IVIG 0.02 mL per kg IM given 1 protective.	Vaccine recommendations in Table 20. 40% of pts with chronic Hep C who developed acute/symptomatic Hep A developed fulminant hepatic failure (NEJM 338:286, 1998)

Hepatitis B—Chronic: For pts co-infected with HIV see Table 12, Sanford Guide to HIV/AIDS Therapy 2008.
Who to treat? Based on status of e antigen and viral quantification. Adapted from Clin Gastro & Hepatology 4:936-962, 2006. Other useful refs: Hepatology 45:507, 2007; AnIM 147:58, 2007; Hep B
Foundation: http://www.hepb.org

	HBV DNA (IU/mL)[1]	**ALT**	**Suggested Management**
HBe Ag-Positive	≥20,000	Elevated or normal	Treat if ALT elevated[2] Treat if biopsy abnormal—even if ALT normal[2]
HBe Ag-Negative	≥2,000	Elevated or normal	Treat if ALT elevated[2] Treat if biopsy abnormal—even if ALT normal[2]

[1] IU/mL equivalent to approximately 5.6 copies/mL; if patient treated, monitor every 6 months if treated with adefovir every 3 mos, if treated with lamivudine.

[2] Treatment duration varies with viral quantification, presence/absence of cirrhosis & drug(s) used. See Clin Gastro & Hepatology 4:936-962, 2006 for details.

* See page 2 for abbreviations. NOTE: All dosage recommendations are for adults (unless otherwise indicated) and assume normal renal function.

TABLE 14A (3)

VIRUS/DISEASE	DRUG/DOSAGE		SIDE EFFECTS/COMMENTS

Hepatitis Viral Infections/Hepatitis B—Chronic *(continued)*

	HBV DNA (IU/mL)[1]		Suggested Management
Documented cirrhosis (positive or negative HBe Ag)	≥2,000 and compensated cirrhosis		Treat with **Adefovir** or **entecavir** (long term)[3]
	<2,000 and compensated cirrhosis		Observe or (**adefovir** or **entecavir** long term)[3]
	Decompensated cirrhosis; any HBV DNA level		Long term therapy with (**lamivudine** or **entecavir** or **adefovir**) + **adefovir**; waiting list for liver transplantation[3]

Comparison of Treatment Options for Chronic Hepatitis B (Patients **not** co-infected with HIV). **Note:** See Table 14B for more dosage details, adverse effects, and cost

	Peg interferon alfa-2A	Telbivudine	Lamivudine	Adefovir	Entecavir
Dose:	180 mcg sc weekly	600 mg po daily	100 mg po daily	10 mg daily	0.5 mg po daily
Parameter:					
Log10 ↓ in serum HBV DNA	4.5	6-6.6 (HBe Ag+)	No data	3.5	6.9
HBV DNA below detection, %	25	60	57	21	67
% ALT normalizes	39	75-86	41-72	48	68
% with improved histology	38	65	49-56	53	72
Resistance develops	No	2-3% after 1 yr	69% after 5 yrs	15% after 4 yrs	0% after 2 yrs

Hepatitis C (up to 3% of world infected, 4 million in US. Co-infection with HIV common—see Sanford Guide to HIV/AIDS Therapy.

Acute
Usually asymptomatic (>75%). Can detect by PCR within 1-3 days; antibody in 36+ days. *(NEJM 345:1452, 2001)*

Follow plasma HCV viral load by PCR:
If clear within 3-4 mos, no treatment:
If persists: PEG IFN + ribavirin as below, albeit controversial *(NEJM 346:1091, 2002)*

15-40% clear infection within 6 mos *(JAMA 297:724, 2007)*.
Sustained viral response with IFN alfa-2b therapy; 32% vs. 4% with placebo, P 0.00007 *(Cochrane Database Sys & Rev CD000369, 2002)*.
Alfa-INF alone effective in early infection *(CID 42:1673, 2006)*.

Chronic: *NEJM 362:2444, 2006*

Genotypes 1, 4, 5 & 6

Treat if: persistent elevated ALT/AST, + HCV RNA plasma viral load, fibrosis &/or inflam on biopsy
+
Pegylated interferon
PEG IFN: Either alfa-2a (Pegasys) 180 mcg subcut. 1x/wk
1x/wk OR
Alfa-2b (PEG-INTRON) 1.5 mcg/kg subcut. 1x/wk
+ **Ribavirin**

	Weight	**Ribavirin Dose**
	<75 Kg	400 mg am & 600 mg pm
	>75 Kg	600 mg am & 600 mg pm

Monitor response by quantification:

	HCV RNA	**Result**	**Action**
After 4 wks rx:		<1 log₁₀ ↓ IU/mL*	Discontinue therapy
After 12 wks rx:		>1 log₁₀ ↓ IU/mL*	
		>2 log₁₀ ↓ IU/mL or undetectable	Treat 48 wks

Genotype 2 or 3 | PEG IFN alfa-2a or 2b—dose as for types 1 & 4 above + **Ribavirin** 400 mg po bid

	Quant. HCV RNA	**Result**	**Action**
After 4 wks rx:		Undetectable →	Treat 12 wks *(NEJM 352:2609, 2005)*
		>1 log₁₀↓	Treat 24 wks (See comment)

In U.S. 90% due to genotype 1. **Sustained viral response (SVR)** tx of genotype 1: 42-51%; SVR to 24-wk rx of genotype 2 or 3: 76-82%.
Avoid alcohol—accelerates HCV disease.
HIV accelerates HCV disease.

See Table 14B for drug adverse effects & cost. Interferon alfa can cause serious depression.

Ribavirin is teratogenic & has dose-related hematologic toxicity.
For drugs in development, see Curr Opin Infect Dis 19:615, 2006.
For genotypes 2 & 3, some use standard Pts results similar & J cost.
NOTE: High viral load = >800,000 IU/mL; Pts with HCV RNA levels <800,000 IU/mL have 15-35% better response rate.
Some would treat 24wks for high titer Genotype 3.

For prevention of acute and chronic infection, see Table 15D, page 172

---

[1] IU/mL equivalent to approximately 5.6 copies/mL; if patient treated, monitor every 6 mos if treated with adefovir; every 3 mos. if treated with lamivudine.
[2] Treatment duration varies with viral quantitation, presence/absence of cirrhosis & drug(s) used. See Clin Gastro & Hepatology 4:936-962, 2006 for details.
[3] HCV RNA quantitation. By WHO international standard 800,000 IU/mL. = 2 million copies/mL. Response to therapy based on log₁₀ fall in IU/mL *(JAMA 297:724, 2007)*.
* See page 2 for abbreviations. NOTE: All dosage recommendations are for adults (unless otherwise indicated) and assume normal renal function.

TABLE 14A (4)

VIRUS/DISEASE	DRUG/DOSAGE	SIDE EFFECTS/COMMENTS
Herpesvirus Infections		
Cytomegalovirus (CMV) Marked ↓ in HIV associated CMV infections & death with Highly Active Antiretroviral Therapy. Initial treatment should optimize HAART.	Primary prophylaxis not generally recommended. Preemptive therapy in pts with ↑ CMV DNA titers in plasma & CD4 <100/mm³. Recommended by some: **valganciclovir** 900mg po q24h (CID 32: 783, 2001). Authors rec: primary prophylaxis be dc if response to HAART with ↑ CD4 >100 for 6 mos. (MMWR 53:98, 2004).	Risk for developing CMV disease correlates with quantity of CMV DNA in plasma, each log₁₀ ↑ associated with 3.1-fold ↑ in disease (JCI 101:497, 1998; CID 28:758, 1999).
Colitis, Esophagitis Dx by biopsy of ulcer base/edge (Clin Gastro Hepatol 2:564, 2004) with demonstration of CMV inclusions & other pathogen(s).	**Ganciclovir** as with retinitis except induction period extended for 3-6wks. Responses less predictable than for retinitis. **Foscarnet** 90 mg/kg q12h another option. **Valganciclovir** when po tolerated & when symptoms not severe enough to interfere with absorption.	No agreement on use of maintenance; may not be necessary except after relapse. **Valganciclovir also likely effective**. Switch to oral valganciclovir when symptoms not severe enough to interfere with absorption.
Encephalitis, Ventriculitis: Treatment not defined. Lumbosacral polyradiculopathy: diagnosis by CMV DNA in CSF	**Ganciclovir** as with retinitis. Disease may develop while taking ganciclovir as suppressive therapy. See Herpes 11(Suppl 2):95A, 2004. **Ganciclovir**, as with retinitis. Consider combination of ganciclovir & foscarnet, esp. if prior CMV rx used. Switch to **valganciclovir** when possible. Suppression continued until CD4 remains >100/mm³ for 6mos.	About 50% will respond; survival ↑ (5.4wks to 14.6wks) (CID 27:345, 1998). Resistance can be demonstrated genotypically.
Mononeuritis multiplex	Not defined	Due to vasculitis & may not be responsive to antiviral therapy
Pneumonia— Seen predominantly in transplants (esp. bone marrow), **rare in HIV**. Treat only when histological evidence resent in IDS pts & other pathogens not identified.	**Ganciclovir/valganciclovir**, as with retinitis. In bone marrow transplant pts, combination therapy with CMV immune globulin.	In bone marrow transplant pts, serial measure of pp65 antigen was useful in establishing early diagnosis of CMV interstitial pneumonia with good results if ganciclovir was initiated within 6 days of antigen positivity (Bone Marrow Transplant 26:413, 2000). For preventive therapy, see Table 10.

* See page 2 for abbreviations. NOTE: All dosage recommendations are for adults (unless otherwise indicated) and assume normal renal function.

TABLE 14A (5)

VIRUS/DISEASE	DRUG/DOSAGE	SIDE EFFECTS/COMMENTS
CMV Retinitis	**For immediate sight-threatening lesions:** Ganciclovir intraocular implant & **valganciclovir** 900 mg po q24h. **For peripheral lesions:** **Valganciclovir** 900 mg po q12h x14-21d, then 900 mg po q24h for maintenance therapy	Differential diagnosis: HIV retinopathy, herpes simplex retinitis, varicella-zoster retinitis (rare, hard to diagnose). (NEJM 346:1119, 2002) Cannot use ganciclovir ocular implant alone as approx. 50% risk of CMV retinitis other eye at 6 mos. & 31% have systemic disease. Risk ↓ with systemic rx but when contralateral retinitis does occur, ganciclovir-resistant mutation often present (JID 189:611, 2004). **Concurrent systemic rx recommended!**
Most common cause of blindness in AIDS patients with <500/mm³ CD4 counts. 19/30 pts (63%) with inactive CMV retinitis who responded to HAART (↑ of ≥60 CD4 cells/ mL) developed immune recovery vitreitis (vision ↓ & floaters with posterior segment inflammation —vitreitis, papillitis & macular changes) an average of 43 wks after rx started (JID 179:697, 1998). Corticosteroid rx (inflammatory reaction of immune recovery vitreitis without reactivation of CMV retinitis, either periocular corticosteroids or short course of systemic steroid.	Ganciclovir 5 mg/kg IV q12h x14-21d, then **valganciclovir** 900 mg po q24h OR Foscarnet 60 mg/kg IV q8h or 90 mg/kg IV q12h x14-21d, then 90-120 mg/kg IV q24h OR Cidofovir 5 mg/kg IV q2wks, then 5 mg/kg every other wk; each dose be administered with IV saline hydration & oral probenecid OR Repeated intravitreal injections with **fomivirsen** (for relapses only, not as initial therapy).	Because of unique mode of action, **fomivirsen** may have a role in pts that become resistant to other therapies. Retinal detachments 50-60% within 1yr of dx of retinitis. (Ophtha 111:2232, 2004) Equal efficacy of IV GCV & FOS. GCV avoids nephrotoxicity of FOS; FOS avoids bone marrow suppression of GCV. Although bone marrow toxicity may be similar to ganciclovir. **Oral valganciclovir should replace both.**
	Post treatment suppression (Prophylactic) If CD4 count <100/mm³: **Valganciclovir** 900mg po q24h.	Pts who discontinue rx should undergo regular eye examination for early detection of relapses. Discontinue if CD4 >100/mm³ x 6 mos (on HAART.)
CMV in Transplant patients: See Table 15E. Use of **valganciclovir** to prevent infections in CMV seronegative recipients who receive organs from a seropositive donor & in seropositive receivers has been highly effective (Ln 365:2105, 2005). Others suggest preemptive rx when pt develops CMV antigenemia or positive PCR post-transplant (Transplant 79:85, 2005).		(See AAC 56:277, 2005 for current status of drugs in development.)
Epstein Barr Virus (EBV)—Mononucleosis (Ln 362:3131, 2003)	No treatment. Corticosteroids for tonsillar obstruction, CNS complications, or threat of splenic rupture.	**HHV-6**—Implicated as cause of roseola (exanthem subitum) & other febrile diseases of childhood (NEJM 352:768, 2005). Fever & rash documented in transplant pts (JID 179:311, 1999). Reactivation in 47% (10/10 U.S. hematopoietic stem cell transplant pts assoc. with delayed monocytes & platelet engraftment (CID 40:932, 2005). Recognized in assoc. with meningoencephalitis in immunocompetent adults. Diagnosis made by PCR in CSF. HHV-6 virus copies in response to **ganciclovir** rx (CID 40:890 & 894, 2005). Foscarnet therapy improved hemodynamic parameters (Am J Hematol 76:156, 2004).
		HHV-7—Ubiquitous virus (~90% of the population is infected by age 3 yrs). No relationship to human disease. Infects CD4 lymphocytes via CD4 receptor, transmitted via saliva.
		HHV-8—The agent of Kaposi's sarcoma, Castleman's disease, & body cavity lymphoma	Localized lesions: radiotherapy, laser surgery or intralesional chemotherapy. Systemic: chemotherapy. Castleman's disease responded to ganciclovir (Blood 103:1632, 2004) & valganciclovir (JID 2006)
Herpes simplex virus (HSV Types 1 & 2)		
Bell's palsy H. simplex most implicated etiology, Other etiologic considerations: VZV, HHV-6, Lyme disease.	As soon as possible after onset of palsy: 1) **Prednisone** 1mg/kg po divided bid x 5 days then taper to 5 mg bid over the next 5 days (total of 10 days prednisone) + 2) **Valganciclovir** 500 mg bid x 5 days **No antiviral treatment.** Effective anti-HIV therapy may help.	Prospective randomized double blind placebo controlled trial compared prednisolone vs acyclovir vs (prednisolone + acyclovir) vs placebo. Best result with prednisolone: 85% recovery with placebo, 96% recovery with prednisolone, 93% with combination of steroid & prednisolone (NEJM 357:1598 & 1653, 2007). Similar study design using valacyclovir showed best outcome with combination of steroid & valacyclovir (Otol Neurol 28:408, 2007).

* See page 2 for abbreviations. NOTE: All dosage recommendations are for adults (unless otherwise indicated) and assume normal renal function.

TABLE 14A (6)

VIRUS/DISEASE	DRUG/DOSAGE	SIDE EFFECTS/COMMENTS
Herpesvirus Infections/Herpes Simplex Virus (HSV Types 1 & 2)		
Encephalitis *(Excellent reviews: CID 35: 254, 2002;* UK experience (EID 9.234, 2003; Eur J Neurol 12:331, 2005; Antiviral Res : 141-148, 2006)	Acyclovir IV 10 mg/kg IV (infuse over 1 hr) q8h x 14-21 days. Up to 20mg/kg q8h in children <12 yrs	HSV-1 is most common cause of sporadic encephalitis. Survival & recovery from neurological sequelae are related to mental status at time of initiation of rx. **Early dx and rx imperative**. Mortality rate reduced from >70% to 19% with acyclovir rx. PCR analysis of CSF for HSV-1 DNA is 100% specific & 75-98% sensitive. 8/33 (25%) CSF samples drawn before day 3 were neg. by PCR neg. PCR assoc. with + protein & < 10 WBC per mm³ in CSF (CID 36:1335, 2003). All were + after 3 days. Relapse after successful rx reported in 7/27 (27%) children. Relapse was associated with a lower total dose of initial acyclovir rx (285 ± 82 mg per kg in relapse group vs. 462 ± 149 mg per kg, p <0.03) (CID 30:185, 2000; Neuropediatrics 35:371, 2004).
Genital Herpes: Sexually Transmitted Treatment Guidelines 2006: www.cdc.gov/std/treatment/2006/genital-ulcers.htm, MMWR Recomm Rep. 2006 Aug 4:55 (RR-11):1–94.		
Primary (initial episode)	Acyclovir (Zovirax or generic) 400 mg po tid x 7–10 days (NB $130 per 10 day course, G $35 per 10 day course) OR Valacyclovir (Valtrex) 1000 mg po bid x 7–10 days ($223 per 10 day course) OR Famciclovir (Famvir) 250 mg po tid x 7–10 days ($161 per 10 day course)	↓ by 2 days time to resolution of signs & symptoms, ↓ by 4 days time to healing of lesions, ↓ by 7 days duration of viral shedding. Does not prevent recurrences. For severe cases only: 5 mg per kg IV q8h times 5–7 days. An ester of acyclovir, which is well absorbed, bioavailability 3–5 times greater than acyclovir. Metabolized to penciclovir, which is active component. Side effects and activity similar to acyclovir. **Famciclovir** 250 mg po tid **equal to acyclovir** 200 mg 5 times per day.
Episodic recurrences	**Acyclovir** 800 mg po bid **x 2 days** or 400 mg po tid **x 5 days** or **Famciclovir** 1000 mg bid **x 1 day** or 125 mg po bid x 5 days or **Valacyclovir** 500 mg po bid **x 3 days** or 1 gm po once daily x 5 days For HIV patients, see Comment	For episodic recurrences in HIV patients: **acyclovir** 400 mg po bid x 5-10 days or **famciclovir** 500 mg po bid x 5-10 days or **valacyclovir** 1 gm po bid x 5-10 days
Chronic daily suppression	**Suppressive therapy reduces the frequency of genital herpes recurrences** by 70–80% among pts who have frequent recurrences (i.e., >6 recurrences per yr) & many report no symptomatic outbreaks. **Acyclovir** 400 mg po bid (cost per yr $662), **or famciclovir** 250 mg po bid (cost per yr $2993), **or valacyclovir** 1 gm po q24h ($3268 per yr): pts with <9 recurrences per yr could use 500 mg po q24h ($1625 per yr) and then use valacyclovir 1 gm po q24h if breakthrough at 500 mg. For HIV patients, see Comment	For chronic suppression in HIV patients: **acyclovir** 400-800 mg po bid or tid or **famciclovir** 500 mg po bid or **valacyclovir** 500 mg po bid

* See page 2 for abbreviations. *NOTE: All dosage recommendations are for adults (unless otherwise indicated) and assume normal renal function.*

TABLE 14A (7)

VIRUS/DISEASE	DRUG/DOSAGE	SIDE EFFECTS/COMMENTS
Herpesvirus Infections/Herpes Simplex Virus (HSV Types 1 & 2)/Genital, Immunocompetent (continued)		
Gingivostomatitis, primary (children)	**Acyclovir** 15 mg/kg po 5x/day x 7 days	Efficacy in randomized double-blind placebo-controlled trial (BMJ 314:1800, 1997).
Kerato-conjunctivitis and recurrent epithelial keratitis	**Trifluridine** (Viroptic), 1 drop 1% solution q2h (max. 9 drops per day) for max. of 21 days (see Table 1, page 12)	In controlled trials, response % > idoxuridine. Suppressive rx with acyclovir (400 mg bid) reduced recurrences of ocular HSV from 32% to 19% (NEJM 339:300, 1998).
Mollaret's recurrent "aseptic" meningitis (usually HSV-2) (Ln 363:1772, 2004)	No controlled trials of antiviral rx & resolves spontaneously. In severe cases, IV or po acyclovir or valacyclovir recommended	Pos. PCR for HSV in CSF confirms dx (CJCMID 23:560, 2004). Daily suppression rx might ↓ frequency of recurrence but no clinical trials.
Mucocutaneous (for genital see previous page) **Oral labial, "fever blisters":** **Normal host:** See Ann Pharmacotherapy 38:705, 2004; JAC 53:703, 2004	Start rx with prodrome symptoms (tingling/burning) before lesions show. **Oral:**	Penciclovir (J Derm Treat 13:67, 2002; JAMA 277:1374, 1997; AAC 46: 2848, 2002); Docosanol (J Am Acad Derm 45:222, 2001). Oral acyclovir 5% cream (AAC 46:2238, 2002). Oral famciclovir (JID 179:303, 1999). Topical fluocinonide (0.05% Lidex gel) q8h times 5 days in combination with famciclovir ↓ lesion size and pain when compared to famciclovir alone (JID 181:1906, 2000).

Oral section detail:

Drug	Dose	Cost	Sx Decrease
Valacyclovir[1]	2 gm po q12h x 1 day	$45	↓ 1 day
Famciclovir[1]	1500 mg po bid x 7 days	$151	↓ 2 days
Acyclovir[APDA]	400 mg po 5 x per day		↓ ½ day
	(q4h while awake) x 5 days	$6 (generic)	

Topical:			
Penciclovir 1% cream	q2h during day x 4 days	$34	↓ 1 day
Acyclovir 5% cream[2]	6x/day (q3h) x 7 days	$49 per 2 gm $115 per 5 gm	↓ ½ day

[1] FDA approved only for HIV pts. [2] Approved for immunocompromised pts. See Table 1, page 24

Herpes Whitlow		
Oral labial or genital: Immunocompromised (includes pts with AIDS) and critically ill pts in ICU setting/large necrotic ulcers in perineum or face. (See Comment)	**Acyclovir** 5 mg per kg IV q8h times 7 days (250 mg per M[2]) or 400 mg po 5 times per day times 14–21 days (see Comment if suspect acyclovir-resistant) **OR Famciclovir:** In HIV infected, 500 mg po bid for 7 days for recurrent episodes of genital herpes **OR Valacyclovir**[APDA]: In HIV-infected, 500 mg po bid for 5–10 days for recurrent episodes of genital herpes or 500 mg po bid for chronic suppressive rx.	**Acyclovir-resistant HSV IV foscarnet** (For dose see Table 14A(15)). Suppressive therapy with famciclovir (500 mg po bid), valacyclovir (500 mg po bid) or acyclovir (400–800 mg po bid) reduces viral shedding and clinical recurrences.
Pregnancy and genital H. simplex	Acyclovir safe even in first trimester. No proof that acyclovir at delivery reduces risk/severity of neonatal Herpes. In contrast, C-section in women with active lesions reduces risk of transmission. Ref: Obstet Gyn 106:845, 2006.	

* See page 2 for abbreviations. NOTE: All dosage recommendations are for adults (unless otherwise indicated) and assume normal renal function.

TABLE 14A (8)

VIRUS/DISEASE	DRUG/DOSAGE	SIDE EFFECTS/COMMENTS
Herpesvirus Infections (continued)		
Herpes simiae (Herpes B virus): **Monkey bite** CID 35:1191, 2002	**Postexposure prophylaxis:** Valacyclovir 1 gm po q8h times 14 days or acyclovir 800 mg po 5 times per day times 14 days. **Treatment of disease:** (1) CNS symptoms absent: Acyclovir 12.5–15 mg per kg IV q8h or ganciclovir 5 mg per kg IV q12h. (2) CNS symptoms present: Ganciclovir 5 mg per kg IV q12h	Fatal human cases of myelitis and hemorrhagic encephalitis have been reported following bites, scratches, or eye inoculation of saliva from monkeys. Initial sx include fever, headache, myalgias. Incubation period of 2–14 days (EID 9:246, 2003). In vitro ACV and ganciclovir less active than other nucleosides (penyclovir or 5-ethyldeoxyuridine may be more active; clinical data needed) (AAC 51:2028, 2007).
Varicella-Zoster Virus (VZV) **Varicella:** Vaccination has markedly ↓ incidence of varicella & morbidity (NEJM 352:450, 2005; NEJM 353:2377, 2005 & NEJM 356:1338, 2007).		
Normal host (chickenpox) Child (2–12 years)	**In general, treatment not recommended.** Might use oral **acyclovir** for healthy persons at ↑ risk for moderate to severe varicella, ie, >12yrs of age, chronic cutaneous or pulmonary diseases; chronic salicylate rx, (↑ risk of Reye syndrome), **acyclovir** dose: 20 mg/kg po qid x 5 days (start within 24 hrs of rash).	Acyclovir slowed development and ↓ number of new lesions and ↓ duration of disease in children: 9 to 7.6 days (PIDJ 21:739, 2002). Oral dose of acyclovir in children should not exceed 80 mg per day or 3200 mg per day
Adolescents, young adults	**Acyclovir** 800mg po 5x/day x 5–7 days (start within 24 hrs of rash) or **valacyclovir**[AP&A] 1000 mg po 3x/day x 5 days). **Famciclovir**[AP&A] 500 mg po 3x/day probably effective but data lacking.	↓ duration of fever, time to healing, and symptoms (AnIM 130:922, 1999).
Pneumonia or chickenpox in 3rd trimester of pregnancy	**Acyclovir** 800 mg po 5 times per day or 10 mg per kg IV q8h times 5 days. Risks and benefits to fetus and mother still unknown. Many experts recommend rx, especially in 3rd trimester. Some would add VZIG (varicella-zoster immune globulin).	Varicella pneumonia associated with 41% mortality in pregnancy. Acyclovir incidence and severity (JID 185:422, 2002). If varicella-susceptible mother exposed and respiratory symptoms develop within 10 days after exposure, start acyclovir.
Immunocompromised host	**Acyclovir** 10–12 mg per kg IV (infused over 1 hr) q8h times 7 days	Disseminated ↑ varicella infection reported during infliximab rx of rheumatoid arthritis (J Rheum 31:2517, 2004). Continuous infusion of high-dose acyclovir (2 mg per kg per hr) successful in 1 pt with severe hemorrhagic varicella (NEJM 336:732, 1997). Mortality high (43%) in AIDS pts (Int J Inf Dis 6:6, 2002).
Prevention—Post-exposure prophylaxis Varicella deaths still occur in unvaccinated persons (MMWR 56 (RR-4):1–40, 2007)	**CDC Recommendations for Prevention:** Since <5% of cases of varicella but >50% of varicella-related deaths occur in adults >20 yrs of age, the CDC recommends a more aggressive approach in this age group: **1st, varicella-zoster immune globulin** (VZIG) (125units/10 kg (22 lbs) body weight IM up to a max. of 625 units; minimum dose is 125 units) is recommended for post-exposure prophylaxis in susceptible persons at greater risk for complications (immunocompromised such as HIV, malignancies, steroid therapy) as soon as possible after exposure (<96 hrs). If varicella develops, initiate treatment quickly (<24 hrs of rash) with **acyclovir** as below. Some would rx presumptively with acyclovir in high-risk pts. **2nd,** susceptible adults should be vaccinated. Check antibody in adults with negative or uncertain history of varicella (10–30% will be Ab-neg.) and vaccinate those who are Ab-neg. **3rd,** susceptible children should receive vaccination. Recommended routinely before age 12–18 mos. but OK at any age.

---

* See page 2 for abbreviations. NOTE: All dosage recommendations are for adults (unless otherwise indicated) and assume normal renal function.

TABLE 14A (9)

VIRUS/DISEASE	DRUG/DOSAGE	SIDE EFFECTS/COMMENTS
Herpesvirus Infections/Herpes Varicella-Zoster Virus (VZV) (continued)		
Herpes zoster (shingles) (See *NEJM 342:635, 2000 & 347:340, 2002*) **Normal host** Effective therapy most evident in pts >50 yrs. (For treatment of post-herpetic neuralgia, see *CID 36: 877, 2003*). New vaccine ↓ herpes zoster & post-herpetic neuralgia (*NEJM 352: 2271, 2005; JAMA 292:157, 2006*).	[**NOTE: Trials showing benefit of therapy: only in pts treated within 3 days of onset of rash**] **Valacyclovir** 1000 mg po tid times 7 days (adjust dose for renal failure)(See *Table 17*), **OR** **Famciclovir** 500 mg tid x 7 days. Adjust dose for renal failure (see *Table 17*) **OR** **Acyclovir** 800 mg po 5 times per day times 7-10 days Add **Prednisone** in pts over 50 yrs old to decrease discomfort during acute phase of zoster. Does not decrease incidence of post-herpetic neuralgia. Dose: 30 mg po bid days 1-7, 15 mg bid days 8-14 and 7.5 mg bid days 15-21.	Valacyclovir ↓ post-herpetic neuralgia more rapidly than acyclovir in pts >50 yrs of age; median duration of zoster-associated pain was 38 days with valacyclovir and 51 days on acyclovir (*AAC 39:1546, 1995*). Toxicity of both drugs similar (*Arch Fam Med 9:863, 2000*). Time to healing more rapid. Reduced post-herpetic neuralgia (PHN) vs placebo in pts >50 yrs of age; duration of PHN similar to famciclovir 63 days, placebo 163 days. Famciclovir similar to acyclovir in reduction of acute pain and PHN (*J Micro Immunol Inf 37:75, 2004*). A meta-analysis of 4 placebo-controlled trials (691 pts) demonstrated that acyclovir accelerated by approx. 2-fold pain resolution by all measures employed and reduced post-herpetic neuralgia at 3 & 6 mos (*CID 22:341, 1996*); med. time to resolution of pain 41 days vs 101 days in those >50 yrs. Prednisone added to acyclovir improved quality of life measurements (↓ acute pain, sleep, and return to normal activity) (*AnIM 125:376, 1996*). In post-herpetic neuralgia, controlled trials demonstrated effectiveness of gabapentin, the lidocaine patch (5%) & opioid analgesic in controlling pain (*Drugs 64:937, 2004; J Clin Virol 29:248, 2004*). Nortriptyline & amitriptyline are equally effective but nortriptyline is better tolerated (*CID 36:877, 2003*). Role of antiviral drugs in rx of PHN unproven (*Neurol 64:21, 2005*) but 8 of 15 pt improved with IV acyclovir 10 mg/kg q 8 hrs x 14 days followed by oral valacyclovir 1 gm 3x a day for 1 month (*Arch Neur 63:940, 2006*).
Immunocompromised host Not severe	**Acyclovir** 800 mg po 5 times per day times 7 days. **Options: Famciclovir** 750 mg po q24h or 500 mg 3 times per day times 7 days **OR valacyclovir** 1000 mg po tid times 7 days, though both are not FDA-approved for this indication)	If progression, switch to IV
Severe: >1 dermatome, trigeminal nerve or disseminated	**Acyclovir** 10-12 mg per kg IV (infusion over 1 hr) q8h times 7-14 days. In older pts, ↓ to 7.5 mg per kg. If nephrotoxicity and pt improving, ↓ to 5 mg per kg q8h.	A common manifestation of immune reconstitution following HAART in HIV-infected children (*J Clin Immun 113:742, 2004*). Rx must be begun within 72 hrs. Acyclovir-resistant VZV occurs in HIV+ pts previously treated with acyclovir. Foscarnet (40 mg per kg IV q8h for 14-26 days) successful in 4/5 pts but 2 relapsed in 7 and 14 days (*AnIM 115:19, 1991*).

---

* See page 2 for abbreviations. *NOTE: All dosage recommendations are for adults (unless otherwise indicated) and assume normal renal function.*

TABLE 14A (10)

VIRUS/DISEASE	DRUG/DOSAGE	SIDE EFFECTS/COMMENTS
Influenza (A & B) (*MMWR* 56:1, 2007) **Suspect or proven acute disease** Rapid diagnostic tests available but sensitivity limited. Antiviral therapy cost-effective without virus testing in febrile pt with typical presentation during influenza season. **Pathogenic avian influenza** (H5N1 emerged in poultry (mainly chickens & ducks) in East & South-east Asia. From Dec 1, 2003 to August 30, 2006, 246 laboratory confirmed cases reported in 10 countries with 144 deaths (see www.cdc.gov/flu/avian). Human-to-human transmission reported; most have had direct contact with poultry. Mortality highest in young age 10-19 (73%) vs. 50% overall and associated with high viral load and cytokine-storm (Nature Medicine Sept, 2006). Human isolates resistant to amantadine/rimantadine. Oseltamivir therapy recommended if avian H5N1 suspected. 1 dose & duration of oseltamivir necessary for maximum effect in mouse model (*JID* 192:665, 2005. *Nature* 435:419, 2005)	If fever & cough; known community influenza activity; and 1st 48 hrs of illness, consider: **For influenza A & B; also avian (H5N1):** **Oseltamivir** 75 mg bid po times 5 days (also approved for rx of children age 1-12 yrs, dose 2 mg per kg up to a total of 75 mg times 5 days) **Zanamivir** 2 inhalations (2 times 5 mg) bid times 5 days	Pts with COPD or asthma, **potential risk of bronchospasm with zanamivir.** All ↓ duration of symptoms by approx. 50% (1-2 days) if given within 36-48 hrs after onset of symptoms (↓ influenced by the duration of sx prior to rx, inhalation of oseltamivir within 1st 12 hrs after fever onset ↓ total median illness duration by 74.6 hrs (*JAC* 51:123, 2003). ↑ risk of pneumonia (*Curr Med Res Opin* 21:761, 2005). **Watch for Emergence of Resistance:** oseltamivir-resistant virus detected after 4 days of rx (*Ln* 364: 733 & 759, 2004). In another study of 296 n cases of adults & children, no oseltamivir-resistant viruses found (*JID* 189:440, 2004). Report of increasing resistance in u up to 18% of children with H5N1 treated with oseltamivir and less responsive H5N1 virus in several patients (J Virology 79(10):1577-86). Less resistance to zanamivir so far. ↑ concern about post-influenza complications including community-acquired MRHSA pneumonia (*CID* 40:1693, 2005). Rimantadine and amantadine no longer recommended by the CDC because of high level resistance emerging since 2005.
Prevention	**Prevention of influenza A & B:** give vaccine or if ≥13 yrs age, consider **oseltamivir** 75 mg po q24h for duration of peak influenza in community or for outbreak control in high-risk populations (*CID* 39:459, 2004.) (Consider for similar populations as immunization recommendations.)	Immunization contraindicated if hypersensitive to hen's eggs. Zanamivir also approved for prophylaxis: 2 inhalations (10 mg) once daily x 10 days (household exposure) or 28 days (community exposure).
Measles While measles in the US is at the lowest rate ever		(*CID* 42: 322, 2006)
Children	No therapy or **vitamin A** 200,000 units po daily times 2 days	Vitamin A may ↓ severity of measles.
Adults	No rx or **ribavirin** IV 20-35 mg per kg per day times 7 days	↓ severity of illness in adults (*CID* 20:454, 1994).
Metapneumovirus (HMPV) A paramyxovirus isolated from pts of all ages, with mild bronchiolitis/bronchospasm to pneumonia (*PIDJ* 23:S215, 2004). Can cause lethal pneumonia in HSCT pts (*Ann Intern Med* 144:344, 2006)	**No proven antiviral therapy** (intravenous ribavirin used anecdotally with variable results)	Human metapneumovirus isolated from 6-21% of children with RTIs (*JID* 190, 20 & 27, 2004; *NEJM* 350:443, 2004 & *PIDJ* 23:436, 2004). Dual infection with RSV assoc. with severe bronchiolitis (*JID* 191:382, 2005).
Monkey pox (orthopox virus) (see *LnID* 4:17, 2004) Outbreak from contact with ill in prairie dogs. Source likely imported Gambian giant rats (*MMWR* 42:642, 2003).	**No proven antiviral therapy.** Cidofovir is active in vitro & in mouse model (*AAC* 46:1329, 2002; *Antiviral Res* 57:13, 2003) (Potential human effect?)	Incubation period of 12 days, then fever, headache, cough, adenopathy, & a vesicular papular rash that pustulates, umbilicates, & crusts on the head, trunk, & extremities. Transmission in healthcare setting rare (*CID* 40:789, 2005; *CID* 41:1742, 2005; *CID* 41:1765, 2005).
Norovirus (Norwalk-like virus, or NLV) Vast majority of outbreaks of non-bacterial gastroenteritis.	**No antiviral therapy.** Replete electrolytes. Transmission by contaminated food, fecal-oral contact with contaminated surfaces, or fomites.	Sudden onset of nausea, vomiting, abdominal or watery diarrhea lasting 12-60 hours. Ethanol-based hand rubs effective (*J Hosp Inf* 60:144, 2005).

* See page 2 for abbreviations. NOTE: All dosage recommendations are for adults (unless otherwise indicated) and assume normal renal function.

TABLE 14A (11)

VIRUS/DISEASE	DRUG/DOSAGE	SIDE EFFECTS/COMMENTS
Papillomaviruses: Warts. For human papillomavirus vaccine, see Table 20C, page 191		
External Genital Warts	**Patient applied:** **Podofilox** 0.15% solution or gel: apply 2x/day x 3 days, 4th day no therapy, repeat cycle 4x; OR **Imiquimod** 5% cream: apply once daily hs 3x/wk for up to 16 wks. **Provider administered:** Cryotherapy with liquid nitrogen; repeat q1-2 wks; OR **Podophyllin resin** 10-25% in tincture of benzoin. Repeat weekly as needed; OR **Trichloroacetic acid** (TCA): repeat weekly as needed; OR surgical removal	**Podofilox:** Inexpensive and safe (pregnancy safety not established). Mild irritation after treatment. **Imiquimod:** Mild to moderate redness & irritation. Safety in pregnancy not established. **Cryotherapy:** blistering and skin necrosis common. Can irritate adjacent skin. **Podophyllin resin:** Must air dry before contacts clothing. Can irritate adjacent skin. **TCA:** caustic. Can cause severe pain on adjacent normal skin. Neutralize with soap or sodium bicarbonate.
Warts on cervix	Need evaluation for evolving neoplasia	Gynecological consult advised.
Vaginal warts	Cryotherapy with liquid nitrogen or **TCA**	
Urethral warts	Cryotherapy with liquid nitrogen or **Podophyllin resin** 10-25% in tincture of benzoin	
Anal warts	Cryotherapy with liquid nitrogen or **TCA** or surgical removal	Advise anoscopy to look for rectal warts.
Skin papillomas	**Topical α-lactalbumin, Oleic acid** (from human milk) applied 1x/day for 3 wks	↓ lesion size & recurrence vs placebo (p <0.001) (NEJM 350:2663, 2004). Further studies warranted.
Parvo B19 Virus (Erythrovirus B19). Review: *NEJM 350:586, 2004.* **Wide range of manifestation. Treatment options for common symptomatic infections:**		
Erythema infectiosum	Symptomatic treatment only	Diagnostic tools: IgM and Igb antibody titers. Perhaps better blood parvovirus PCR.
Arthritis/arthralgia	Nonsteroidal anti-inflammatory drugs (NSAID)	Dose of IVIG not standardized; suggest 400 mg/kg IV of commercial IVIG for 5 or 10 days or 1000 mg/kg IV for 3 days.
Transient aplastic crisis	Transfusions and oxygen	Most dramatic anemias in pts with pre-existing hemolytic anemia.
Fetal hydrops	Intrauterine blood transfusion	Bone marrow shown erythrocyte maturation arrest with giant pronormoblasts.
Chronic infection with anemia	IVIG and transfusion	
Chronic infection without anemia	perhaps **IVIG**	
Papovavirus/Polyomavirus		
Progressive multifocal leukoencephalopathy (PML) Serious demyelinating disease due to JC virus in immunocompromised pts	No specific therapy for JC virus. *Two general approaches:* 1. In HIV pts: **HAART** 2. Stop or decrease *immunosuppressive therapy.*	Failure of treatment with interferon alfa-2b, cytarabine, cidofovir and topotecan. Immunosuppressive natalizumab temporarily removed from market due to reported associations with PML.
BK virus induced nephropathy in immunocompromised pts e.g., hemorrhagic cystitis, urethral stenosis, interstitial nephritis	Decrease immunosuppression if possible. Suggested antiviral therapy based on anecdotal data. If progressive renal dysfunction: 1. **Fluoroquinolone** IV 2. **IVIG** 500 mg/kg IV 3. **Leflunomide** 100 mg po daily x 3 days, then 10-20 mg po daily; 4. **Cidofovir** only if refractory to all of the above (see Table 14B for dose).	Use PCR to monitor viral "load" in urine and/or plasma.

* See page 2 for abbreviations. NOTE: All dosage recommendations are for adults (unless otherwise indicated) and assume normal renal function.

TABLE 14A (12)

VIRUS/DISEASE	DRUG/DOSAGE	SIDE EFFECTS/COMMENTS
Rabies (see Table 20E, pages 196; see MMWR 54-RR-3:1, 2005, CDC Guidelines for Prevention and Control 2006, MMWR/55/RR-5,2006) Rabid dogs account for 50,000 cases per yr worldwide. Most cases in the U.S. are cryptic, i.e., no documented evidence of bite or contact with a rabid animal (CID 35:738, 2003). 70% assoc. with 2 rare bat species (EID 9:151, 2003). An organ donor with early rabies infected 4 recipients (2 kidneys, liver & artery) who all died of rabies avg. 13 days after transplant (NEJM 352:1103, 2005).	**Mortality 100% with rare survivors those who receive rabies vaccine before the onset of illness/symptoms** (CID 36:61, 2003). A 15-year-old female who developed rabies 1 month post-bat bite survived after drug induction of coma (+ other rx) for 7 days; did not receive immunoprophylaxis (NEJM 352:2508, 2005).	Corticosteroids ↑ mortality rate and ↓ incubation time in mice. Therapies that have failed alter symptoms develop include rabies vaccine, rabies immuno-globulin, rabies virus neutralizing antibody, ribavirin, alfa interferon, & ketamine.
Respiratory Syncytial Virus (RSV) Major cause of morbidity in neonates/infants.	Hydration, supplemental oxygen. Routine use of ribavirin not recommended. Ribavirin therapy associated with small increases in O₂ saturation. No consistent decrease in need for mech. ventilation or ICU stays. High-cost, aerosol administration & potential toxicity (Red Book of Pediatrics, 2006).	In adults, RSV accounted for 10.6% of hospitalizations for pneumonia, 11.4% for COPD, 7.2% for asthma & 5.4% for CHF in pts >65 yrs of age (NEJM 352:1749, 2005). RSV caused 11% of clinically important respiratory illnesses in military recruits (CID 41:311, 2005).
Prevention of RSV in: (1) Children <24 mos. old with chronic lung disease of prematurity (formerly broncho-pulmonary dysplasia) requiring supple-mental O₂ or (2) Premature infants (<32 wks gestation) and <6 mos. old at start of RSV season or (3) Children with selected congenital heart diseases	**Palivizumab** (Synagis) 15 mg per kg IM q month Nov.-April Cost: 200 mg $1672. Ref: Red Book of Pediatrics, 2006.	Expense argues against its use, but in 2004 approx. 100,000 infants received drug annually in U.S. (PIDJ 23:1051, 2004). Significant reduction in RSV hospitalization in children with congenital heart disease (Expert Opin Biol Ther 7.1471-80, 2007)
Rhinovirus See Ln 361:51, 2003. Found in 1/2 of children with community-acquired pneumonia, rx in pathogenesis unclear (CID 39:681, 2004). Antiviral Kleenex may reduce spread (Med Lett 47:3, 2005).	No antiviral rx indicated (Ped Ann 34:53, 2005). Symptomatic rx: • ipratropium bromide nasal (2 sprays per nostril tid) • clemastine 1.34 mg 1-2 tab po bid-tid (OTC)	Sx relief: ipratropium nasal spray ↓ rhinorrhea and sneezing vs placebo (AnIM 125:89, 1996). Clemastine (an antihistamine) ↓ sneezing, rhinorrhea but associated with dry nose, mouth & throat in 6-19% (CID 22:656, 1996). Oral **pleconaril** given within 24 hrs of onset reduced duration (1 day) & severity of "cold symptoms" in DBPCT (p < .001) (CID 36:1523, 2003). Echinacea didn't work (CID 38:1367, 2004 & 40:807, 2005)—put to rest!
Rotavirus Leading recognized cause of diarrhea-related illness among infants and children world-wide and kills 1/2 million children annually.	No antiviral rx available, oral hydration life-saving. In one study, **Nitazoxanide 7.5 mg/kg 2x/d x3 days** reduced duration of illness from 75 to 31 hrs in Egyptian children. Impact on rotavirus or other parameters not measured. (Lancet 368:100 & 124, 2006) Too early to recommend routine use (Lancet 368:100, 2006)	Two live-attenuated vaccines highly effective (85 and 98%) and safe in preventing rotavirus diarrhea and hospitalization (NEJM 354:, 1 & 23, 2006)
SARS-CoV: See page 135.		
Smallpox (NEJM 346:1300, 2002). **Contact vaccinia** (JAMA 288:1901, 2002)	Smallpox Vaccine (If within 4 days of exposure): ± cidofovir (dosage uncertain) ± cdofovir (dosage uncertain) From vaccination. Progressive vaccinia—vaccinia immune globulin may be of benefit. To obtain immune globulin, contact CDC: 770-488-7100. (CID 39:759, 776 & 819, 2004)	
West Nile virus: See page 136.		

---

* See page 2 for abbreviations. NOTE: All dosage recommendations are for adults (unless otherwise indicated) and assume normal renal function.

TABLE 14B – ANTIVIRAL DRUGS (OTHER THAN RETROVIRAL)

DRUG NAME(S) GENERIC (TRADE)	DOSAGE/ROUTE/COST*	COMMENTS/ADVERSE EFFECTS*
CMV (See SANFORD GUIDE TO HIV/AIDS THERAPY)		
Cidofovir (Vistide)	5 mg per kg IV 1x week times 2, then q2 weeks. (375 mg $888) Properly timed IV prehydration with normal saline and **Probenecid must be used with each cidofovir infusion**: 2 gm po 3 hrs before each dose and further 1 gm doses 2 & 8 hrs after completion of the cidofovir infusion. Renal function (serum creatinine and urine protein) must be monitored prior to each dose (see pkg insert for details).	**Adverse effects: Nephrotoxicity**: dose-dependent proximal tubular injury (Fanconi-like syndrome): proteinuria, glycosuria, bicarbonaturia, phosphaturia, polyuria (nephrogenic diabetes insipidus: Ln 350:413, 1997). ↑ creatinine. Nephrotic syndrome reported. Probenecid, probenecid dosing intervals allowed use. 25% of pts dc IV cidofovir due to nephrotoxicity. Other toxicities: nausea 48%, fever 31%, alopecia 16%, myalgia 16%, probenecid hypersensitivity 16%, neutropenia 29%. Iritis and uveitis reported; also ↓ intraocular pressure. **Comment:** Recommended dosage, frequency or infusion rate must not be exceeded. Dose must be reduced or discontinued if changes in renal function occur during rx. For ↑ of 0.3-0.4 mg per dL in serum creatinine, cidofovir dose must be ↓ from 5 to 3 mg per kg. discontinue cidofovir if ↑ of 0.5 mg per dL above baseline or 3+ proteinuria develops (for 2+ proteinuria, observe pts carefully and consider discontinuation).
Foscarnet (Foscavir)	90 mg per kg IV q12h (induction) 90 mg per kg q24h (maintenance) Dosage adjust. with renal dysfunction *(see Table 17)* (6 gm: NB $185, G $138)	**Adverse effects: Major clinical toxicity is renal impairment (1/3 of patients)** ↑ creatinine, proteinuria, nephrogenic diabetes insipidus. ↓ K⁺, ↓ Ca⁺⁺, ↓ Mg⁺⁺↑? Toxicity ↑ with other nephrotoxic drugs (ampho B, aminoglycosides or pentamidine (especially severe ↓ Ca⁺⁺). Adequate hydration may ↓ toxicity. Other: headache, mild (100%); fatigue (100%), nausea (80%), fever (25%). CNS: seizures. Hematol↓ WBC, ↓ Hgb. Hepatic: liver function tests ↑. Neuropathy. Penile and oral ulcers.
Ganciclovir (Cytovene)	IV: 5 mg per kg q12h times 14 days (induction) 5 mg per kg q24h or 6 mg per kg 5 times per wk (maintenance) Dosage adjust. with renal dysfunction *(see Table 17)* (500 mg IV $60) Oral: 1.0 gm tid with food (fatty meal) (500 mg cap: NB $11, G $9)	**Adverse effects:** Absolute neutrophil count below 500 per mm³ in 15%, thrombocytopenia 21%, anemia 6%. Fever 48%. GI 50%: nausea, vomiting, diarrhea, abdominal pain 19%, rash 10%. Retinal detachment 11% (relationship to ganciclovir ?). Confusion, headache, psychiatric disturbances and seizures. Neutropenia may respond to granulocyte colony stimulating factor (G-CSF or GM-CSF). Severe myelosuppression may be ↑ with coadministration of zidovudine or azathioprine. 32% dc/interrupted rx, principally for neutropenia. Hematologic less frequent than with IV. Granulocytopenia 18%, anemia 12%, thrombocytopenia 6%, GI, skin same as with IV. Retinal detachment 8%.
Ganciclovir (Vitrasert)	Intraocular implant (~$5,400 per device + cost of surgery).	**Adverse effects:** Late retinal detachment (7/30 eyes). Does not prevent CMV retinitis in good eye or visceral dissemination. **Comment:** Replacement every 6 months recommended.
Valganciclovir (Valcyte)	900 mg (two 450 mg tabs) po bid times 21 days for induction, followed by 900 mg po q24h. Take with food. (450 mg cap $37, ~$2,196 for 60 caps)	A prodrug of ganciclovir with better bioavailability. ~60% with food. **Adverse effects:** Similar to ganciclovir.
Herpesvirus (non-CMV) Acyclovir (Zovirax) or generic	Doses: see Table 14A 400 mg tab G $0.23 (or $170/yr for chronic suppression) IV 500 mg G $9.60 Suspension 200 mg per 5 mL, 473 mL, $133 Ointment 5% 15 gm $133	**po:** Generally well-tolerated with occ. diarrhea, vertigo, arthralgia. Less frequent rash, fatigue, insomnia, fever, menstrual abnormalities, acne, sore throat, muscle cramps, lymphadenopathy. **IV:** Phlebitis, caustic with vesicular lesions with IV infiltration. CNS (1%): lethargy, tremors, confusion, hallucinations, delirium, seizures, coma—all reversible. Renal (5%): ↑ creatinine, hematuria. With high doses may crystallize in renal tubules → obstructive uropathy (rapid infusion, dehydration, renal insufficiency and ↑ dose ↑ risk). Adequate pre-hydration may prevent such nephrotoxicity. Hepatic: ↑ ALT, AST. Uncommon: neutropenia, rash, diaphoresis, hypotension, headache, nausea.

* See page 2 for abbreviations. *NOTE: All dosage recommendations are for adults (unless otherwise indicated) and assume normal renal function.* Cost = average wholesale price from 2007 RED BOOK, Thomson Healthcare, Inc.

TABLE 14B (2)

DRUG NAME(S) GENERIC (TRADE)	DOSAGE/ROUTE/COST*	COMMENTS/ADVERSE EFFECTS
Herpesvirus (non-CMV) *(continued)*		
Famciclovir (Famvir)	250 mg cap $5.40 500 mg cap $10.60	Metabolized to penciclovir. **Adverse effects:** similar to acyclovir; included headache, nausea, diarrhea, and dizziness but incidence does not differ from placebo. May be taken without regard to meals. Dose should be reduced if CrCl <60 mL per min (see package insert & Table 14A, page 139 & Table 17, page 155).
Penciclovir (Denavir)	Topical 1% cream 1.5 gm $34	Well tolerated.
Trifluridine (Viroptic)	1 drop 1% solution q2h (max. 9 drops per day) for max. of 21 days (7.5 mL 1% solution $121)	Mild burning (5%), palpebral edema (3%), punctate keratopathy, stromal edema
Valacyclovir (Valtrex)	500 mg cap $5.90, 1000 mg caplet (capsule-shaped tablet $11.35)	An ester pro-drug of acyclovir that is well-absorbed; bioavailability 3-5 times greater than acyclovir. **Adverse effects** similar to acyclovir (see JID 186:S40, 2002). Thrombotic thrombocytopenic purpura/hemolytic uremic syndrome reported in pts with advanced HIV disease and transplant recipients participating in clinical trials at doses of 8 gm per day.
Hepatitis		
Adefovir dipivoxil (Hepsera)	10 mg per day q24h (with normal CrCl); see Table 17A if renal impairment. Cost $28ea = $868 per month	Adefovir dipivoxil is a prodrug of adefovir. It is an acyclic nucleotide analog with activity against hepatitis B (HBV) at 0.2-2.5 mM (IC$_{50}$). See Table 9 for Cmax & T1/2. Active against YMDD mutant lamivudine-resistant strains and EN resistant strains. No cross-resistance. Primarily renal excretion—adjust dose. No food interactions. Remarkably few side effects. No nephrotoxicity at 10 mg per day. Monitor renal function, esp. with pts with pre-existing or other risks for renal impairment. Lactic acidosis reported with nucleoside analogs, esp. in women. Pregnancy Category C. Hepatitis may exacerbate when treatment discontinued; 6-25% of pts developed ALT ↑ 10 times normal within 12 wks; usually responds to re-treatment and hepatic decompensation has occurred.
Entecavir (Baraclude)	0.5 mg per day q24h. If refractory to lamivudine: 1 mg per day q24h. per month) 0.5 = $25.60 ea = $766/mo	A nucleoside analog active against HBV including lamivudine-resistant mutants. Minimal adverse effects reported: headache, fatigue, dizziness, & nausea reported in 22% of pts. Potential for lactic acidosis but not reported to date. Adjust dosage in renal impairment (see Table 17, page 155).
Interferon alfa is available as alfa-2a, alfa-2b (Intron-A)	3 million units: (Intron $49, Infergen 9 mcg $88)	**Adverse effects:** Flu-like syndrome common, esp. during 1st week of rx. Never 98%, fatigue 89%, myalgia 73%, headache 71%. GI anorexia 46%, diarrhea 29%, CNS dizziness 21%, rash 18%, later profound fatigue & psychiatric symptoms in up to ⅓ of pts (J Clin Psych 64:708, 2003) (depression, anxiety, emotional lability and agitation), alopecia. ↑ TSH, autoimmune thyroid disorders with hypo- or
PEG interferon alfa-2b (PEG-Intron)	0.5-1.5 mcg per kg subcut. q wk (120 mcg) $460)	hyperthyroidism. Graves disease reported (J Intern Med 53:26, 2005). Hemato: ↓ WBC 49%, ↓ Hgb 27%, ↓ platelets 35%. Consider prophylactic antidepressant in pts with history of depression. Acute reversible hearing loss and/or tinnitus in up to 1/3 (J Clin Rheum, e30, June 2005).
Peglyated-40k interferon alfa-2a (Pegasys)	180 mcg subcut. q wk times 48 wks (180 mcg) $477)	hearing loss and/or tinnitus in up to 1/3 (J Clin Rheum, e30, June 2005). Optic neuropathy (retinal hemorrhage, cotton wool spots, ↓ in color vision) reported (Am J Ophthalmol 138:18:1806, 2004). Cryoglobulinemia assoc. with HCV usually responds to IFN rx but exacerbations with vasculitis also reported with rx (Clin Rheum, e30, June 2005). Side-effects ↑ with ↑ doses and dose reduction necessary in up to 46% receiving chronic rx for HBV.
Lamivudine (3TC) (Epivir-HBV)	**Adverse effects:** See Table 14D, page 157. NOTE: 100 mg q24h times 1 yr for hepatitis B.	Attachment of IFN to polyethylene glycol (PEG) prolongs half-life and allows weekly dosing. Better efficacy data with similar adverse effects profile as compared to regular formulation. (100 mg tab $7, $205 per month)

* See page 2 for abbreviations. NOTE: All dosage recommendations are for adults (unless otherwise indicated) and assume normal/renal function.
Cost = average wholesale price from 2007 RED BOOK, Thomson Healthcare, Inc.

TABLE 14B (3)

DRUG NAME(S) GENERIC (TRADE)	DOSAGE/ROUTE/COST*	COMMENTS/ADVERSE EFFECTS
Hepatitis (continued)		

Ribavirin–Interferon alfa-2b combination pack (Rebetron)
 	
or
 	
PEG IFN + ribavirin in combination
	Combination kit contains 2 wk. supply of IFN and 42, 70, or 84 caps of 200 mg ribavirin.
	Dose: IFN 3 million units subcut. 3 times per wk AND ribavirin 400 mg po q a.m. + 600 mg po q p.m. (<75 kg) or 600 mg po bid (≥75 kg). Rebetron (1000 mg per day ribavirin dose pack)
	
	Dose changes:
	
	          Ribavirin Interferon
	Hgb: <10 ↓ to 200 mg q a.m., No change
	           400 mg q p.m.
	    <8.5 DC DC
	WBC: <1500 ↓ to 1.5 million units subcut. 3 times per wk
	    <1000 DC
	Abs. PMNs: <750 ↓ to 1.5 million units subcut. 3 times per wk
	         <500 DC
	Platelets: <50,000 No change
	          <25,000 DC
		Ribavirin: Hemolytic anemia common but usually responds to ↓ ribavirin dosage (see package insert). Ribavirin plasma level correlates with degree of anemia but also with efficacy against HBV (JAIDS 39:401, 2005); 1 Japanese study suggests levels between 3000 to 3500 ng per mL 8 wks after initiating rx optimal (Intervirol 48:138, 2005).
		Erythropoietin (Epoetin alfa) effective in ↑ Hgb levels & quality of life while allowing adequate dosage of ribavirin to be maintained (Pharmacother 25:862, 2005). Pure red cell aplasia 2° to anti-erythropoietin antibodies reported (Am J Gastro 100:1415, 2005). **Since ribavirin is teratogenic, drug must not be used during pregnancy or within 6 months of pregnancy.** Also should not be used in pts with endstage renal failure, severe heart disease, or hemoglobinopathies. ARDS reported (Chest 124:406, 2003).
		Interferon alfa: Severe psychiatric effects, esp. depression, most common (23–36%) reason for discontinuation of rx. Suicidal behavior reported. Preemptive rx with antidepressants effective in 1 open-label study (J Hpt 42:793, 2005). Hyper- & hypothyroidism, alopecia (30%) including reversible alopecia universalis (J Chemother 17:212, 2005), & pulmonary disease reported (Mayo Clin Proc 74:367, 1999). Uncommon side-effects include exacerbation of psoriasis (Chemotherapy 51:167, 2005) & other rheumatological conditions (Rheumatol 44:1016, 2005), sexual dysfunction with ↓ testosterone levels (J Endo 186:345, 2005), ↑ risk of lipoatrophy 2° to mitochondrial toxicity when administered with nucleoside analogs to HIV-co-infected pts (Antivir Ther 10:557, 2005), & sarcoidosis (ArDerm 141:865, 2005)

Ribavirin (Rebetol)	Use with pegylated interferons [alfa-2a & 2b] for treatment of hepatitis C. Available as 200 mg capsules. Dose: <75 kg BW = 2 caps in a.m. & 3 caps in p.m.; >75 kg BW 3 caps in a.m. & 3 caps in p.m. Cost: 200 mg $10.60	Side-effects as above, esp. hemolytic anemia (during 1st 1–2 wks of rx) with hemoglobin ↓ of 3–4 gm. Should not be used with CrCl <50 mL per min & cautiously with cardiac disease.
Influenza A Amantadine (Symmetrel) or Rimantadine (Flumadine)	**Currently not recommended by the CDC for Influenza A because of high level resistance found in 2005 isolates.** Amantadine and rimantadine doses are the same (rimantadine approved only for prophylaxis in children, not treatment). Amantadine 100 mg po bid—>65 y.o. 100 mg q24h. G: 100 mg cap $1. 50 mg/5 mL syrup, 473 mL, $21.35. Rimantadine 100 mg tab/syrup $2.	**Side-effects/toxicity:** CNS (nervousness, anxiety, difficulty concentrating, and lightheadedness). Symptoms occurred in 6% on rimantadine vs 14% on amantadine. They usually ↓ after 1st week and disappear when drug dc. GI (nausea, anorexia). Some serious side-effects—delirium, hallucinations, and seizures—are associated with high plasma drug levels resulting from renal insufficiency, esp. in older pts. In pts with impaired renal function, dosage of both drugs should be reduced (amantadine, creatinine clearance <50 mL per min; rimantadine: CrCl <10 mL per min); see package inserts and Table 17, pages 183 & 184. Both drugs teratogenic in animals and **contraindicated during pregnancy** (Med Lett 39:72, 1997).

* See page 2 for abbreviations. NOTE: All dosage recommendations are for adults (unless otherwise indicated) and assume normal renal function.
Cost = average wholesale price from 2007 Red Book, Thomson Healthcare, Inc.

TABLE 14B (4)

DRUG NAME(S) GENERIC (TRADE)	DOSAGE/ROUTE/COST*	COMMENTS/ADVERSE EFFECTS
Influenza A and B—For both drugs, initiate within 48 hrs of symptom onset		
Zanamivir (Relenza) For pts ≥12 yrs of age	2 inhalations (2 times 5 mg) bid times 5 days. Powder is inhaled using specially designed breath-activated device. Each medication-containing blister contains 5 mg of zanamivir. $64.50 per course	Active by inhalation against neuraminidase of both influenza A and B and inhibits release of virus from epithelial cells of respiratory tract. Approx. 4–17% of inhaled dose absorbed into plasma. Excreted by kidney but with low absorption, dose reduction not necessary in renal impairment. Minimal side-effects: <3% cough, sinusitis, diarrhea, nausea and vomiting. **Reports of respiratory adverse events in pts with or without h/o airways disease, should be avoided in pts with underlying respiratory disease.**
Oseltamivir (Tamiflu)	75 mg po bid for treatment [pediatric suspension (12 mg per mL) approved for treatment, not prevention, in children age 1–12 at dose of 2 mg per kg (up to 75 mg) bid times 5 days] For prevention: 75 mg po q24h for duration of peak of flu epidemic. $84 per 5 day course	Well absorbed (80% bioavailable) from GI tract as ethyl ester of active compound GS 4071. T½ 6–10 hrs; excreted unchanged by kidney. Adverse effects in 15% include diarrhea 1.6%, nausea 0.5%, vomiting, headache (J Am Ger Soc 50:608, 2002). Nausea ↓ with food. Also available as 12 mg per mL, oral suspension.
Respiratory Syncytial Virus (RSV) and other		
Palivizumab (Synagis) Used for prevention of RSV infection in high-risk children	15 mg per kg IM q month 100 mg vial (for 1 injection) $1672	A monoclonal antibody directed against the F glycoprotein on surface of virus; side-effects are nominal, occ. ↑ ALT. Preferred over polyclonal immune globulin in high risk infants & children.
Ribavirin (Virazole)	1.1 gm per day (6 gm vial for inhalation $1700)	**Ribavirin side-effects:** Anemia, rash, conjunctivitis. Read package insert. Avoid procedures that lead to drug precipitation in ventilator tubing with subsequent dysfunction. Significant teratogenicity in animals. **Contraindicated in pregnant women and partners.** Pregnant health care workers should avoid direct care of pts receiving aerosolized ribavirin.
Warts (See C/D S37, 1999)		
Interferon alfa-2b or alfa-n3	Apply 1 million units into lesion	Interferon alfa-2b 3 million units per 0.5 mL, interferon alfa-n3 5 million units per 1 mL. Cost: $10
Podofilox (Condylox) Imiquimod (Aldara)	3.5 mL 0.5% solution for topical application. $128 Cream applied 3 times per week to maximum of 16 wks. 250 mg packets $18 each G	**Side-effects:** Local reactions—pain, burning, inflammation in 50%. No systemic effects. Mild erythema, erosions, itching and burning

* See page 2 for abbreviations. NOTE: All dosage recommendations are for adults (unless otherwise indicated) and assume normal renal function.
Cost = average wholesale price from 2007 Red Book, Thomson Healthcare, Inc.

TABLE 14C - SUMMARY OF SUGGESTED ANTIVIRAL AGENTS AGAINST TREATABLE PATHOGENIC VIRUSES

Virus	Acyclovir	Amantadine	Adefovir Entecavir Lamivudine Tenofovir	Cidofovir	Famciclovir	Foscarnet	Ganciclovir	αInterferon Or PEG INF	Oseltamivir	Ribavirin	Rimantadine	Valacyclovir	Valganciclovir	Zanamivir
Adenovirus	-	-	-	+	-	-	±	-	-	-	-	-	±	-
BK virus	-	-	-	+	-	-	-	-	-	-	-	-	-	-
Cytomegalovirus	±	-	-	+++	±	+++	+++	-	-	-	-	±	+++	-
Hepatitis B	-	-	+++	-	-	-	-	+++	-	±	-	-	-	-
Hepatitis C	-	-	-	-	-	-	-	+++*	-	+++*	-	-	-	-
Herpes simplex virus	+++	-	-	++	+++	++	++	-	-	-	-	+++	++	-
Influenza A Influenza B	-	±**	-	-	-	-	-	-	+++	-	±**	-	-	+++
Respiratory Syncytial Virus	-	-	-	-	-	-	-	-	-	+	-	-	-	-
Varicella-zoster virus	+++	-	-	-	++	++	+	-	-	-	-	+++	+	-

* 1st line rx = an IFN + Ribavirin ** not CDC recommended due to high prevalence of resistance

- = no activity; ± = possible activity; + = active, 3rd line therapy (least active clinically)

++ = Active, 2nd line therapy (less active clinically); +++ = Active, 1st line therapy (usually active clinically)

TABLE 14D – ANTIRETROVIRAL THERAPY IN TREATMENT-NAÏVE ADULTS

(See the 2008 SANFORD GUIDE TO HIV/AIDS THERAPY, Table 6, for additional information regarding treatment and complications of antiretroviral agents)

The U.S. Dept of Health & Human Services (DHHS) updated guidelines for treatment of adults and adolescents with HIV-1 infection in late 2007. These, and guidelines for pediatric patients and pregnant women, can be found at www.aidsinfo.nih.gov. Since the previous edition, the first of 2 new classes of antiretrovirals (CCR5 co-receptor antagonist and integrase inhibitor) were approved in the US. Whenever starting antiretroviral therapy, **resistance testing** should be performed to help guide choice of agents. Note that **immune reconstitution syndromes** may result from initiation of antiretroviral therapy, and may require medical intervention. For additional explanation and other acceptable alternatives relating to these tables, see www.aidsinfo.nih.gov.

The following concepts guide therapy:
- The goal of rx is to inhibit maximally viral replication, allowing re-establishment & persistence of an effective immune response that will prevent or delay HIV-related morbidity.
- The lower the viral RNA can be driven, the lower the rate of accumulation of drug resistance mutations & the longer the therapeutic effect will last.
- To achieve maximal & durable suppression of viral RNA, combinations of potent antiretroviral agents are required, as is a high degree of adherence to the chosen regimens.
- Treatment regimens must be tailored to the individual as well as to the virus. Antiretroviral drug toxicities can compromise adherence in the short term & can cause significant negative health effects over time. Carefully check for specific risks to the individual, for renal or hepatic dysfunction, & for possible pharmacokinetic interactions. **Interactions between the antiretrovirals selected & between those & concurrent drugs, & adjust doses as necessary for body weight, for renal or hepatic dysfunction, & for possible pharmacokinetic interactions.**

A. When to start therapy? (see www.aidsinfo.nih.gov for additional indications: pregnancy, nephropathy, HBV co-infection requiring rx)

HIV Symptoms	CD4 cells/µl	Start Treatment	Comment
Yes	Any	Yes	
No	<200	Yes	*New DHHS recommendation.
No	≥200 – <350	Yes*	*Maybe if CD4 decreasing rapidly &/or viral load > 100,000 copies/mL. Whether there is long-term
No	≥350	No*	immunological benefit of starting ART at CD4 <350 remains a topic of investigation (CID 44:441, 2007).

B. Acute HIV Infection. The benefits of ARV treatment in acute HIV infection are uncertain, but may include improved immunological response to the virus and decreased potential for transmission. However, treatment also exposes the patient to risks of drug adverse events, and the optimal duration of rx is unknown. Therefore, treatment is considered optional and is best undertaken in a research setting. Optimal regimens in this setting have not yet been defined. An observational study of acute or early HIV-1 infection showed comparable results from either PI-based or NNRTI-based regimens (CID 42:1024, 2006), although some feel that the higher barrier to resistance of PIs might be advantageous (JAMA 296:827, 2006).

C. Approach to constructing ARV regimens for treatment naïve adults. (From Guidelines for the Use of Antiretroviral Agents in HIV-1-Infected Adults and Adolescents at www.aidsinfo.nih.gov. See that document for explanations, qualifications and further alternatives.)

Design a regimen consisting of
[either an NNRTI **OR** a Protease Inhibitor] **PLUS** [a dual-NRTI component]

- See section D of this table for specific regimens and tables which follow for drug characteristics, usual doses, adverse effects and additional details
- Selection of components will be influenced by many factors, such as
  - Co-morbidities (e.g., lipid effects of PIs, liver or renal disease, etc)
  - Pregnancy (e.g., avoid efavirenz—pregnancy class D)
  - HIV status (e.g., avoid nevirapine in women with CD4 >250)
  - Results of viral resistance testing
  - Potential drug interactions or adverse drug effects
  - Convenience of dosing

Co-formulations increase convenience, but sometimes prescribing the two constituents individually is preferred, as when dose-adjustments are needed for renal disease.

TABLE 14D (2)

Preferred components by class (alphabetical order)

	Protease Inhibitor	Dual-NRTI
NNRTI		
Efavirenz	Atazanavir + ritonavir or	Tenofovir/ Emtricitabine (co-formulated) or
	Fosamprenavir + ritonavir (twice-daily regimen) or	Zidovudine/ Lamivudine (co-formulated)
	Lopinavir/ritonavir (co-formulated, twice-daily regimen)	

Alternative components by class

	Protease Inhibitor	Dual-NRTI
NNRTI		
Nevirapine	Atazanavir or	Abacavir/Lamivudine (co-formulated) or
	Fosamprenavir or	Didanosine + (emtricitabine or lamivudine)
	Fosamprenavir + ritonavir (once-daily regimen) or	
	Lopinavir/ritonavir	
	(co-formulated, once-daily regimen)	

D. **Suggested Initial Therapy Regimens for Untreated Chronic HIV-1 Infection** Doses & use assume normal renal & hepatic function unless otherwise stated. *(For pregnancy, see below; also, Table 6B of The Sanford Guide to HIV/AIDS Therapy 2008 for additional explanation & alternatives, see www.aidsinfo.nih.gov)*

1. **Preferred Regimens**

Regimen	Pill strength (mg)	Usual Daily Regimen (oral)	No. pills/ day	Cost/mo (Avg. Whole-sale Price)	Comment (See also Individual agents & Table 14E)
a. (Tenofovir + Emtricitabine) + Efavirenz	(300 + 200) + 600	(Combination—Truvada 1 tab q24h) + 1 tab q24h at bedtime, empty stomach	2	$1247	Analysis at 48-wks of ongoing trial reported superior virus suppression, higher CD4 & fewer AEs of tenofovir/ emtricitabine/ efavirenz as compared to ZDV/3TC/efavirenz (NEJM 354:251, 2006). Tenofovir reports of renal toxicity (CID 42:283, 2006). Avoid efavirenz
OR					in pregnancy or in women who might become pregnant
(Tenofovir + Emtricitabine + Efavirenz)	(300 + 200 + 600)	Combination—Atripla 1 tab q24h at bedtime, empty stomach	1	$1439	(Pregnancy Category D). Food may ↑ serum efavirenz concentration, which can lead to ↑ adverse events. See section F.2 re how to stop efavirenz.
b. (Zidovudine + Lamivudine) + Efavirenz	(300 + 150) + 600	(Combination—Combivir 1 tab bid) + 1 tab q24h at bedtime, empty stomach	3	$1238	Good efficacy; low pill burden; low AE profile. Avoid efavirenz in pregnancy or in women who might become pregnant (Pregnancy Category D). Food may ↑ serum efavirenz concentration, which can lead to ↑ adverse events. See section F.2 re how to stop efavirenz.

TABLE 14D (3)

	Regimen	Pill strength (mg)	Usual Daily Regimen (oral)	No. pills/day	Cost/mo (Avg. Whole-sale Price)	Comment (See also Individual agents & Table 14E)
c.	(Zidovudine + Lamivudine) + Lopinavir / Ritonavir	(300 + 150) + 200/50	(Combination—Combivir 1 tab bid) + (Combination—Kaletra 2 tabs bid) without regard to food	6	$1514	Good virologic efficacy & durable effect. Tolerable AEs. Preferred regimen is to use lopinavir/ritonavir twice daily. As an alternative regimen, lopinavir/ritonavir can be given as 4 tabs once daily in rx-naive pts.
d.	(Zidovudine + Lamivudine) + Atazanavir + Ritonavir	(300 + 150) + 300 + 100	(Combination—Combivir 1 tab bid) + 1 cap q24h + 1 cap q24h both with food	4	$1955	Lower potential for lipid derangement by (unboosted) atazanavir than w/other PIs. May ↑ EKG PR interval & bilirubin. Acid-lowering agents can markedly ↓ absorption; avoid with PPIs & give 2hr before or 10hr after H2-blockers. As an alternative regimen, atazanavir can be used without ritonavir, at a dose of 400 mg q24h with food, in combination therapy for Rx-naive patients.
e.	(Zidovudine + Lamivudine) + Fosamprenavir + Ritonavir	(300 + 150) + 700 + 100	(Combination—Combivir 1 tab bid) + 1 tab bid fed or fasting + 1 cap bid fed or fasting	6	$2002	Can take without regard to meals. Skin rash, GI symptoms. Fosamprenavir contains sulfa moiety. Alternative fosamprenavir regimens available for rx-naive pts, including fosamprenavir without ritonavir & once-daily fosamprenavir/ritonavir regimens (see label for use & doses).

2. **Alternative Regimens** (For additional alternatives, see *Comments section above, also Tables 6A-6C of The Sanford Guide to HIV/AIDS Therapy* 2008 and *www.aidsinfo.nih.gov*)

	Regimen	Pill strength (mg)	Usual Daily Regimen (oral)	No. pills/day	Cost/mo (Avg. Whole-sale Price)	Comment (See also Individual agents & Table 14E)
a.	Didanosine EC + Lamivudine + Efavirenz	400 + 300 + 600	1 cap q24h at bedtime, fasting + 1 tab q24h + 1 tab q24h at bedtime, empty stomach **Didanosine dosage shown for ≥60 kg**	3	$1191	Low pill burden. Efficacy & durability under study. Potential didanosine AEs (pancreatitis, peripheral neuritis). Avoid efavirenz in pregnancy or in women who might become pregnant (**Pregnancy Category D**). Food may ↑ serum efavirenz concentration, which can lead to ↑ adverse events. Can substitute emtricitabine 200 mg po q24h for lamivudine 300 mg po q24h.
b.	(Abacavir + Lamivudine) + Efavirenz	(600 + 300) + 600	(Combination—Epzicom 1 tab q24h) without regard to food + 1 tab q24h at bedtime, empty stomach	2	$1387	Low pill burden. **Risk of abacavir hypersensitivity reaction (see Comment Table 14E).** Comparison of abacavir/lamivudine with tenofovir/emtricitabine as backbone in rx-naive pts under study. Avoid efavirenz in pregnancy or in women who might become pregnant (**Pregnancy Category D**). Food may ↑ serum efavirenz concentration, which can lead to ↑ adverse events.

TABLE 14D (4)

3. **Triple nucleoside regimen:** Due to inferior virologic activity, use only when preferred or alternative regimen not possible. Seek expert advice about alternatives.

Regimen	Pill strength (mg)	Usual Daily Regimen (oral)	No. pills/day	Cost/mo (Avg. Whole-sale Price)	Comment (See also individual agents)
a. (Zidovudine + Lamivudine + Abacavir)	(300 + 150 + 300)	**(Combination–Trizivir** 1 tab bid)	2	$1301	Reduced activity as compared with preferred or alternative regimens. Potentially serious abacavir AEs (see comments for individual agents.)

4. **During pregnancy. Expert consultation mandatory.** Timing of rx initiation & drug choice must be individualized. Viral resistance testing should be performed. Long-term effects of agents unknown. Certain drugs hazardous or contraindicated. (*See Table 8A of the Sanford Guide to HIV/AIDS Therapy*). For additional information & alternative options, see www.aidsinfo.nih.gov. For regimens to prevent perinatal transmission, see *Table 8A of the Sanford Guide to HIV/AIDS Therapy*.

Regimen	Pill strength (mg)	Usual Daily Regimen (oral)	No. pills/day	Cost/mo (Avg. Whole-sale Price)	Comment (See also individual agents)
a. (Zidovudine + Lamivudine) + Nevirapine	(300 + 150) + 200	(Combination–Combivir 1 tab bid) + 1 tab bid fed or fasting [after 14-day lead-in period of 1 tab q24h]	4	$1167	See especially nevirapine **Black Box warnings—** among others ↑ risk of **potentially fatal hepatotoxicity** in women with CD4 >250. Avoid in this group, unless benefits clearly > risks; monitor intensively if drug must be used.
b. (Zidovudine + Lamivudine) + Lopinavir/ritonavir	(300 + 150) + 200/50	(Combination—Combivir 1 tab bid) + 2 tabs bid without regard to food	6	$1514	Optimal dose in 3rd trimester unknown. May need to monitor levels as 1 dose may be required. Once-daily dosing of lopinavir/ritonavir not recommended.

5. **Alternative Regimen (DHHS 2006: www.aidsinfo.nih.gov)**

Regimen	Pill strength (mg)	Usual Daily Regimen (oral)	No. pills/day	Cost/mo (Avg. Whole-sale Price)	Comment (See also individual agents)
a. (Zidovudine + Lamivudine) + Saquinavir + Ritonavir	(300 + 150) + 500 + 100	(Combination–Combivir 1 tab bid) + 2 tabs bid + 1 cap bid	8	$2116	Use saquinavir tabs only in combination with ritonavir. Certain drugs metabolized by CYP3A are contra-indicated with saquinavir/ritonavir. (Original DHHS recommendations were based on saquinavir soft gel caps, which are no longer available, plus ritonavir).

156

TABLE 14D (5)

E. **Selected Characteristics of Antiretroviral Drugs**

1. **Selected Characteristics of Nucleoside or Nucleotide Reverse Transcriptase Inhibitors (NRTIs)**
   All agents have Black Box warning: Risk of lactic acidosis/hepatic steatosis. Also, labels note risk of fat redistribution/accumulation with ARV rx. For combinations, see warnings for component agents.

Generic/Trade Name	Pharmaceutical Prep. (Avg. Wholesale Price)	Usual Adult Dosage & Food Effect	% Absorbed, po	Serum T½, hrs	Intracellular T½, hrs	Elimination	Major Adverse Events/Comments (See Table 14E)
Abacavir (ABC; Ziagen)	300 mg tabs or 20 mg/ml oral solution ($471/month)	300 mg po bid or 600 mg po q24h. Food OK	83	1.5	20	Liver metab., renal excretion of metabolites, 82%	**Hypersensitivity reaction:** fever, rash; N/V, malaise, diarrhea, abdominal pain, respiratory symptoms. (Severe reactions may be ↑ with 600 mg dose) **Do not rechallenge!** Report to 800-270-0425. **See Comment Table 14E.**
Abacavir/lamivudine/zidovudine (Trizivir)	Film-coated tabs ABC 300 mg + 3TC 150 mg + ZDV 300 mg ($1301/month)	1 tab po bid (not recommended for wt <40 kg or CrCl <50 mL/min or impaired hepatic function)			*(See individual components)*		*(See Comments for individual components)* Note: **Black Box warnings** for ABC hypersensitivity reaction & others. Should only be used for regimens intended to include these 3 agents. Black Box warning—limited data for VL >100,000 copies/mL.
Didanosine (ddI; Videx or Videx EC)	125, 200, 250, 400, enteric-coated caps; 100, 167, 250mg powder for oral solution. (Videx EC); (Tablets discontinued in US in 2006.)	≥60kg: Usually 400mg enteric-coated po q24h 0.5 hr before or 2hrs after meal. Do not crush! 250mg EC po q24h. Food ↓ levels. See Comment	30–40	1.6	25–40	Renal excretion, 50%	**Pancreatitis,** peripheral neuropathy, lactic acidosis & hepatic steatosis (rare but life-threatening, esp. combined with stavudine in pregnancy). Retinal, optic n. changes. **If ddI + TDF is used,** reduce dose of ddI-EC from 400mg to 250mg EC po q24h (or from 250mg EC to 200mg EC for adults <60kg). **This combination is generally avoided, but if needed, monitor for increased toxicity & possible decrease in efficacy of this combination; may result in decreased CD4.**
Emtricitabine (FTC, Emtriva)	200mg caps; 10mg per mL oral solution. ($346/month)	200mg po q24h. Food OK	93 (caps), 75 (oral sol'n)	Approx. 10	39	Renal excretion 86%, minor biotransformation, 14% excretion in feces	Well tolerated; headache, nausea, vomiting & diarrhea occasionally; skin rash rarely. Skin hyperpigmentation. Differs only slightly in structure from lamivudine (5-fluoro substitution). **Exacerbation of Hep B reported in pts after stopping FTC.** Monitor FTC in Hep B pts; some may need anti-HBV therapy.

TABLE 14D (6)

Generic/Trade Name	Pharmaceutical Prep. (Avg. Wholesale Price)	Usual Adult Dosage & Food Effect	% Absorbed, po	Serum T½, hrs	Intracellular T½, hrs	Elimination	Major Adverse Events/Comments (See Table 14E)
Emtricitabine/tenofovir disoproxil fumarate (Truvada)	Film-coated tabs: FTC 200mg + TDF 300mg ($728/month)	1 tab po q24h for CrCl ≥50 ml/min. Food OK	92/25	10/17	—	Primarily renal/renal	See Comments for individual agents Black Box warning—Exacerbation of HepB after stopping FTC.
Emtricitabine/tenofovir /efavirenz (Atripla)	Film-coated tabs: FTC 200 mg + TDF 300 mg + efavirenz 600 mg ($1439 per month)	1 tab po q24h on an empty stomach, preferably at bedtime. Do not use if CrCl <50ml/min	(See individual components)				Not recommended for pts <18yrs. (See warnings for individual components). Exacerbation of Hep B reported in pts discontinuing component drugs. Pregnancy category D- may cause fetal harm. Avoid in pregnancy or in women who may become pregnant.
Lamivudine (3TC; Epivir)	150, 300mg tabs; 10mg/ml oral solution ($347/month)	150mg po bid or 300mg po q24h. Food OK	86	5-7	18	Renal excretion, minimal metabolism	Use HIV dose, not Hep B dose. Usually well-tolerated. Risk of exacerbation of Hep B after stopping 3TC. Monitor at least several months after stopping 3TC in Hep B pts; some may need anti-HBV therapy.
Lamivudine/abacavir (Epzicom)	Film-coated tabs: 3TC 300mg + abacavir 600mg ($868/month)	1 tab po q24h, Food OK. Not recommended for CrCl <50ml/min or impaired hepatic function	86/86	5-7/1.5	16/20	Primarily renal/ metabolism	See Comments for individual agents. Note abacavir hypersensitivity Black Box warnings (severe reactions may be somewhat more frequent with 600 mg dose) and 3TC Hep B warnings.
Lamivudine/ zidovudine (Combivir)	Film-coated tabs: 3TC 150mg + ZDV 300mg ($719/month)	1 tab po bid. Not recommended for CrCl <50 ml/min or impaired hepatic function Food OK.	86/64	5-7/ 0.5-3	—	Primarily renal/ metabolism with renal excretion of glucuronide	See Comments for individual agents See Black Box warning—exacerbation of Hep B in pts stopping 3TC
Stavudine (d4T, Zerit)	15, 20, 30, 40 mg capsules; 1 mg per mL oral solution ($340/month 40 mg caps)	≥60 kg: 40 mg po bid <60 kg: 30 mg po bid Food OK	86	1.2-1.6	3.5	Renal excretion, 40%	Highest incidence of lipoatrophy, hyperlipidemia, & lactic acidosis of all NRTIs. Pancreatitis. Peripheral neuropathy. (See didanosine comments.)

TABLE 14D (7)

Generic/Trade Name	Pharmaceutical Prep. (Avg. Wholesale Price)	Usual Adult Dosage & Food Effect	% Absorbed, po	Serum T½, hrs	Intracellular T½, hrs	Elimination	Major Adverse Events/Comments (See Table 14E)
Tenofovir disoproxil fumarate (TDF, Viread)—a nucleotide	300 mg tabs ($503/month)	CrCl ≥50 ml/min: 300 mg po q24h. Food OK, high-fat meal ↑ absorption	39 (with food) 25 (fasted)	17	>60	Renal excretion	Headache, N/V. **Cases of renal dysfunction reported:** avoid concomitant nephrotoxic agents. Monitor CrCl esp. in those with preexisting renal dysfunction. Must adjust dose of ddI (↓↓) if used concomitantly but best to avoid this combination (see ddI Comments). Atazanavir & lopinavir/ritonavir ↑ tenofovir concentrations; monitor for adverse effects. **Black Box warning—exacerbations of Hep B reported after stopping tenofovir.** Monitor several months after stopping TDF in Hep B pts; some may need anti-HBV Rx.
Zalcitabine (ddC, Hivid)	0.375, 0.75 tabs ($273/month)	0.75 mg po q8h. Food OK	85	2	3	Renal excretion, 70%	**Peripheral neuropathy,** stomatitis, rarely life-threatening lactic acidosis, pancreatitis. **Not recommended.**
Zidovudine (ZDV, AZT, Retrovir)	100 mg caps, 300 mg tabs; 10 mg per mL IV solution; 10 mg/mL oral syrup ($387/month)	300 mg po q12h. Food OK	64	1.1	11	Metabolized to glucuronide & excreted in urine	Bone marrow suppression, GI intolerance, headache, insomnia, malaise, myopathy.

2. **Selected Characteristics of Non-Nucleoside Reverse Transcriptase Inhibitors (NNRTIs)**

Generic/Trade Name	Pharmaceutical Prep. (Avg. Wholesale Price)	Usual Adult Dosage & Food Effect	% Absorbed, po	Serum T½, hrs	Elimination	Major Adverse Events/Comments
Delavirdine (Rescriptor)	100, 200 mg tabs ($304/month)	400 mg po three times daily. Food OK	85	5.8	Cytochrome P450 (3A inhibitor). 51% excreted in urine (<5% unchanged), 44% in feces	Rash severe enough to stop drug in 4.3%. ↑ AST/ALT, headaches. **Not recommended.**

TABLE 14D (8)

Generic/Trade Name	Pharmaceutical Prep. (Avg. Wholesale Price)	Usual Adult Dosage & Food Effect	% Absorbed, po	Serum T½, hrs	Elimination	Major Adverse Events/Comments
Efavirenz (Sustiva) **(Pregnancy Category D)**	50, 100, 200 mg capsules; 600 mg tablet ($519/month)	600 mg po q24h at bedtime, without food. Food may ↑ serum conc. which can lead to ↑ in risk of adverse events.	42	40–55 See Comment	Cytochrome P450 (3A mixed inducer/ inhibitor). 14–34% of dose excreted in urine as glucuroni- dated metabolites, 16–61% in feces	Rash severe enough to d/c use of drug in 1.7%. High fre- quency of diverse CNS AEs: somnolence, dreams, confusion, agitation. Serious psychiatric symptoms. False-pos. cannabinoid screen. **Pregnancy Category D—may cause fetal harm—avoid in pregnant women or those who might become pregnant.** (Note: No single method of contraception is 100% reliable). Very long tissue T½: **If rx is to be discontinued, stop efavirenz 1–2 wks before stopping companion drugs.** Otherwise, risk of developing efavirenz resistance, as after 1–2 days only efavirenz in blood &/or tissue. Some authorities bridge this gap by adding a PI to the NRTI backbone if feasible after efavirenz is discontinued. (CID 42:401, 2006)
Nevirapine (Viramune)	200 mg tabs; 50 mg per 5 mL oral suspension ($448/month)	200 mg po q24h x14 days & then 200 mg po bid (see Comments & **Black Box warning)**. Food OK	>90	25–30	Cytochrome P450 (3A4, 2B6) inducer. 80% of dose excreted in urine as glucuronidated metabolites, 10% in feces	**Black Box warning—fatal hepatotoxicity.** Women with CD4 >250 esp. vulnerable, inc. pregnant women. Avoid in this group unless benefits clearly > risks (www.fda.gov/cder/drug/advisory/nevirapine.htm). If used, intensive monitoring required. Men with CD4 >400 also at ↑ risk. Rash severe enough to stop drug in 7%, **severe or life-threatening skin reactions** in 2%. Do not restart if any suspicion of such reactions. 2wk dose escalation period may ↓ skin reactions. As with efavirenz, because of long T½, consider continuing companion agents for several days if nevirapine is discontinued.

TABLE 14D (9)

3. **Selected Characteristics of Protease Inhibitors (PIs).**

All PIs: Glucose metabolism: new diabetes mellitus or deterioration of glucose control; fat redistribution; possible hemophilia bleeding; hypertriglyceridemia or hypercholesterolemia. Exercise caution re: potential drug interactions & contraindications. QTc prolongation has been reported in a few pts taking PIs; some PIs can block HERG channels in vitro (*Lancet* 365:682,2005*).* Observ. study found ↑ risk of MI with PI exposure (*NEJM* 356:1723, 2007).

Generic/Trade Name	Pharmaceutical Prep. (Avg. Wholesale Price)	Usual Adult Dosage & Food Effect	% Absorbed, po	Serum T½, hrs	Elimination	Major Adverse Events/Comments (See Table 14E)
Atazanavir (Reyataz)	100, 150, 200, 300 mg capsules ($875/month)	400 mg po q24h with food (exception is atazanavir 300 mg po q24h + ritonavir 100 mg po q24h when combined with either efavirenz 600 mg po q24h or TDF 300 mg po q24h). Take with food 2 hrs or 1 hr post buffered ddI. Ritonavir-boosted dose also recommended for ARV tx-experienced pts.	Good oral bioavailability; food enhances bioavailability & ↓ pharmacokinetic variability. Absorption ↓ by antacids, H₂-blockers, proton pump inhibitors. Avoid with PPIs. Give 2hr before or 10hr after H₂-blockers, or boost with ritonavir (see 2006 *drug label changes*).	Approx. 7	Cytochrome P450 (3A4, 1A2 & 2C9 inhibition) & UGT1A1 inhibitor. 13% excreted in urine (7% unchanged). 70% excreted in feces (20% unchanged)	No ↑ lipids in available studies. Asymptomatic unconjugated hyperbilirubinemia common; jaundice especially likely in Gilbert's syndrome (*JID* 192:1381, 2005). Headache, rash, GI symptoms. Prolongation of PR interval (1st degree AV block) reported. Caution in pre-existing conduction system disease. Efavirenz & tenofovir ↓ atazanavir exposure: use atazanavir/ritonavir regimen; also, atazanavir ↑ tenofovir concentrations—watch for adverse events.
Darunavir (Prezista)	300 mg tablet ($900 per month)	(600 mg darunavir (2 tabs) + 100 mg ritonavir) po bid, with food	82% absorbed (taken with ritonavir). Food ↑ absorption.	Approx 15 hr (with ritonavir)	Metabolized by CYP3A4 and is a CYP3A inhibitor	Contains sulfa moiety. Rash, nausea, headaches seen. Coadmin of certain drugs cleared by CYP3A is contraindicated (see label). Use with caution in pts with hepatic dysfunction. May cause hormonal contraception failure.
Fosamprenavir (Lexiva)	700 mg tablet; 50 mg/ml oral suspension ($966/month when used with ritonavir)	1400 mg (two 700 mg tabs) po bid OR with ritonavir: [1400 mg fosamprenavir (2 tabs) + ritonavir 200 mg] po q24h OR [700 mg fosamprenavir (1 tab) + ritonavir 100 mg] po bid OR [1400 mg fosamprenavir (2 tabs) + ritonavir 100 mg] po q24h	Bioavailability not established. Food OK.	7.7 Amprenavir	Hydrolyzed to amprenavir, then acts as cytochrome P450 (3A4 substrate, inhibitor, inducer)	Amprenavir prodrug. Contains sulfa moiety. Potential for serious drug interactions (see label). Rash, including Stevens-Johnson syndrome. Once daily regimen: (1) not recommended for PI-experienced pts, (2) additional ritonavir needed if given with efavirenz (see label). Boosted twice daily regimen is recommended for PI-experienced pts.

TABLE 14D (10)

Generic/Trade Name	Pharmaceutical Prep. (Avg. Wholesale Price)	Usual Adult Dosage & Food Effect	% Absorbed, po	Serum T½, hrs	Elimination	Major Adverse Events/Comments (See Table 14E)
Indinavir (Crixivan)	100, 333, 400 mg capsules ($305/month) Store in original container with desiccant	Two 400 mg caps (800 mg) po q8h, without food or with light meal. Can take with enteric-coated Videx. [If taken with ritonavir (e.g., 800 mg indinavir + 100 mg ritonavir po q12h), no food restrictions]	65	1.2–2	Cytochrome P450 (3A4 inhibitor)	**Maintain hydration. Nephrolithiasis,** nausea, inconsequential ↑ of indirect bilirubin (jaundice in Gilbert syndrome), ↑ AST/ALT, headache, asthenia, blurred vision, metallic taste, hemolysis. ↑ urine WBC (>100/hpf) has been assoc. with nephritis/medullary calcification, cortical atrophy.
Lopinavir + ritonavir (Kaletra)	(200 mg lopinavir + 50 mg ritonavir) film-coated tablets and (100 mg ritonavir) film-coated tablets. Tabs do not need refrigeration. Oral solution: (80 mg lopinavir + 20 mg ritonavir) per mL. Refrigerate, but can be kept at room temperature ($77°F) x2 mos. ($795/month)	(400 mg lopinavir + 100 mg ritonavir)—2 tabs po bid. Higher dose may be needed in non-tx-naive pts when used with efavirenz, nevirapine, or unboosted fosamprenavir. [Dose adjustment in concomitant drugs may be necessary; see Table 22B & Table 22C, Table 22D & package label.]	No food effect with tablets.	5–6	Cytochrome P450 (3A4 inhibitor)	Nausea/vomiting/diarrhea, ↑ AST/ ALT, pancreatitis. Oral solution 42% alcohol. Lopinavir + ritonavir can be taken as a single daily dose of 4 tabs (total 800 mg lopinavir + 200 mg ritonavir), except in treatment-experienced pts or those taking concomitant efavirenz, nevirapine, or nelfinavir. (High concentration of oral solution.)
Nelfinavir (Viracept)	625, 250 mg tabs; 50 mg/gm oral powder ($726/month)	Two 625 mg tabs (1250 mg) po bid, with food	20–80 Food ↑ exposure & ↓ variability	3.5–5	Cytochrome P450 (3A inhibitor)	Do not use in pregnancy. Diarrhea. Coadministration of drugs with life-threatening toxicities & which are cleared by CYP3A is contraindicated.
Ritonavir (Norvir)	100 mg capsules; 600 mg per 7.5 mL solution. Refrigerate caps but not solution. Room temperature for 1 mo. is OK. ($10.29/capsule)	Full dose (not recommended): 6 caps (600 mg) po bid, with food. Escalate to full dose: 300 mg bid x2 days; 400 mg bid x3 days; 500 mg bid x2 days; then full dose. "Booster drug"—see Comment	Food ↑ absorption	3–5	Cytochrome P450. Potent 3A & 2D6 inhibitor	Nausea/vomiting/diarrhea, extremity & circumoral paresthesias, hepatitis, pancreatitis, taste perversion, ↑ CPK & uric acid. **With rare exceptions, used exclusively to enhance pharmacokinetics of other PIs, using lower ritonavir doses. Black Box warning—** potentially fatal drug interactions. Many drug interactions—see Table 22B & Table 22C.

TABLE 14D (11)

Generic/Trade Name	Pharmaceutical Prep. (Avg. Wholesale Price)	Usual Adult Dosage & Food Effect	% Absorbed, po	Serum T½, hrs	Elimination	Major Adverse Events/Comments (See Table 14E)
Saquinavir (Invirase—hard gel caps or tabs) + **ritonavir**	Saquinavir 200 mg caps, 500 mg film-coated tabs; ritonavir 100 mg caps ($790/month)	[2 tabs saquinavir (1000 mg) + 1 cap ritonavir (100 mg)] po bid with food	Erratic, 4 (saquinavir alone)	1–2	Cytochrome P450 (3A inhibitor)	Nausea, diarrhea, headache, ↑ AST/ ALT. Avoid rifampin with saquinavir + ritonavir: ↑ hepatitis risk. **Black Box warning**—Invirase to be used only with ritonavir.
Tipranavir (Aptivus)	250 mg caps. Refrigerate unopened bottles. Use opened bottles within 2 mo. ($1073/month)	[500 mg (two 250 mg caps) + ritonavir 200 mg] po bid with food	Absorption low, ↑ with high fat meal, ↓ with Al⁺⁺ & Mg⁺⁺ antacids.	5.5–6	Cytochrome 3A but with ritonavir, most of drug is eliminated in feces.	Contains sulfa moiety. **Black Box warning—reports of fatal/nonfatal intracranial hemorrhage**; hepatitis, fatal hepatic failure. Use cautiously in liver disease, esp. hepB, hepC; contraindicated in Child-Pugh class B-C. Monitor LFTs. Coadministration of certain drugs contraindicated (see label). **For highly ART-experienced pts or for multiple-PI resistant virus.**

4. **Selected Characteristics of Fusion Inhibitors**

Generic/Trade Name	Pharmaceutical Prep. (Avg. Wholesale Price)	Usual Adult Dosage	% Absorbed	Serum T½, hrs	Elimination	Major Adverse Events/Comments (See Table 14E)
Enfuvirtide (T20, Fuzeon)	Single-use vials of 90mg/mL, when reconstituted. Vials should be stored at room temperature. Reconstituted vials can be refrigerated for 24 hrs only. ($2,334 per month)	90 mg (1 ml) subcut. bid. Rotate injection sites, avoiding those currently inflamed.	84	3.8	Catabolism to its constituent amino acids with subsequent recycling of the amino acids in the body pool. Elimination pathway(s) have not been performed in humans. Does not alter the metabolism of CYP3A4, CYP2D6, CYP1A2, CYP2C19 or CYP2E1 substrates.	Local reaction site reactions 98%, 4% discontinue; erythema/induration –80–90%, nodules/cysts –80%. **Hypersensitivity reactions reported** (fever, rash, chills, N/V, ↓ BP, &/or ↑ AST/ALT)—do not restart if occur. Including background regimens; peripheral neuropathy 8.9%, insomnia 11.3%, ↓ appetite 6.3%, myalgia 5%, lymphadenopathy 2.3%, eosinophilia –10%, ↑ incidence of bacterial pneumonias. Alone offers little benefit to a failing regimen (NEJM 348:2249, 2003).

TABLE 14D (12)

5. Selected Characteristics of CCR-5 co-receptor antagonists

Generic/ Trade name	Pharmaceutical Prep. (Avg. Wholesale Price)	Usual Adult Dosage (po) & Food Effect	% Absorbed po	Serum T½, hrs	Elimination	Major Adverse Effects/Comments
Maraviroc (Selzentry)	150 mg, 300 mg film-coated tabs ($848/mo, for 300 mg bid dose)	Without regard to food: 150 mg bid if concomitant meds include CYP3A inhibitors 300 mg bid without significantly interacting meds 600 mg bid if concomitant meds include CYP3A inducers (without strong CYP3A inhibitors)	Est. 33% with 300 mg dosage	14-18	CYP3A and P-glycoprotein substrate. Metabolites (via CYP3A) excreted feces > urine.	Black Box Warning: Hepatotoxicity; may be preceded by rash; ↑ eos or IgE. Data lacking in hepatic/renal insufficiency; ↑concen with either could ↑ risk of ↓BP. Currently for treatment-experienced patients with multi-resistant strains. Document CCR-5-tropic virus before use, as treatment failures assoc. with appearance of CXCR-4 or mixed-tropic virus.

6. Selected Characteristics of Integrase Inhibitors

Generic/ Trade name	Pharmaceutical Prep. (Avg. Wholesale Price)	Usual Adult Dosage (po) & Food Effect	% Absorbed po	Serum T½, hrs	Elimination	Major Adverse Effects/Comments
Raltegravir (Isentress)	400 mg film-coated tablets	400 mg bid, without regard to food	Not established	~9	Glucuronidation via UGT1A1, with excretion into feces and urine.	For treatment-experienced adults with multiply-resistant virus. Generally well tolerated, with nausea, diarrhea, headache, fever similar to placebo. CK ↑/rhabdomyolysis reported, with unclear relationship to drug.

TABLE 14E– ANTIRETROVIRAL DRUGS AND ADVERSE EFFECTS
(www.aidsinfo.nih.gov)

DRUG NAME(S): GENERIC (TRADE)	ADVERSE EFFECTS
Nucleoside Reverse Transcriptase Inhibitors (NRTI)	**Black Box warning for all nucleoside/nucleotide RTIs: lactic acidosis/hepatic steatosis, potentially fatal.** Also carry Warnings that fat redistribution has been observed.
Abacavir (Ziagen)	**Most common:** Headache 7-13%, nausea 7-19%, diarrhea 7%, malaise 7-12%. **Most significant: Black Box warning—Hypersensitivity reaction** in 8% with malaise, fever, GI upset, rash, lethargy & respiratory symptoms most commonly reported; myalgia, arthralgia, edema, paresthesia less common. **Rechallenge contraindicated; may be life-threatening.** Severe HR may be more common with once-daily dosing. **HLA-B*5701** allele predicts ↑ risk of HR in Caucasian pop., excluding pts with B*5701 markedly ↓ ↓ HR incidence in W. Australian Cohort (CID 43:99, 2006). We recommend test for allele before using abacavir, if possible, and avoiding drug in any pt with B*5701; but absence of allele cannot guarantee safety, esp. in non-Caucasian populations. Vigilance is essential in all groups.
Didanosine (ddI) (Videx)	**Most common:** Diarrhea 28%, nausea 6%, rash 9%, headache 7%, fever 12%, hyperuricemia 2% **Most significant: Pancreatitis 1-9%. Black Box warning—Cases of fatal and nonfatal pancreatitis** have occurred in pts receiving ddI, especially when used in combination with ddI or d4T + hydroxyurea. Fatal lactic acidosis in pregnancy with ddI + d4T. Peripheral neuropathy in 20%. 12% required dose reduction. Rarely, retinal changes.
Emtricitabine (FTC, Emtriva)	**Most common:** Headache, diarrhea, nausea, rash, skin hyperpigmentation. Well-tolerated. **Most significant:** Potential for lactic acidosis (as with other NRTIs), **exacerbation of hepatitis B on stopping drug; monitor clinical/labs for several months after stopping.** Anti-HBV rx may be warranted if FTC stopped.
Lamivudine (3TC) (Epivir)	Well tolerated. Headache 35%, nausea 33%, diarrhea 18%, abdominal pain 9%, insomnia 11% (all in combination with ZDV). Pancreatitis more common in pediatrics (15%). **Black Box warning.** Make sure to use HIV dosage, not Hep B dosage. **Exacerbation of hepatitis B on stopping drug; monitor clinical/labs for several months after stopping. Anti-HBC rx may be warranted if 3TC stopped.**
Stavudine (d4T) (Zerit)	**Most common:** Diarrhea, nausea, vomiting, headache **Most significant: Peripheral neuropathy** 15-20%. Pancreatitis 1%. Appears to produce lactic acidosis more commonly than other NRTIs. **Black Box warning—Fatal & nonfatal pancreatitis with d4T + ddI + hydroxyurea. Fatal lactic acidosis/steatosis in pregnant women receiving d4T + ddI.** Motor weakness in the setting of lactic acidosis mimicking the clinical presentation of Guillain-Barré syndrome (including respiratory failure) (rare).
Zalcitabine (ddC) (Hivid)	**Most common:** Oral ulcers 13%, rash 8% **Most significant: Black Box warning—peripheral neuropathy** 22-35%. Severe continuous pain, slowing reversible when ddC stopped; ↑ risk with diabetes. **Hepatic failure in pts with hep B.** Esophageal ulcers. **Pancreatitis 1%.** (No longer available)
Zidovudine (ZDV, AZT) (Retrovir)	**Most common:** Nausea 50%, anorexia 20%, vomiting 17%, **headache 62%.** Also reported: asthenia, insomnia, myalgias, nail pigmentation. Macrocytosis expected with all dosage regimens. **Most significant: Black Box warning—hematologic toxicity, myopathy. Anemia** (<8 gm, 1%); **granulocytopenia** (<750, 1.8%). Anemia may respond to epoetin alfa if endogenous serum erythropoietin levels are ≤500 mIU–International Units per mL
Nucleotide Reverse Transcriptase Inhibitor (NtRTI) Black Box warning for all nucleoside/nucleotide RTIs: lactic acidosis/hepatic steatosis, potentially fatal. Also carry Warnings that fat redistribution has been observed.	
Tenofovir (TDF) (Viread)	**Most common:** Diarrhea 11%, nausea 8%, vomiting 5% (generally well tolerated) **Most significant: Black Box warning—Severe exacerbations of hepatitis B reported in pts who stop tenofovir. Monitor carefully if drug is stopped;** anti-HBV rx may be warranted if TDF stopped. Possible ↑ bone demineralization. Reports of Fanconi syndrome & renal injury induced by tenofovir (CID 37:e174, 2003; JAIDS 35:269, 2004). Modest decline in CrCl with TDF may be greater than with NRTIs (CID 40:1194, 2005). Avoid other nephrotoxic drugs. Monitor CrCl especially with pre-existing disease.
Non-Nucleoside Reverse Transcriptase Inhibitors (NNRTI)	
Delavirdine (Rescriptor)	**Most common:** Nausea, diarrhea, vomiting, headache **Most significant: Skin rash** has occurred in 18%; can continue or restart drug in most cases. Stevens-Johnson syndrome and erythema multiforme have been reported rarely. ↑ in liver enzymes in <5% of patients.

TABLE 14E (2)

DRUG NAME(S): GENERIC (TRADE)	ADVERSE EFFECTS
Non-Nucleoside Reverse Transcriptase Inhibitors (NNRTI) *(continued)*	
Efavirenz (Sustiva)	**Most common: CNS side-effects 52%;** symptoms include dizziness, insomnia, somnolence, impaired concentration, psychiatric sx, and abnormal dreams; symptoms are worse after 1st or 2nd dose and improve over 2-4 weeks; discontinuation rate 2.6%. Rash 26% vs. 17% in comparators); often improves with oral antihistamines; discontinuation rate 1.7%. Can cause false-positive urine test results for cannabinoid with CEDIA DAU multi-level THC assay. **Most significant:** Serious neuropsychiatric symptoms, including severe depression 2.4 %, suicidal ideation 0.7%. Elevation in liver enzymes. **Teratogenicity reported in primates; avoid in pregnancy (avoid in 1st day and 1st trimester). In pregnant women or those who might become pregnant** (see 2008 SANFORD GUIDE TO HIV/AIDS THERAPY, Table 8). NOTE: No single method of contraception 100% reliable. Contraindicated with certain drugs metabolized by CYP3A4.
Nevirapine (Viramune)	**Most common: Rash 37%;** occurs during 1st 6 wks of therapy. Follow recommendations for 14-day lead-in period to ↓ risk of rash (see Table 14D). Women experience 7-fold ↑ in risk of severe rash (CID 32:124, 2001). 50% resolve within 2wks of dc drug and 80% by 1mo. 6.7% discontinuation rate. **Most significant: Black Box warning—Severe life-threatening skin reactions reported:** 2/3 during first 12wks of rx. For severe rashes, D/C drug immed & do not restart. In clinical trial, use of prednisone ↑ risk of rash. **Black Box warning—Life-threatening hepatotoxicity reported** (Hep 35:182, 2002). Overall 1% develop hepatitis. Pts with pre-existing ↑ in ALT or AST &/or history of chronic Hep B or C ↑ susceptible (AJM 35:182, 2002). For preg women, ↑ risk. Avoid in this group unless no other option. Men with CD4 >400 also at ↑ risk. Monitor pts intensively (Clinical & LFTs), esp. during first 12wks of rx. If clinical hepatotoxicity, severe skin or hypersensitivity reactions occur, dc drug, & **never rechallenge**
Protease Inhibitors (PI)	Abnormalities in glucose metabolism, dyslipidemias, fat redistribution syndromes are potential problems. Pts taking PI may be at ↑risk for developing osteopenia/osteoporosis. Spontaneous bleeding in HIV+ pts with hemophilia being treated with PI. Rheumatoid complications have been reported with PI (An Rheum Dis 61:82, 2002). **Caution for all PIs**—Coadministration with certain drugs dependent on CYP3A for elimination & for which ↑ levels can cause serious toxicity may be contraindicated. Potential of some PIs for QTc prolongation suggested (Lancet 365:682,2005).
Atazanavir (Reyataz)	**Most common:** Asymptomatic unconjugated hyperbilirubinemia in up to 60% of pts, jaundice in 7-9%, especially in Gilbert syndrome (JID 192:1381, 2005). Moderate to severe events: Diarrhea 1-3%, nausea 6-14%, abdominal pain 4%, headache 6%, rash 5-7%. **Most significant:** ↑ PR interval (1st degree AV block) reported; rarely 2° AV block. QTc ↑ with torsades reported (AIDS 20:2131,2006; NEJM 355:2158,2006). Acute interstitial nephritis (Am J Kid Dis 44:e81,2004) and urolithiasis (Clin Infect Dis 55:e94,2012). Potential for major drug interactions. Use caution in pts with hepatic dysfunction.
Darunavir (Prezista)	**Most common:** Skin rash 20% (moderate or worse in 3-8%), nausea, headache, diarrhea. **Most significant:** Rarely Stevens-Johnson syndrome. Pro-drug of amprenavir. Contains sulfa moiety.
Fosamprenavir (Lexiva)	**Most common:** ↑ in indirect bilirubin 10-15% [22.5 mg per dL], with overt jaundice more likely in those with Gilbert syndrome (JID 192:1381, 2005). Nausea 12%, vomiting 4%, diarrhea 5%. Rare rash 1st day. Metabolized to amprenavir. **Most significant:** Rarely Stevens-Johnson syndrome, erythema multiforme. May cause failure of hormonal contraceptives.
Indinavir (Crixivan)	**Most significant: Kidney stones.** Indinavir crystals in collecting system. Nephrolithiasis in 12% of adults. ↑ In pts. Prevent (minimize) by good hydration (≥48oz. water/day) (AAC 42:332, 1998). Tubulointerstitial nephritis/renal cortical atrophy reported in assoc. with asympt ↑ urine WBC. Severe hepatitis reported (LD 349:924, 1997). Hemolytic anemia reported.
Lopinavir/Ritonavir (Kaletra)	**Most common: GI: diarrhea** 14-24%, nausea 2-16%, lipid abnormalities in up to 20-40%. More diarrhea with q24h dosing. **Most significant:** Pancreatitis, inflammatory edema of the legs (AIDS 16:673, 2002) Oral solution contains alcohol. Note high drug concentration in oral solution.
Nelfinavir (Viracept)	**Most common: Mild-moderate diarrhea** 20%. For diarrhea: Oat bran tabs, calcium, or oral anti-diarrheal agents (e.g., loperamide, diphenoxylate/atropine sulfate). **Most significant:** Potential for drug interactions
Ritonavir (Norvir)	**Most common:** ↓ bitter aftertaste ↓ by taking with choc milk, Ensure, or Advera; nausea 23%, ↓ by initial dose escalation (titration) regimen; vomiting 13%; diarrhea 15%. Circumoral paresthesias 5-6%. ↑ dose >100mg q12h assoc. with ↑ GI side-effects & ↑ in lipid abnormalities. **With rare exceptions, used in low doses to enhance levels of other antiretrovirals** because of ↑ toxicity/interactions with full-dose ritonavir. **Most significant:** Hepatic (AJM 129:670, 1998). **Black Box warning** relates to drug-drug interactions—inhibits P450 CYP3A & CYP2D6 system—may be life-threatening (see Table 22). Rarely Stevens-Johnson syndrome, anaphylaxis.

TABLE 14E (3)

DRUG NAME(S): GENERIC (TRADE)	ADVERSE EFFECTS
Protease inhibitors (PI) (continued)	
Saquinavir (Invirase / hard cap, tablet)	**Most common: Diarrhea,** abdominal discomfort, nausea, headache.
	Black Box Warning—Invirase & Fortovase are not bioequivalent. (NOTE: Fortovase discontinued in 2006.) **Use Invirase only with ritonavir.**
Tipranavir (Aptivus)	**Most common:** Nausea & vomiting, diarrhea, abdominal pain. Rash in 8-14%, more common in women, & 33% in women taking ethinyl estradiol. Major lipid effects. **Most serious: Black Box warnings**—associated with fatal/non-fatal intracranial hemorrhage (can inhibit platelet aggregation in vitro); caution in those with bleeding risk. Associated with hepatitis & fatal hepatic failure. Risk of hepatotoxicity ↑ in HepB or HepC co-infection. Potential for major drug interactions. Contains sulfa moiety.
Fusion Inhibitor: Enfuvirtide (T20, Fuzeon)	**Most common:** local injection site reactions (98% at least 1 local ISR, 4% dc because of ISR) (pain & discomfort, induration, erythema, nodules & cysts, pruritus, & ecchymosis). Diarrhea 32%, nausea 23%, fatigue 20%. **Most significant:** ↑ rate of bacterial pneumonia (6.7 pneumonia events per 100 pt yrs), **hypersensitivity reactions** ≤1% (rash, fever, nausea & vomiting, rigors, hypotension, & ↑ serum liver transaminases), can occur with re-exposure.
CCR-5 co-receptor antagonist: Maraviroc (Selzentry)	**Most common:** With ARV background: cough 13%, fever 12%, rash 10%, abdom. pain 8%. Also, dizziness, myalgia, arthralgias. ↑ Risk of URI, HSV infection. **Most significant: Black box warning-Hepatotoxicity.** May be preceded by allergic features. Use with caution in pt with HepB or C. Cardiac ischemia/infarction in 1.3%. May cause ↓BP, syncope. Significant interactions with CYP3A inducers/inhibitors. Long-term risk of malignancy unknown.
Integrase Inhibitor: Raltegravir	**Most common:** Diarrhea, headache, nausea. LFT ↑ may be more common in pts co-infected with HBV or HCV **Most significant:** Hypersensitivity can occur. ↑CK with myopathy or rhabdomyolysis reported, with unclear relationship to drug.

TABLE 15A – ANTIMICROBIAL PROPHYLAXIS FOR SELECTED BACTERIAL INFECTIONS*

CLASS OF ETIOLOGIC AGENT/DISEASE/CONDITION	PROPHYLAXIS: AGENT/DOSE/ROUTE/DURATION	COMMENTS
Group B streptococcal disease (GBS), neonatal: Approaches to management [CDC Guidelines, MMWR 51(RR-11):1, 2002]:		
Pregnant women—Intrapartum antimicrobial prophylaxis procedures: 1. Screen all pregnant women with vaginal & rectal swab for GBS at 35–37 wks gestation (unless other indications for prophylaxis exist: GBS bacteriuria during this pregnancy, previously delivered infant with invasive GBS disease), even then cultures may be useful for susceptibility testing). Use transport medium; GBS survive at room temp; up to 96 hrs. **If at high risk for drug allergy: culture positive.** 2. Rx during labor if previously delivered infant with invasive GBS infection, or if any GBS bacteria during this pregnancy (MMWR 53:506, 2004). 3. Rx if GBS status unknown but if any of the following are present: (a) delivery at <37 wks gestation [see MMWR 51(RR-11):1, 2002 algorithm for threatened preterm delivery], or (b) duration of ruptured membranes ≥18 hrs, or (c) intrapartum temp. ≥100.4°F (≥38.0°C).	**Prophylactic regimens during labor:** **Pen G** 5 million units IV (load) then 2.5 million units IV q4h. **Pen-allergic: Ampicillin** 2 gm IV (load) then 1 gm IV q4h. **Pen-allergic: Pts not at high risk for anaphylaxis: Cefazolin** 2 gm IV initial dose, then 1 gm IV q8h **Pts at high risk for anaphylaxis:** GBS susceptible to clinda & erythro: **Clindamycin** 900 mg IV q8h **or erythromycin** 500 mg IV q6h. Vancomycin if at high risk for anaphylaxis when alternative to clindamycin or erythromycin needed (e.g. GBS resistant or unknown susceptibility). Continue treatment until delivery.
		Careful observation of signs & symptoms. 96% of infants will show clinical signs of infection during the 1st 24 hrs whether mother received intrapartum antibiotics or not (Pediatrics 106:244, 2000). For gestational age <35 wks of intrapartum antibiotics <4 hrs, lab evaluation (CBC, diff, blood culture) & 24h of observation recommended. See algorithm MMWR 51(RR-11):1, 2002
Neonate not given prophylaxis		
Preterm, premature rupture of the membranes in Group B strep-negative women	IV **ampicillin** 2 gm q6h + IV **erythromycin** 250 mg q6h) for 48 hrs followed by po **amoxicillin** 250 mg q8h + po **erythromycin** base 333 mg q8h times 5 days. (Note: May require additional antibiotics for therapy of specific existing infections)	Antibiotic rx reduced infant respiratory distress syndrome (50.6% to 40.8%, p = 0.03), necrotizing enterocolitis (5.8% to 2.3%, p = 0.03) and prolonged pregnancy (2.9 to 6.1 days, p < 0.001) vs placebo. In 1 large study (4809 pts), po erythromycin rx improved neonatal outcomes vs placebo (11.2% vs 14.4% poor outcomes, p = 0.02 for single births) but not co-AM-CL or both drugs in combination (Lancet 357:979, 2001). Decreases infant mortality. (JAMA 278:989, 1997)
Post-splenectomy bacteremia. Likely agents: Pneumococcus (90%), meningococcus, H. influenzae type b (also at rx of fatal malaria, severe babesiosis, and Capnocytophaga spp). Ref. 2006 Red Book 27th Ed, Amer Acad Pediatrics	**Immunizations:** Ensure admin of pneumococcal vaccine, H. influenzae B & quadrivalent meningococcal vaccines at recommended times (see Table 20). In addition, adults: Table 20C children with sickle cell anemia, thalassemia, & perhaps others, daily antimicrobial prophylaxis to age 5—see Comments	Antimicrobial prophylaxis until age 5: Amox 20mg/kg/day or Pen V-K 125 mg bid Over age 5: Consider Pen V-K 250 mg bid for at least 1 yr in children post-splenectomy. Some recommend prophylaxis until at least age 18. Maintain immunizations plus self-administer AM-CL when rx for febrile illness while seeking physician assistance. Pen. allergy: TMP-SMX or clarithro are options, but resistance in S. pneumo may be significant in some areas, particularly among pen-resistant isolates
Sexual Exposure		
Sexual assault survivor [likely agents and risks; see NEJM 332:234, 1995; MMWR 55(RR-11):1, 2006]	(**Ceftriaxone** 125 mg IM) + **metronidazole** 2 gm po single dose) + (**azithromycin** 1 gm po single dose) or **doxycycline** 100 mg po bid times 7 days) [MMWR 55(RR-11):1, 2006]	Obtain expert advice re: forensic tests & specimens, pregnancy, physical trauma, psychological support. If decision is to proceed with spec. collection, at initial exam. Test for gonococci & chlamydia, wet mount for T. vaginalis (& culture vaginal swab). Serologic evaluation for syphilis, Hep B, HIV; others as appropriate. Initiate post-exposure protocols for HIV & hepatitis B as appropriate (see Table 15D). Follow-up exam for STD at 1–2 wks. Retest syphilis & HIV serology at 6, 12, 24 wks if negative earlier
Sexual contacts, likely agents: N. gonorrhoeae, C. trachomatis	[(**Ceftriaxone** 125 mg IM once) or **cefixime** 400 mg po once)] for GC, **plus** (**doxycycline** 100 mg po bid times 7 days) or (**azithromycin** 1 gm po once)] for Chlamydia	Be sure to check for syphilis since all regimens may not eradicate incubating syphilis. Consider also T. vaginalis. Identify & rx contacts as appropriate to suspected STD [see Table 1, page 21]
Syphilis exposure	[(**Ceftriaxone** 125 mg IM once, **plus** (**doxycycline** 100 mg po once)] for Chlamydia	Presumptive rx for exposure within 3 mos.—as tests may be negative. See Table 1, page 21 Make effort to rx syphilis
Sickle-cell disease. Likely agents: S. pneumoniae (see post-splenectomy, above) Ref. 2006 Red Book 27th Ed, Amer Acad Pediatrics	Children <5 yrs: **Penicillin V** 125 mg po bid ≥5 yrs: **Penicillin V** 250 mg po bid (Alternative in children: Amoxicillin 20 mg per kg per day)	Start prophylaxis by 2 mos. (Pediatrics 106:367, 2000). Age-appropriate vaccines, including pneumococcal, Hib, influenza, meningococcal. Treating infections, consider possibility of penicillin non-susceptible pneumococci.

* See page 2 for abbreviations

TABLE 15B – ANTIBIOTIC PROPHYLAXIS TO PREVENT SURGICAL INFECTIONS IN ADULTS*
(CID 38:1706, 2004; Am J Surg 189:395, 2005)

Surgical Procedures: To be optimally effective, **antibiotics must be started in the interval: 2 hrs before time of surgical incision** (NEJM 326:281, 1982; or even closer to incision time (JAC 58:645, 2006). For most procedures the number of doses needed for optimal coverage is not defined. Most applications employ a single dose (Treat Guide Med Lett. 4:83, 2006) although FDA-approved product labeling is often for 2 or more doses. If the surgical procedure lasts >3 hrs, additional intraoperative doses should be given at approx. 3-hr intervals. A recent consensus statement from the National Surgical Infection Prevention Project (CID 38:1706, 2004) advises antibiotic prophylaxis be started within 1 hr before incision (except vancomycin & quinolones), be supplemented intraoperatively if the procedure lasts more than 2 half-lives of the prophylactic agent, and in most cases not be extended beyond 24 hrs. (Note: The dose/route/durations listed below for adults with normal renal function & not intolerant of these agents are for the most part those approved in FDA product labeling. For single dose regimens, the dosage & route are the same.) See Table 15C for regimens to reduce risk of endocarditis.
General Comments: In some centers, ↑ resistance may render certain regimens (e.g., quinolones) unacceptable. Pharmacokinetic considerations suggest that surgical prophylaxis dosing may yield suboptimal serum/tissue levels in pts with high BMI (see Surgery 136:738, 2004 for cefazolin; Eur J Clin Pharm 54:622, 1998 for vancomycin), although clinical implications uncertain.

TYPE OF SURGERY	PROPHYLAXIS	COMMENTS
Cardiovascular Surgery		
Antibiotic prophylaxis in cardiovascular surgery has been proven beneficial only in the following procedures:	**Cefazolin** 1–2 gm IV as a single dose or q8h for 1–2 days or **cefuroxime** 1.5 gm IV as a single dose or q12h for total of 6 gm or **vancomycin** 1 gm IV as a single dose or q12h for 1–2 days.	Single infusion just before surgery probably as effective as multiple doses. Not needed for cardiac catheterization. For prosthetic heart valves, customary to stop prophylaxis either after removal of retrosternal drainage catheters or just a 2nd dose after coming off bypass. Vancomycin may be preferable in hospitals with ↑ freq of MRSA or in high-risk pts (CID 38: 1555, 2004); or those colonized with MRSA (CID 38:1706, 2004); however, does not cover Gm-neg
• Reconstruction of abdominal aorta		
• Procedures on the leg that involve a groin incision	Consider **intranasal mupirocin** evening before, day of surgery & for 5 days post-op in pts with pos. nasal culture for S. aureus.	bacilli, therefore would add cefazolin. Meta-analysis failed to demonstrate overall superiority of vancomycin over β-lactam prophylaxis for cardiac surgery (CID 38: 1357, 2004). A meta-analysis of 7 placebo-controlled randomized studies of prophylaxis for placement of
• Any vascular procedure that inserts prosthesis/foreign body		permanent pacemakers, sig. ↓ in incidence of infection (Circulation 97: 1796, 1998). Intranasal mupirocin ↓ sternal wound infections from S. aureus in 1850 pts. used historical controls (An Thor Surg 71:1572, 2001); in another trial, it ↓ nosocomial S. aureus infections only in nasal
• Lower extremity amputation for ischemia		carriers (NEJM 346:1871, 2002). One study of 0.12% chlorhexidine gluconate gel to nares and
• Cardiac surgery		oral rinse showed ↓ deep surg site and lower resp infections (JAMA 296:2460, 2006)
• Permanent Pacemakers (see Comment)		
Gastric, Biliary and Colonic Surgery		
Gastroduodenal/Biliary		
Gastroduodenal, includes percutaneous endoscopic gastrostomy (high-risk only, see Comments)	**Cefazolin** or **cefotetan** or **cefotaxime** or **cefuroxime** 1.5 gm IV as a single dose give additional doses q12h for 2–3 days).	**Gastroduodenal-** High-risk is marked obesity, obstruction, ↓ gastric acid or ↓ motility. Meta-analysis supports use in percutaneous endoscopic gastrostomy (Am J Gastro 95:3133, 2000). **Biliary** high-risk: age >70, acute cholecystitis, non-functioning gallbladder, obstructive jaundice or common duct stones. With cholangitis, treat as infection, not prophylaxis (CID 38:1706,
Biliary, includes laparoscopic cholecystectomy (high-risk only, see Comments)	In biliary surgery, **cefazolin** 1 gm or **cefotaxime** 1 gm (± repeat dosing at 12 & 24 hrs) were equivalent (AAC 40:70, 1996).	2004). TC-CL 3.1 gm q4–6h IV, or AM-SB 3 gm q6h IV.
Endoscopic retrograde cholangiopancreatography	No rx without obstruction. If obstruction: **Ciprofloxacin** 500–750 mg po 2 hrs prior to procedure or **Ceftizoxime** 1.5 gm IV 1 hr prior to procedure and	Most studies show that **achieving adequate drainage** will prevent postprocedural cholangitis or sepsis and no further benefit from prophylactic antibiotics. Meta-analysis suggested antibiotics may ↓ bacteremia, but not sepsis/cholangitis (Endoscopy 31:718, 1999).
Controversial: No benefit from single dose piperacillin in randomized placebo-controlled trial, AHM (125:442, 1996 (see Comments)	**PIP-TZ** 4.5 gm IV 1 hr prior to procedure	Oral CIP as cephalosporins in 2 studies & less expensive about resistance increasing (CID 23:380, 1996).

* See page 2 for abbreviations

TABLE 15B (2)

TYPE OF SURGERY	PROPHYLAXIS	COMMENTS
Gastric, Biliary and Colonic Surgery (continued)		
Colorectal	Oral antibiotics for elective surgery (see Comments) **Parenteral regimens** (emergency or elective) [**Cefazolin** 1–2 gm IV + **metronidazole** 0.5 gm IV] or **cefoxitin** or **cefotetan** 1–2 gm IV (if available) or **AM-SB** 3 gm IV or **ERTA 1** 1 gm IV [NEJM 355:2640, 2006 study found ertapenem more effective than cefotetan, but associated with non-significant ↑ risk of C. difficile].	**Oral regimens: Neomycin + erythromycin** Pre-op day: (1) 10am 4L polyethylene glycol electrolyte solution (Colyte, GoLYTELY) po over 2hr. (2) Clear liquid diet only. (3) 1pm, 2pm & 11pm, neomycin 1gm + erythro base 1gm po. (4) NPO after midnight. Alternative regimens have been less well studied: GoLYTELY 1–6pm, then neomycin 2gm po + metronidazole 2gm po at 7pm & 11pm. Oral agents effective as parenteral: parenteral not in addl'n to oral not required but often used (AmJSurg 189:395, 2005). [Alternative: Neomycin + metronidazole. GoLYTELY 1–6 pm, then neomycin 2 gm PO + metronidazole 2 gm PO at 7 pm and 11 pm.]. Many used both parenteral + oral regimens for elective procedures (AmJSurg 189:395, 2005), but recent ↓ enthusiasm for mechanical bowel preparation. Meta-analysis did not support mech bowel prep in preventing anastomotic leaks with elective colorectal surg (Cochran Database Syst Rev (3), 2007).
Ruptured viscus: See Peritoneum/Peritonitis, Secondary, Table 1, page 42.		
Head and Neck Surgery (Ann Otol Rhinol Laryngol 101 Suppl:16, 1992) **Cefazolin** 2 gm IV (single dose) or [**clindamycin** 600–900 mg IV (single dose)] + **gentamicin** 1.5 mg per kg IV (single dose)]		Antimicrobial prophylaxis in head & neck surg appears efficacious only for procedures involving oral/pharyngeal mucosa (e.g., laryngeal or pharyngeal tumor) but even with prophylaxis, wound infection rate high (41% in 1 center) (Head Neck 23:447, 2001). Uncontaminated head & neck surg does not require prophylaxis.
Neurosurgical Procedures [Prophylaxis not effective in ↓ infection rate with intracranial pressure monitors in retrospective analysis of 215 pts (J Neurol Neurosurg Psych 69:381, 2000)]		
Clean, non-implant; e.g., craniotomy Clean, contaminated (cross sinuses, or naso/oropharynx) CSF shunt surgery	**Cefazolin** 1–2 gm IV once. Alternative: **vanco** 1 gm IV once. **Clindamycin** 900 mg IV (single dose) **Cefazolin** 1–2 gm IV once. Alternative: **vanco** 1 gm IV once.	Reference: Ln 344:1547, 1994. British recommend amoxicillin-clavulanate 1.2 gm IV ^{M&b} or (cefuroxime 1.5 gm IV + metronidazole 0.5 gm IV). Meta-analysis suggests benefit (Cochrane Database (4) 2006)
Obstetric/Gynecologic Surgery		
Vaginal or abdominal hysterectomy	**Cefazolin** 1–2 gm or **cefoxitin** 1–2 gm or **cefotetan** 1–2 gm or **cefuroxime** 1.5 gm all IV 30 min. before surgery	1 study found cefotetan superior to cefazolin (CID 20:677, 1995). For prolonged procedures, doses can be repeated q4–8h for duration of procedure. Ampicillin-sulbactam is considered an acceptable alternative (CID:43:322, 2006).
Cesarean section for premature rupture of membranes or active labor	**Cefazolin** once, administer IV as soon as umbilical cord clamped. (See Comments)	Prophylaxis decreases risk of endometritis/wound infection in elective as well as non-elective C-section; single dose equivalent to multiple dose regimens (Cochrane Database System Rev 2002, issue 3, & 1999, issue 1). Study suggests pre-incision cefazolin may be superior to post-clamp dosing in preventing endomyometritis (Am J Obstet Gynecol 196:455.e1, 2007). Larger studies needed to assess effect on neonates.
Abortion	1st trimester: aqueous **pen G** 2 mU IV or **doxycycline** 300 mg po. 2nd trimester: **Cefazolin** 1 gm IV	Meta-analysis showed benefit of antibiotic prophylaxis in all risk groups. One regimen was doxy 100 mg orally 1 hr before procedure, then 200 mg after procedure (Ob Gyn 87:884, 1996).
Orthopedic Surgery [Most pts with prosthetic joints do not require prophylaxis for routine dental procedures, but individual considerations prevail for high-risk procedures & prostheses (J Am Dental Assn 134:895, 2003; Med Lett 47:59, 2005)]		
Hip arthroplasty, spinal fusion	Same as cardiac	Customarily stopped after "Hemovac" removed. NSIPP workgroup recommends stopping prophylaxis within 24 hrs of surgery (CID 38:1706, 2004).
Total joint replacement (other than hip)	**Cefazolin** 1–2 gm IV pre-op (± 2nd dose) or **vancomycin** 1 gm IV on call to OR	NSIPP workgroup recommends stopping prophylaxis within 24 hrs of surgery (CID 38:1706, 2004).
Open reduction of closed fracture with internal fixation	**Ceftriaxone** 2 gm IV or IM once	3.6% vs 8.3% (for placebo) infection found in Dutch trauma trial (Ln 347:1133, 1996)

* See page 2 for abbreviations

TABLE 15B (3)

TYPE OF SURGERY	PROPHYLAXIS	COMMENTS
Peritoneal Dialysis Catheter Placement	**Vancomycin** single 1 gm IV dose 12 hrs prior to procedure	Effectively reduced peritonitis during 14 days post-placement in 221 pts: vanco 1%, cefazolin 7%, placebo 12% (p=0.02) (Am J Kidney Dis 36:1014, 2000).
Urologic Surgery/Procedures Antimicrobials not recommended in pts with sterile urine. Pts with pre-operative bacteriuria should be treated.	Recommended antibiotic to pts with pre-operative bacteriuria. **Cefazolin** 1 gm IV q8h times 1–3 doses perioperatively, followed by oral antibiotics (**nitrofurantoin** or **TMP-SMX**) until catheter is removed or for 10 days. Modify based on susceptibility test results. Prophylaxis usually given for GU implants (Treat Guide Med Lett 4:83, 2006).	
Transrectal prostate biopsy	**Ciprofloxacin** 500 mg po 12 hrs prior to biopsy and repeated 12 hrs after 1st dose	Bacteremia 7% with CIP vs 37% gentamicin (Urology 38:84, 1991; review in JAC 39:115, 1997). Levo 500 mg 30–60 min. before procedure was effective in low-risk pts; additional doses were given for ↑ risk (J Urol 168:1021, 2002). ↑ Fluoroquinolone resistance in enteric gram-negatives is a concern.
Other Breast surgery, herniorrhaphy	**P Ceph 1,2**, dosage as Gynecologic Surgery, above	Meta-analysis did not show clear evidence of benefit from prophylaxis in elective inguinal hernia repair (Cochrane Database System Rev 2004, issue 4).

* See page 2 for abbreviations

TABLE 15C – ANTIMICROBIAL PROPHYLAXIS FOR THE PREVENTION OF BACTERIAL ENDOCARDITIS IN PATIENTS WITH UNDERLYING CARDIAC CONDITIONS*

In 2007, the American Heart Association guidelines for the prevention of bacterial endocarditis were updated. The resulting document (*Circulation 2007; 115:1* and http://circ.ahajournals.org), which was also endorsed by the Infectious Diseases Society of America, represents a significant departure from earlier recommendations.

• Antibiotic prophylaxis for dental procedures is now directed at individuals who are likely to suffer the most devastating consequences should they develop endocarditis.

Prophylaxis to prevent endocarditis is no longer specified for gastrointestinal or genitourinary procedures. The following is adapted from and reflects the new AHA recommendations. See original publication for explanation and precise details.

SELECTION OF PATIENTS FOR ENDOCARDITIS PROPHYLAXIS

FOR PATIENTS WITH ANY OF THESE HIGH-RISK CARDIAC CONDITIONS ASSOCIATED WITH ENDOCARDITIS:	WHO UNDERGO DENTAL PROCEDURES INVOLVING:	WHO UNDERGO INVASIVE RESPIRATORY PROCEDURES INVOLVING:	WHO UNDERGO INVASIVE PROCEDURES OF THE GI OR GU TRACTS:	WHO UNDERGO PROCEDURES INVOLVING INFECTED SKIN AND SOFT TISSUES:
Prosthetic heart valves Previous infective endocarditis Congenital heart disease with any of the following: • Completely repaired cardiac defect using prosthetic material (Only for 1ˢᵗ 6 months) • Partially corrected but with residual defect near prosthetic material • Uncorrected cyanotic congenital heart disease • Surgically constructed shunts and conduits Valvulopathy following heart transplant	Any manipulation of gingival tissue, dental periapical regions, or perforating the oral mucosa. **PROPHYLAXIS RECOMMENDED** (see *Dental Procedures Regimens* table below) (Prophylaxis is not recommended for routine anesthetic injections through non-infected area), dental x-rays, shedding of primary teeth, adjustment of orthodontic appliances or placement of orthodontic brackets or removable appliances.)	Incision of respiratory tract mucosa **CONSIDER PROPHYLAXIS** (see *Dental Procedures Regimens* table) Or For treatment of established infection **PROPHYLAXIS RECOMMENDED** (see *Dental Procedures Regimens* table for oral flora, but include anti-staphylococcal coverage when *S. aureus* is of concern)	PROPHYLAXIS is no longer recommended solely to prevent endocarditis, **but the following approach is reasonable:** For patients with enterococcal UTIs • treat before elective GU procedures • include enterococcal coverage in peri-operative regimen for non-elective procedures For patients with existing GU or GI infections or those who receive peri-operative antibiotics to prevent surgical site infections or sepsis • it is reasonable to include agents with anti-enterococcal activity in peri-operative coverage§	Include coverage against staphylococci and β-hemolytic streptococci in treatment regimens

§ Agents with anti-enterococcal activity include penicillin, ampicillin, amoxicillin, piperacillin, vancomycin and others. Check susceptibility if available. *(See Table 5 for highly resistant organisms.)*

PROPHYLACTIC REGIMENS FOR DENTAL PROCEDURES

SITUATION	AGENT	REGIMEN†
Usual oral prophylaxis	Amoxicillin	Adults 2 gm, children 50 mg per kg orally, 1 hour before procedure
Unable to take oral medications	Ampicillin‡ OR	Adults 2 gm, children 50 mg per kg, IV or IM, within 30 min before procedure.
Allergic to penicillins	Cephalexin‡ OR	Adults 2 gm, children 50 mg per kg orally, 1 hour before procedure.
	Clindamycin OR	Adults 600 mg, children 20 mg per kg, orally, 1 hour before procedure
	Azithromycin or clarithromycin	Adults 500 mg, children 15 mg per kg, orally, 1 hour before procedure
Allergic to penicillins and unable to take oral medications	Cefazolin‡ OR	Adults 1 gm, children 50 mg per kg, IV or IM, within 30 min before procedure
	Clindamycin	Adults 600 mg, children 20 mg per kg, IV or IM, within 30 min before procedure

† Children's dose should not exceed adult dose. AHA document lists all doses at 30-60 min before procedure.
‡ AHA lists cefazolin or ceftriaxone (at appropriate doses) as alternatives.
‡ Cephalosporins should not be used in individuals with immediate-type hypersensitivity reaction (urticaria, angioedema, or anaphylaxis) to penicillins or other β-lactams. AHA proposes ceftriaxone as potential alternative to cefazolin; and other 1ˢᵗ or 2° generation cephalosporin in equivalent doses as potential alternatives to cephalexin.

* See page 2 for abbreviations

TABLE 15D – MANAGEMENT OF EXPOSURE TO HIV-1 AND HEPATITIS B AND C*

OCCUPATIONAL EXPOSURE TO BLOOD, PENILE/VAGINAL SECRETIONS OR OTHER POTENTIALLY INFECTIOUS BODY FLUIDS OR TISSUES WITH RISK OF TRANSMISSION OF HEPATITIS B/C AND/OR HIV-1 (E.G., NEEDLESTICK INJURY)

[Adapted from MMWR 50(RR-11):1, 2001; NEJM 348:826, 2003 and MMWR 54(RR-9)1: 2005 (available at www.aidsinfo.nih.gov).]

Free consultation for occupational exposures, call (PEPline) 1-888-448-4911.

General steps in management:
1. Wash clean wounds/flush mucous membranes immediately (use of caustic agents or squeezing the wound is discouraged; data lacking regarding antiseptics).
2. Assess risk by doing the following: (a) Characterize exposure; (b) Determine/evaluate source of exposure by medical history, risk behavior, & testing for hepatitis B/C, HIV; (c) Evaluate and test exposed individual for hepatitis B/C & HIV.

Hepatitis B Exposure *[Adapted from CDC recommendations; MMWR 50(RR-11), 2001]*

Exposed Person	Exposure Source		
	HBs Ag+	HBs Ag–	Status Unknown
Unvaccinated	Give HBIG 0.06 mL per kg IM & initiate HB vaccine	Initiate HB vaccine	Initiate HB vaccine and if possible, check HBs Ag of source person. Consider HBIG if source high risk.
Vaccinated (antibody status unknown)	Do anti-HBs on exposed person: If titer ≥10 milli-International units per mL, no rx If titer <10 milli-International units per mL, give HBIG + 1 dose HB vaccine[†]	No rx necessary	Do anti-HBs on exposed person: If titer ≥10 milli-International units per mL, no rx If titer <10 milli-International units per mL, give 1 dose of HB vaccine (plus 1 dose HBIG if source high risk)

For known vaccine series responder (titer ≥10 milli-International units per mL), monitoring of levels or booster doses not currently recommended. Known non-responder (<10 milli-International units per mL) to 1° series HB vaccine & exposed to either HBsAg+ source or suspected high-risk source–rx with HBIG & re-initiate vaccine series or give 2 doses HBIG 1 month apart. For non-responders after a 2nd vaccine series, 2 doses HBIG 1 month apart is preferred approach to new exposure [MMWR 40(RR-13):21, 2001].
† Follow-up to assess/address vaccine response and to complete series

Hepatitis C Exposure
Determine antibody to hepatitis C for both exposed person and, if possible, exposure source. If source +, follow-up HCV testing advised. **No recommended prophylaxis**; immune serum globulin not effective. Monitor for early infection, as therapy may ↓ risk of progression to chronic hepatitis. See page 137 and discussion in Clin Micro Rev 16:546, 2003.
Case-control study found risk factors for occup. transmission: injury from needle that had been in art/vein, deep injury, male HCW, source VL >6 mil. copies/mL (CID 41:1423, 2005).

---

* See page 2 for abbreviations

TABLE 15D(2)

HIV: Occupational exposure management [Adapted from MMWR 54 (RR-9), 2005]

- The decision to initiate post-exposure prophylaxis (PEP) for HIV is a clinical judgment that should be made in concert with the exposed healthcare worker (HCW). It is based on:
  1. The exposure type of the source patient having HIV infection: 1. with history of high-risk activity—injection drug use, sexual activity with multiple partners (either heterosexual or homosexual), receipt of blood products 1978–1985, with clinical signs suggestive of advanced HIV (unexplained wasting, night sweats, thrush, seborrheic dermatitis, etc.).
  2. Type of exposure (approx. 1 in 300–400 needlesticks from infected source will transmit HIV).
  3. Limited data regarding efficacy of PEP (PEP with ZDV alone reduced transmission by >80% in 1 retrospective case-controlled study—NEJM 337:1485, 1997).
  4. Significant adverse effects of PEP drugs & potential for drug interactions.
  5. Substances considered potentially infectious include: blood, tissues, semen, vaginal secretions, CSF, synovial, pleural, peritoneal, pericardial and amniotic fluids; and other visibly bloody fluids.
     Fluids normally considered low risk for transmission, unless visibly bloody, include: urine, vomitus, stool, sweat, saliva, nasal secretions, tears and sputum (MMWR 54(RR-9), 2005)
- If source person is **known positive** (i.e. source person is **known to be infected** and **status of exposure warrants PEP**, antiretroviral drugs should be started **immediately** (ASAP or within hours). If source person is HIV antibody negative, drugs can be stopped **unless source is suspected of having acute HIV infection**. The HCW should be re-tested at **3–4 weeks, 3 & 6 months whether PEP is used or not** (not the vast majority of seroconversions will occur by 3 months; delayed conversions after 6 months are exceedingly rare). Tests for HIV RNA should not be used for dx of HIV infection in HCW because of false-positives (esp. at low titers) & these test are only approved for established HIV infection [a possible exception is if it develops signs of acute HIV (mononucleosis-like) syndrome within the 1st 4–6 wks of exposure when antibody tests might still be negative].
- PEP for HIV is usually given for **4wks** and monitoring of adverse effects recommended: baseline **complete blood count, renal and hepatic panel** to be **repeated at 2 weeks**, 50–75% of HCW on PEP demonstrate mild side-effects (nausea, diarrhea, myalgias, headache, etc.) but in up to ⅓ severe enough to discontinue PEP (Antivir Ther 3:195, 2000). Consultation with infectious diseases/HIV specialist valuable when questions regarding PEP arise. **Seek expert help in special situations, such as pregnancy, renal impairment, treatment-experienced source.**

3 Steps to HIV Post-Exposure Prophylaxis (PEP) After Occupational Exposure: [For latest CDC recommendations, see MMWR 54(RR-9), 2005 available at www.aidsinfo.nih.gov]

Step 1: Determine the exposure code (EC)

```
Is source material blood, bloody fluid, semen/vaginal fluid or other normally sterile fluid or tissue?
        |                                                                           |
       Yes                                                                        No → No PEP
        |
   What type of exposure occurred?
        |                                           |
   Mucous membrane or skin integrity          Percutaneous exposure
   compromised (e.g., dermatitis, open wound)        |
        |                                         Severity
      Volume                                    |              |
   |           |                          Less severe:     More severe: Large-bore hollow needle, deep puncture,
 Intact skin                              Solid needle, scratch   visible blood, needle used in blood vessel of source
   No PEP†                                      |                        |
                                               EC2                      EC3
   |               |
 Small: Few drops   Large: Major splash and/or
        |              long duration
       EC1               |
                        EC2
```

† Exceptions can be considered when there have been prolonged, high-volume contact.

Step 2: Determine the HIV Status Code (HIV SC)

```
                          What is the HIV status of the exposure source?
        |                              |                              |                        |
   HIV negative                   HIV positive                   Status unknown           Source unknown
        |                    |                     |             HIV SC unknown           HIV SC unknown
     No PEP          Low titer exposure:    High titer exposure: advanced AIDS, primary
                     asymptomatic,          HIV, high viral load or low CD4 count
                     low CD4 count,               |
                     & high VL (<1500       HIV SC 2
                     copies per mL.)
                          |
                     HIV SC 1
```

* See page 2 for abbreviations

TABLE 15D(3)

Step 3: Determine Post-Exposure Prophylaxis (PEP) Recommendation

EC	HIV SC	PEP
1	1	Consider basic regimen[*] [a] [e]
1	2	Recommend basic regimen[*] [b]
2	1	Recommend basic regimen[*]
2	2	Recommend expanded regimen[†]
3	1 or 2	Recommend expanded regimen[†]
1, 2, 3	Unknown	If exposure setting suggests risks of HIV exposure, consider basic regimen[*] [e]

[*] Based on estimates of ↓ risk of infection after mucous membrane exposure in occupational setting compared with needlestick.
[a] Modification of CDC recommendations:
[b] Or consider expanded regimen[†]
[e] In high risk circumstances, consider expanded regimen[†] on case-by-case basis.

Around the clock, urgent expert consultation available from:
National Clinicians' Post-Exposure Prophylaxis Hotline
(PEPline) at 1-888-448-4911 (1-888-HIV-4911)

Regimens: (Treat for 4 weeks, monitor for drug side-effects every 2 weeks)

Basic regimen: ZDV + 3TC, or FTC + TDF, or as an alternative d4T + 3TC.

Expanded regimen Basic regimen + one of the following: lopinavir/ritonavir (preferred), or (as alternatives) atazanavir/ritonavir or fosamprenavir/ritonavir. Efavirenz can be considered (except in pregnancy or potential for pregnancy—**Pregnancy Category D**); but CNS symptoms might be problematic. [**Do not use nevirapine**: serious adverse reactions including hepatic necrosis reported in healthcare workers (MMWR 49:1153, 2001).]

Other regimens can be designed. If possible, use antiretroviral drugs for which resistance is unlikely based on susceptibility data or treatment history of source (if known). Seek expert consultation if ARV-experienced source or in pregnancy or potential for pregnancy.

NOTE: Some authorities feel that an expanded regimen should be employed whenever PEP is indicated (NEJM 349:1091, 2003; Eur J Epidemiol 19:577 2004). Expanded regimens are likely to be advantageous with ↑ numbers of ART-experienced source pts or when there is doubt about exact extent of exposures in decision algorithm. Mathematical model suggests that under some conditions, completion of full course basic regimen is better than prematurely discontinued expanded regimen (CID 39:395, 2004). However, while expanded PEP regimens have ↑ adverse effects, there is not necessarily ↑ discontinuation (CID 40:205, 2005).

POST-EXPOSURE PROPHYLAXIS FOR NON-OCCUPATIONAL EXPOSURES TO HIV-1
From MMWR 54(RR-2):1, 2005—DHHS recommendations

Because the risk of transmission of HIV via sexual contact or sharing needles by injection drug users may reach or exceed that of occupational needlestick exposure, it is reasonable to consider PEP in persons who have had a non-occupational exposure to blood or other potentially infected fluids (e.g., genital/rectal secretions, breast milk) from an HIV+ source. Risk of HIV acquisition per exposure varies with the act: (for needle sharing and receptive anal intercourse, 20.5%; approximately 10-fold lower with insertive vaginal or anal intercourse, 0.05-0.07%). Overt or occult traumatic lesions may ↑ risk in survivors of sexual assault.

For pts at risk of HIV acquisition through non-occupational exposure to HIV+ source material having occurred ≤72 hours before evaluation, DHHS recommendation is to treat for 28 days with an antiretroviral **expanded regimen**, using preferred regimens [efavirenz (not in pregnancy or pregnancy risk—**Pregnancy Category D**) + (3TC or FTC) + (ZDV or TDF)] or [lopinavir/ritonavir + (3TC or FTC) + ZDV] or one of several alternative regimens [see Table 14D & MMWR 54(RR-2):1, 2005]. Failures of prophylaxis have been reported, and may be associated with longer interval from exposure to start of PEP (CID 41:1507, 2005); this supports prompt initiation of PEP.

Areas of uncertainty: (1) expanded regimens are not proven to be superior to 2-drug regimens, (2) when PEP is indicated is unknown, decision to treat and regimen selection must be individualized based on assessment of specific circumstances.

Evaluate for exposures to Hep B, Hep C (see *Occupational PEP* above), and bacterial sexually-transmitted diseases (see Table 15A) and treat as indicated. DHHS recommendations for sexual exposures to HepB and bacterial pathogens are available in MMWR 55(RR-11), 2006. Persons who are unvaccinated or who have not responded to full HepB vaccine series should receive HepB immune globulin preferably within 24-hours of percutaneous or mucosal exposure to blood or body fluids of an HBsAg-positive person, along with HepB vaccine, with follow-up to complete vaccine series. Unvaccinated or not-fully-vaccinated persons exposed to a source with unknown HepBsAg-status should receive vaccine and complete vaccine series. See MMWR 55(RR-11), 2006 for details and recommendations in other circumstances.

* See page 2 for abbreviations

TABLE 15E – PREVENTION OF OPPORTUNISTIC INFECTION IN HUMAN STEM CELL TRANSPLANTATION (HSCT) OR SOLID ORGAN TRANSPLANTATION (SOT) FOR ADULTS WITH NORMAL RENAL FUNCTION*

General comments: Medical centers performing transplants will have detailed protocols for the prevention of opportunistic infections which are representative of the resources and patients represented at those sites. Regimens continue to evolve and protocols adopted by an institution may differ from those of other centers. Care of transplant patients should be guided by physicians with expertise in this area. References. *MMWR 49(RR-10):1, 2000; CID 33:526, 2001; COID 17:353, 2004*

OPPORTUNISTIC INFECTION (at risk)	TYPE OF TRANSPLANT	PROPHYLACTIC REGIMENS	COMMENTS/REFERENCES
CMV (Recipient + OR Donor +/Recipient −)	HSCT	**Preemptive therapy:** Monitor ≥ 1x/wk. (days 100–100) for CMV-antigenemia or viremia by PCR test (Note: culture alone not sufficiently sensitive); start rx when + (Ganciclovir 5mg/kg IV q12h 7–14 days, then 5mg/kg IV q24h 5 days/wk to day 100 or ≥ 3wks, whichever longer) [MMWR 49(RR-10):1, 2000]. Some use oral valganciclovir 900mg bid (monitoring tests should be done in order to reduce numbers of patients who are treated, for some centers [EBMT 35:999, 2005; COID 17:353, 2004; BMT 37:693, 2006]). Recent papers showed that 2wks valganciclovir 900mg po bid comp to ganciclovir 5mg/kg IV bid as preemptive therapy in allo-HSCT [BMT 37:851, 2006] & that valganciclovir 900mg bid for 2wks then 900mg q24h for ≥ 7days after neg. assay was effective [BMTI 37: 851, 2006]. **OR**	
		Prophylaxis: (for high-risk pts, see *CID 35:999, 2002*, or where CMV detection tests not available): From engraftment to day 100, rx with ganciclovir IV 5 mg per kg q12h for 7 days, then 5 mg per kg q24h 5–6 days per week.	
		General Comments: Review in *CMR 16:647, 2003*. Role of valganciclovir in CMV prevention is under investigation.	
	SOT	**Kidney, kidney/pancreas, heart:** Valganciclovir 900 mg po q24h, start by day 10 & continue through day 100 of transplant.	
		Liver: Ganciclovir 1 gm po q8h, start by day 10 & continue through day 100.	
		Lung: Ganciclovir 5 mg per kg q12h IV for 5–7 days, then valganciclovir 900 mg po q24h or 6 months (or at least 3 mos.).[1] Some centers have added CMV immune globulin 150 mg per kg within 72 hrs of transplant, & at 2, 4, 6, & 8 wks post-transplant, then 100 mg per kg at wk. 12 & 16.	
		Comments: For recs by US & Cndtn transplantation societies, see *Am. J. Transpl 4(Suppl 10):51, 2004 & 5:218, 2005.* For lung, see *Transpl 80:157, 2005.* Universal prophylaxis approach (above) favored by most, there are proponents of preemptive therapy in liver transplant [CID 40:704 & 709, 2005; Transpl 79:85 & 1428, 2005]. Some add CMV Ig for high-risk SOTs also. (Note: Valganciclovir not approved by FDA for liver or lung transplantation, but some use it. ↑ Bioavailability of valganciclovir may [??] ↑ risk of resistance [CID 45: 448, 2007].	
Hepatitis B-induced cirrhosis	Liver	See Table 14A, page 137. An interesting phenomenon of "reverse seroconversion" has been described in pts with HBV reactivation in bone marrow transplantation: loss of HbsAb and appearance of HbsAg with viremia [CID 41:1277, 2005].	
Herpes simplex (seropositive)	HSCT	Acyclovir 250mg per meter-squared IV q12h or 200mg po 3x/day from conditioning to engraftment or resolution of mucositis.	
	SOT	Acyclovir 200 mg po 3x/day to 400mg bid–start early post transplant [ClinMicroRev 10:86, 1997].	
		Comment: Do not select acyclovir if receiving CMV prophylaxis. One study found pts receiving higher dose acyclovir or valacyclovir for ≥1 yr to prevent VZV reactivation in HSCT had ↓ HSV and ↓ acyclovir-resistant HSV than cohort treated for 30 days [JID 196:266, 2007].	
Aspergillus sp.	Lung/ Heart-lung	No controlled trials to determine optimal management, but regimens of an aerosolized liposomal ampho-based ampho B preparation & an oral anti-aspergillus agent have been used [Am J Transpl 4(Suppl 10):110, 2004]. Randomized trial suggested nebulized ABLC better tolerated than nebul. ampho B deoxycholate [Transpl 77:232, 2004]. Another study found nebulized liposomal amphotericin and nebul. amphotericin deoxycholate to be comparably effective in lung transplantation [Transpl Infect Dis. 9: 121, 2007]. Multi-station study of voriconazole vs fluconazole to prevent invasive aspergillus in progress [CID 39:S176, 2004]. Von assoc.	
	HSCT	Itraconazole w/po solution led to non-significant ↓ invasive aspergillus compared with fluconazole [AnIM 138:705, 2003] or significant ↓ infection with ↑ toxicity/intolerance [Blood 103:1527, 2004]. Study of voriconazole vs fluconazole to prevent invasive fungal infections in progress [CID 39:S176, 2004]. Von assoc. with ↑ risk of zygomycosis [JID 191:1350, 2005]. Posaconazole approved for prophylaxis of invasive Aspergillus and candida in high-risk, severely immunocompromised pts (eg. HSCT w/GVHD) at a dose of 200 mg three times daily. In comparative trial, posaconazole overall similar to fluconazole in preventing invasive fungal infections, but more effective in preventing Aspergillus [NEJM 356: 335, 2007].	
Candida sp. (CID 38:161, 2004)	Liver	Fluconazole 200–400 mg po 1 time per day starting before transplant & continuing up to 3 mos. in high-risk pts. Optimal duration unknown. Concerns for ↑ non-albicans candida with fluconazole prophylaxis [Transpl 75:2023, 2003]. Liver Transpl 12: 850, 2006	
	HSCT	Fluconazole 400 mg po 1 time per day from day 0 to engraftment or ANC >1000. Micafungin has also been approved for prophylaxis of Candida infections in HSCT (at recommended dose of 50 mg q24h, CID 39:1407, 2004). Posaconazole oral susp. 200 mg three times daily approved for prophylaxis in high-risk pts.	
Coccidioides immitis	All	Fluconazole 400 mg po q24h [Transpl Inf Dis 5:3, 2003] or 200-400 mg po q24h [Am J Transpl 4:1, 2006] have been used in liver and renal transplant patients, respectively, with prior coccidioidomycosis	

* See page 2 for abbreviations

TABLE 15E(2)

OPPORTUNISTIC INFECTION (at risk)	TYPE OF TRANSPLANT	PROPHYLACTIC REGIMENS	COMMENTS/ REFERENCES
Pneumocystis carinii (P. jiroveci) & Toxoplasma gondii	All	TMP-SMX, 1 SS tab po q24h or 1 DS tab po 1x/day to 3–7days/wk. Dur: 6 mo–1yr renal; ≥6mo for allogenic HSCT; ≥1yr to life for heart, lung, liver [Am J Transpl 4(Suppl.10)135, 2004]. Breakthrough pneumocystis infections reported with atovaquone doses <1500mg/day (CID 38:e76, 2004). For toxo D+/R− heart transplants, 3 mos pyrimethamine/sulfa prior to lifetime TMP-SMX prophylaxis has been suggested [see Am J Transpl 4(Suppl.10):142, 2004 for intensive pyri-sulfa regimen & alternatives].	
Trypanosoma cruzi	Heart	May be transmitted from organs or transfusions. Inspect peripheral blood smear of suspected cases for parasites (MMWR 55:798, 2006) If known Chagas' disease in donor or recipient, contact CDC for nifurtimox (phone 404-639-3670).	

TABLE 16 – PEDIATRIC DOSAGES OF SELECTED ANTIBACTERIAL AGENTS*

[Adapted from: (1) Nelson's Pocket Book of Pediatric Antimicrobial Therapy, 2006–2007, 16th Ed., J. Bradley & J. Nelson, eds., Alliance for World Wide Editing, Buenos Aires, Argentina, and (2) 2006 Red Book, 27th Ed., American Academy of Pediatrics, pages 700–718]

DRUG	DOSES IN MG PER KG PER DAY OR MG PER KG AT FREQUENCY INDICATED[1]				
	BODY WEIGHT <2000 gm		BODY WEIGHT >2000 gm		>28 DAYS OLD
	0–7 days	8–28 days	0–7 days	8–28 days	
Aminoglycosides, IV or IM (check levels; some dose by gestational age + wks of life; *see Nelson's Pocket Book, p. 25*)					
Amikacin	7.5 q18–24h	7.5 q12h	10 q12h	10 q12h	10 q8h
Gent/tobra	2.5 q18–24h	2.5 q12h	2.5 q12h	2.5 q12h	2.5 q8h
Aztreonam, IV	30 q12h	30 q8h	30 q8h	30 q6h	30 q6h
Cephalosporins					
Cefaclor					20–40 div tid
Cefadroxil					30 div bid (max 2gm per day)
Cefazolin	25 q12h	25 q12h	25 q12h	25 q8h	25 q8h
Cefdinir					7 q12h or 14 q24h
Cefepime	30 q12h	30 q12h	30 q12h	30 q12h	150 div q8h
Cefixime					8 as q24h or div bid
Cefotaxime	50 q12h	50 q8h	50 q12h	50 q8h	50 q8h (75 q6h for meningitis)
Cefoxitin			20 q12h		80–160 div q6h
Cefpodoxime					10 div bid (max 400mg per day)
Cefprozil					15–30 div bid (max 1gm per day)
Ceftazidime	50 q12h	50 q8h	50 q12h	50 q8h	50 q8h
Ceftibuten					4.5 bid
Ceftizoxime					33–66 q8h
Ceftriaxone	25 q24h	50 q24h	25 q24h	50 q24h	50 q24h (meningitis 100)
Cefuroxime IV	50 q12h	50 q8h	50 q8h	50 q8h	50 q8h (80 q8h for meningitis)
po					10–15 bid (max 1gm per day)
Cephalexin					25–50 div q6h (max 4gm per day)
Loracarbef					15–30 div bid (max 2gm per day)
Chloramphenicol IV	25 q24h	25 q24h	25 q24h	15 q12h	12.5–25 q6h (max 2–4gm per day)
Clindamycin IV	5 q12h	5 q8h	5 q8h	5 q6h	7.5 q6h
po					
Ciprofloxacin po[2]					20–30 div bid (max 1.5gm per day)
Ertapenem IV	No data	No data	No data	No data	15 q12h (max. 1g/day)
Imipenem[3] IV			25 q12h	25 q8h	15–25 q6h (max 2–4gm per day)
Linezolid	10 q12h	10 q8h	10 q8h	10 q8h	10 q8h to age 12
Macrolides					
Erythro IV & po	10 q12h	10 q12h	10 q12h	13 q12h	10 q6h
Azithro po/IV	5 q24h	10 q24h	5 q24h	10 q24h	10 q24h
Clarithro					7.5 q12h (max. 1gm per day)
Meropenem IV	20 q12h	20 q8h	20 q12h	20 q8h	60–120 div q8h (120 for meningitis)
Metro IV & po	7.5 q24h	7.5 q12h	7.5 q12h	15 q12h	7.5 q6h
Penicillins					
Ampicillin	50 q12h	50 q8h	50 q8h	50 q6h	50 q6h
AMP-sulbactam					100–300 div q6h
Amoxicillin po			30 div bid		25–50 div tid
Amox-Clav po			30 div bid	30 div bid	45 or 90 (AM/CL-HD) div bid if over 12wks
Dicloxacillin					12–25 div q6h
Mezlocillin	75 q12h	75 q8h	75 q12h	75 q8h	75 q6h
Nafcillin, oxacillin IV	25 q12h	25 q8h	25 q8h	37 q6h	37 q6h (to max. 8–12 gm per day)
Piperacillin, PIP-tazo IV	50 q12h	100 q12h	100 q12h	100 q8h	100 q6h
Ticarcillin, T.clav IV	75 q12h	75 q8h	75 q8h	75 q6h	75 q6h
Tinidazole					> Age 3: 50mg/kg for 1 dose
Penicillin G, U/kg IV	50,000 q12h	75,000 q8h	50,000 q8h	50,000 q6h	50,000 units/kg per day
Penicillin V					25–50mg per kg per day div q6–8h
Rifampin IV, po	10 q24h	10 q24h	10 q24h	10 q24h	10 q24h
Sulfisoxazole po					120–150mg per kg per day div q4–6h
TMP-SMX po, IV; UTI: 8–12 TMP component div bid; Pneumocystis: 20 TMP component div q6h					
Tetracycline po (age 8 or older)					25–50 div q6h (>7yr old)
Doxycycline po, IV (age 8 or older)					2–4 div bid to max of 200 (>7yr old)
Vancomycin IV	12.5 q12h	15 q12h	18 q12h	22 q12h	40 div q6–8h; 60 for meningitis

[1] May need higher doses in patients with meningitis: *see CID 39:1267, 2004*

[2] With exception of cystic fibrosis, anthrax, and complicated UTI, not approved for use under age 18.

[3] Not recommended in children with CNS infections due to risk of seizures.

* *See page 2 for abbreviations*

TABLE 17A – DOSAGE OF ANTIMICROBIAL DRUGS IN ADULT PATIENTS WITH RENAL IMPAIRMENT

Adapted from a combination of DRUG PRESCRIBING IN RENAL FAILURE, 5th Ed., Aronoff et al (Eds), American College of Physicians, 2007 and selected package inserts. For review of Continuous Renal Replacement Therapy: CID 41:1159, 2005.

UNLESS STATED, ADJUSTED DOSES ARE % OF DOSE FOR NORMAL RENAL FUNCTION.

Drug adjustments are based on the patient's estimated endogenous creatinine clearance, which can be calculated as:

	Ideal body weight for men:	50.0 kg + 2.3 kg per inch over 5 feet
[140–age](ideal body weight in kg) for men (x 0.85 for women)	Ideal body weight for women:	45.5 kg + 2.3 kg per inch over 5 feet
(72)(serum creatinine, mg per dL)		

For alternative methods to calculate estimated CrCl, see NEJM 354:2473, 2006.

NOTE: For summary of drugs requiring NO dosage adjustment with renal insufficiency, see Table 17B, page 185.

ANTIMICROBIAL	HALF-LIFE (NORMAL/ ESRD) hr	DOSE FOR NORMAL RENAL FUNCTION§	METHOD * (see footnote)	ADJUSTMENT FOR RENAL FAILURE Estimated creatinine clearance (CrCl), mL/min			HEMODIALYSIS, CAPD* (see footnote)	COMMENTS & DOSAGE FOR CRRT†
				>50–90	10–50	<10		
ANTIBACTERIAL ANTIBIOTICS								
Aminoglycoside Antibiotics:		**Traditional multiple daily doses—adjustment for renal disease**						
Amikacin	1.4–2.3/17–150	7.5 mg per kg q12h or 15 mg per kg once daily (see below)	I	7.5 mg/kg q12h	7.5 mg/kg q24h **Same dose for CRRT†**	7.5 mg/kg q48h	HEMO: ½ of normal renal function dose AD* CAPD: 15–20 mg lost per L of dialysate per day (see Comment)	High flux hemodialysis membranes lead to unpredictable aminoglycoside clearance, measure post-dialysis drug levels for efficacy and toxicity. With CAPD, pharmacokinetics highly variable—**check serum levels.**
Gentamicin, Tobramycin	2–3/20–60	1.7 mg per kg q8h. Once daily dosing below	I	100% of q8h	100% of q12–24h **Same dose for CRRT†**	100% of q48h	HEMO: ½ of normal renal function dose AD* CAPD: 3–4 mg lost per L dialysate per day	Usual method for CAPD. 2 liters of dialysis fluid placed qid x 8 liters per day (give 8Lx20 mg lost per L = 160 mg of amikacin supplement IV per day)
Netilmicin^NUS	2–3/35–72	2.0 mg per kg q8h. Once daily dosing below	I	100% of q12h	100% of q12–24h **Same dose for CRRT†**	100% of q48h	HEMO: ½ of normal renal function dose AD* CAPD: 3–4 mg lost per L dialysate per day	Adjust dosing weight for obesity: [ideal body weight + 0.4(actual body weight – ideal body weight)] (CID 25:112, 1997).
Streptomycin	2–3/30–80	15 mg per kg (max. of 1.0 gm) q24h. Once daily dosing below	D, I	q24h	q24–72h **Same dose for CRRT†**	q72–96h	HEMO: ½ of normal renal function dose AD* CAPD: 20–40 mg lost per L dialysate per day	

ONCE-DAILY AMINOGLYCOSIDE THERAPY: ADJUSTMENT IN RENAL INSUFFICIENCY (see Table 10D for OD dosing/normal renal function)

Creatinine Clearance (mL per min.)	60–80	40–60	30–40	20–30	10–20	<10–0
Drug	Dose q24h (mg per kg)			Dose q48h (mg per kg)		Dose q72h and AD*
Gentamicin/Tobramycin	5.1	4	3.5	2.5	4	3
Amikacin/Kanamycin/streptomycin	15	12	7.5			
Isepamicin^NUS	8	8	8	7.5	8	
			q48h		q72h	q96h
Netilmicin^NUS	6.5	5	4	3	2.5	

§ CRRT = continuous renal replacement therapy.   * AD = after dialysis.   † AD* refers to timing of dose. "Dose AD" refers to dose.   CAPD = Continuous ambulatory peritoneal dialysis.

TABLE 17A (2)

ANTIMICROBIAL	HALF-LIFE (NORMAL/ ESRD) hr	DOSE FOR NORMAL RENAL FUNCTIONS	METHOD * (see footnote)	ADJUSTMENT FOR RENAL FAILURE Estimated creatinine clearance (CrCl), mL/min			HEMODIALYSIS, CAPD* (see footnote)	COMMENTS & DOSAGE FOR CRRT[†]
				>50-90	10-50	<10		
ANTIBACTERIAL ANTIBIOTICS (Continued)								
Carbapenem Antibiotics								
Doripenem	1/18	500 mg IV q8h	D&I	500 mg IV q8h	**31-50:** 250 mg IV q8h **10-30:** 250 mg q12h	No data	No data	
Ertapenem	4/>4	1.0 gm q24h	D	1.0 gm q24h	0.5 gm q24h (CrCl <30)	0.5 gm q24h	HEMO: Dose as for CrCl <10; if dosed <6 hrs prior to HD, give 150 mg supplement AD*	
Imipenem (see Comment)	1/4	0.5 gm q6h	D&I	250-500 mg q6-8h	250 mg q6-12h; **Dose for CRRT[†]: 0.5-1 gm bid** (AAC 49:2421, 2005)	125-250 mg q12h	HEMO: Dose AD* CAPD: Dose for CrCl <10	↑ potential for seizures if recommended doses exceeded in pts with CrCl <20 mL per min. See pkg insert, esp. for pts <70 kg
Meropenem	1/6-8	1.0 gm q8h	D&I	1.0 gm q8h	1.0 gm q12h **Same dose for CRRT[†]**	0.5 gm q24h	HEMO: Dose AD* CAPD: Dose for CrCl <10	
Cephalosporin Antibiotics: DATA ON SELECTED PARENTERAL CEPHALOSPORINS								
Cefazolin	1.9/40-70	1.0–2.0 gm q8h	D&I	q8h	q12h **Same dose for CRRT[†]**	q24-48h	HEMO: Extra 0.5-1 gm AD* CAPD: 0.5 gm q12h	
Cefepime	2.2/18	2.0 gm q8h (max. dose)	D&I	2 gm q8h	2 gm q12-24h **Same dose for CRRT[†]**	1 gm q24h	HEMO: Extra 1 gm AD* CAPD: 1-2 gm q48h	
Cefotaxime, Ceftizoxime	1.7/15-35	2.0 gm q8h	I	q8-12h	q12-24h **Same dose for CRRT[†]**	q24h	HEMO: Extra 1 gm AD* CAPD: 0.5-1 gm q24h	Active metabolite of cefotaxime in ESRD. ↓ dose further for hepatic & renal failure.
Cefotetan	3.5/13-25	1-2 gm q12h	D	100%	1-2 gm q24h **Same dose for CRRT[†]**	1-2 gm q48h	HEMO: Extra 1 gm AD* CAPD: 1 gm q24h	CRRT dose: 750 mg q12h
Cefoxitin	0.8/13-23	2.0 gm q8h	I	q8h	q8-12h **Same dose for CRRT[†]**	q24-48h	HEMO: Extra 1 gm AD* CAPD: 1 gm q24h	May falsely increase serum creatinine by interference with assay.
Ceftazidime	1.2/13-25	2 gm q8h	I	q8-12h	q12-24h **Same dose for CRRT[†]**	q24-48h	HEMO: Extra 1 gm AD* CAPD: 0.5 gm q24h	Volume of distribution increases with infection.
Ceftobiprole	3-4/No data	500 mg IV q8-12h	I	500 mg IV q8h	**30-50:** 500 mg q12h **<30:** No data	No data	No data	
Cefuroxime sodium	1.2/17	0.75-1.5 gm q8h	I	q8h	q8-12h **Same dose for CRRT[†]**	q24h	HEMO: Dose AD* CAPD: Dose for CrCl <10	
Fluoroquinolone Antibiotics								
Ciprofloxacin	3-6/6-9	500-750 mg po (or 400 mg IV) q12h	D	100%	50-75% CRRT 400 mg IV q24h	50%	HEMO: 250 mg po or 200 mg IV q12h CAPD: 250 mg po or 200 mg IV q8h	
Gatifloxacin[NUS]	7-14/11-40	400 mg po/IV q24h	D	400 mg q24h	400 mg, then 200 mg q24h **Same dose for CRRT[†]**	400 mg, then 200 mg q24h	HEMO: 200 mg q24h AD* CAPD: 200 mg q24h	

† CRRT = continuous renal replacement therapy. * AD = after dialysis. "Dose AD" refers to timing of dose. CAPD = Continuous ambulatory peritoneal dialysis.
§ Supplement is to replace drug lost via dialysis; extra drug beyond continuation of regimen used for CrCl <10 mL per min.

TABLE 17A (3)

ANTIMICROBIAL	HALF-LIFE (NORMAL/ESRD) hr	DOSE FOR NORMAL RENAL FUNCTIONS	METHOD * (see footnote)	ADJUSTMENT FOR RENAL FAILURE — Estimated creatinine clearance (CrCl), mL/min			HEMODIALYSIS, CAPD† (see footnote)	COMMENTS & DOSAGE FOR CRRT†
				>50-90	10-50	<10		
ANTIBACTERIAL ANTIBIOTICS/Fluoroquinolone Antibiotics *(Continued)*								
Gemifloxacin	7/>7	320 mg po q24h	D	320 mg q24h	160 mg q24h	160 mg q24h	HEMO: 160 mg q24h AD* CAPD: 160 mg q24h	
Levofloxacin	4-8/76	750 mg q24h IV, PO	D&I	750 mg q24h	20-49: 750 mg q48h	<20: 750 mg once, then 500 mg q48h	HEMO/CAPD: Dose for CrCl <20	CRRT† 750 mg once, then 500 mg q48h
Macrolide Antibiotics								
Clarithromycin	5-7/22	0.5-1.0 gm q12h	D	100%	75%	50-75%	HEMO: Dose AD* CAPD: None	CRRT† as for CrCl 10-50
Erythromycin	1.4/5-6	250-500 mg q6h	D	100%	100%	50-75%	HEMO/CAPD/CRRT: None	Ototoxicity with high doses in ESRD
Miscellaneous Antibacterial Antibiotics								
Colistin base	<6/>48	80-160 mg q8h	D	160 mg q12h	160 mg q24h	160 mg q36h	HEMO: 80 mg AD* HEMO & CAPD: 4-6 mg per kg q48h (after dialysis if possible)	LnID 6:589, 2006; CVVH: 2.5mg/kg q48h
Daptomycin	9.4/30	4-6 mg per kg per day	I	4-6 mg per kg per day	CrCl <30, 4-6 mg per kg q48h			
Linezolid	5-6/6-8	600 mg po/IV q12h	None	600 mg q12h	600 mg q12h	600 mg q12h AD*	HEMO: Dose AD* CAPD & CRRT: No dose adjustment	Accumulation of 2 metabolites—risk unknown (JAC 56:172, 2005)
Metronidazole	6-14/7-21	7.5 mg per kg q6h	D	100%	100%	50%	HEMO: Dose AD* CAPD: Dose for CrCl <10	Same dose for CRRT†
Nitrofurantoin	0.5/1	50-100 mg	D	100%	Avoid	Avoid	Not applicable	
Sulfamethoxazole	10/20-50	1.0 gm q8h	I	q12h	q18h Same dose for CAVH	q24h	HEMO: Extra 1 gm AD* CAPD: 1 gm q24h	
Teicoplanin[NUS]	45/62-230	6 mg per kg per day	I	q24h	q48h Same dose for CRRT†	q72h	HEMO: Dose for CrCl <10 CAPD: Dose for CrCl <10	
Telithromycin	10/15	800 mg q24h	D	800 mg q24h	600 mg q24h (<30 mL per min)	600 mg q24h	HEMO: 600 mg AD* CAPD: No data	No data
Telavancin	7.8/17.9	10 mg/kg q24h	D&I	10 mg/kg q24h	30-50: 7.5 mg/kg q24h; <30: 10 mg/kg q48h	<30: 10 mg/kg q48h	HEMO: No data CAPD: No data	No data
Trimethoprim (TMP)	11/20-49	100-200 mg q12h	I	q12h	>30 q12h; 10-30 q18h Same dose for CRRT†	q24h	HEMO: Dose AD* CAPD: q24h	CRRT† dose q18h
Trimethoprim-sulfamethoxazole-DS								
Treatment	As for TMP	5 mg per kg IV q24h	D	100%	50%	Not recommended		

---

† CRRT = continuous renal replacement therapy. * AD = after dialysis. "Dose AD" refers to timing of dose. CAPD = Continuous ambulatory peritoneal dialysis.
Supplement is to replace drug lost via dialysis; extra drug lost for CrCl <10 mL. per min.

TABLE 17A (4)

ANTIBACTERIAL ANTIBIOTICS/Miscellaneous Antibacterial Antibiotics (Continued)

ANTIMICROBIAL	HALF-LIFE (NORMAL/ESRD) hr	DOSE FOR NORMAL RENAL FUNCTIONS	METHOD (see footnote)	ADJUSTMENT FOR RENAL FAILURE — Estimated creatinine clearance (CrCl), mL/min			HEMODIALYSIS, CAPD* (see footnote)	COMMENTS & DOSAGE FOR CRRT‡
				>50-90	10-50	<10		
Prophylaxis	As for TMP	1 tab po q24h or 3 times per week	No change	100%	100%	100%		
Vancomycin†	6/200-250	1 gm q12h	D&I	1 gm q12h	1 gm q24-96h	1 gm q4-7 days	HEMO/CAPD: Dose for CrCl <10	CAVH/CVVH: 500 mg q24-48h. New hemodialysis membranes ↑ clear. of vanco; check levels
Penicillins								
Amoxicillin	1.0/5-20	250-500 mg q8h	I	100%	q8-12h	q24h	HEMO: Dose AD* CAPD: 250 mg q12h	IV amoxicillin not available in the U.S. CRRT* dose for CrCl 10-50
Ampicillin	1.0/7-20	250 mg-2 gm q6h	I	q6h	q6-12h	q12-24h		
Amoxicillin/Clavulanate²	1.3 AM/1.0 · · 5-20/4.3	500/125 mg (see Comments)	D&I	q8h	250-500 mg AM component q12h	250-500 mg AM component q24h	HEMO: As for CrCl <10, extra dose after dialysis	If CrCl ≤30 per mL, do not use 875/125 or 1000/62.5 AM/CL
Ampicillin (AM)/Sulbactam (SB)	1.0 (AM)/1.0 (SB) 9.0 (AM)/10.0 (SB)	2 gm AM + 1.0 gm SB q6h	I	q6h	q8-12h	q24h	HEMO: Dose AD* CAPD: 2 gm AM/1 gm SB q24h	CRRT dose: 1.5 AM/0.75 SB q12h
Aztreonam	2.0/6-8	2 gm q8h	D	100%	50-75% Same dose for CRRT†	25%	HEMO: Dose 0.5 gm AD* CAPD: Dose for CrCl <10	Technically is a β-lactam antibiotic.
Penicillin G	0.5/6-20	0.5-4 million U q4h	D	100%	75% Same dose for CRRT†	20-50%	HEMO: Dose for CrCl <10 CAPD: Dose for CrCl <10	1.7 mEq potassium per million units. ↑s potential of seizure. 10 million units per day max. dose in ESRD
Piperacillin	1.0/3.3-5.1	3-4 gm q4-6h	I	q4-6h	q6-8h Same dose for CRRT†	q8h	HEMO: 2 gm q8h plus 1 gm extra AD* CAPD: Dose for CrCl <10	1.9 mEq sodium per gm
Pip/Tazo(T)	0.71-1.2 (both)/2-6	3.375 – 4.5 gm q6-8h	D&I	100%	2.25 gm q6h <20: q8h Same dose for CRRT†	2.25 gm q8h	HEMO: Dose for CrCl <10 + 0.75 gm AD* CAPD: 4.5 gm q12h; CRRT: 4.5 gm q48h	
Ticarcillin	1.2/13	3 gm q4h	D&I	1-2 gm q4h	1-2 gm q8h Same dose for CRRT†	1-2 gm q12h	HEMO: Extra 3.0 gm AD* CAPD: Dose for CrCl <10	5.2 mEq sodium per gm
Ticarcillin/Clavulanate²	1.2/11-16	3.1 gm q4h	D&I	3.1 gm q4h	3.1 gm q8-12h Same dose for CRRT†	2.0 gm q12h	HEMO: Extra 3.1 gm AD* CAPD: 3.1 gm q12h	See footnote 2
Tetracycline Antibiotics								
Tetracycline	6-10/57-108	250-500 mg qid	I	q8-12h	q12-24h	q24h	HEMO/CAPD/CAVH: None	Avoid in ESRD

¹ If renal failure, use EMIT assay to measure levels; levels overestimated by RIA or fluorescent immunoassay.

² Clavulanate cleared by liver, not kidney. Hence as dose of combination decreased, a deficiency of clavulanate may occur (JAMA 285:386, 2001).

‡ CRRT = continuous renal replacement therapy. • AD = after dialysis. "Dose AD" refers to timing of dose. CAPD = Continuous ambulatory peritoneal dialysis.

‡ Supplement is to replace drug lost via dialysis; extra drug beyond continuation of regimen used for CrCl <10 mL per min.

TABLE 17A (5)

ANTIMICROBIAL	HALF-LIFE (NORMAL/ESRD) hr	DOSE FOR NORMAL RENAL FUNCTIONS	METHOD* (see footnote)	ADJUSTMENT FOR RENAL FAILURE — Estimated creatinine clearance (CrCl), mL/min			HEMODIALYSIS, CAPD* (see footnote)	COMMENTS & DOSAGE FOR CRRT[†]
				>50-90	10-50	<10		
ANTIFUNGAL ANTIBIOTICS								
Amphotericin B & Lipid-based ampho B	24h-15 days/unchanged	Non-lipid: 0.4-1.0 mg/kg/day; ABLC: 3-6 mg/kg/day; ABCC: 5mg/kg/day; LAB: 3-5 mg/kg/day	I	q24h	q24h / **Same dose for CRRT[†]**	q24h	HEMO/CAPD/CRRT: No dose adjustment	For ampho B, toxicity lessened by saline loading; risk amplified by concomitant cyclosporine A, aminoglycosides, or pentamidine
Fluconazole	37/100	100-400 mg q24h	D	100%	50%	50%	HEMO: 100% of recommended dose AD*; CAPD: Dose for CrCl <10	CRRT: 200-400 mg q24h
Flucytosine	3-6/75-200	37.5 mg per kg q6h	I	q12h	q12-24h / **Same dose for CRRT[†]**	q24h	HEMO: Dose AD*; CAPD: 0.5-1.0 gm q24h	Goal is peak serum level >25 mcg per mL and <100 mcg per mL
Itraconazole, po soln	21/25	100-200 mg q12h	D	100%	100% / **Same dose for CRRT[†]**	50%	HEMO/CAPD: oral solution: 100 mg q12-24h	
Itraconazole, IV	21/25	200 mg IV q12h	–	200 mg IV bid	Do not use IV itra if CrCl <30 due to accumulation of carrier, cyclodextrin / For CRRT[†]: 4mg/kg po q12h		If CrCl <50 mL per min, accum. of IV vehicle (cyclodextrin). Switch to po or DC	
Terbinafine	36-200/?	250 mg po per day	–	q24h	Use has not been studied. Recommend avoidance of drug.			
Voriconazole, IV	Non-linear kinetics	6 mg per kg IV q12h times 2, then 4 mg per kg q12h	–	No change				
ANTIPARASITIC ANTIBIOTICS								
Pentamidine	3-12/73-18	4 mg per kg per day	I	q24h	q24h / **Same dose for CRRT[†]**	q24-36h	HEMO: As for CrCl <10 plus 0.75 g AD; CAPD: Dose for CrCl <10	
Quinine	5-16/5-16	650 mg q8h	I	650 mg q8h	650 mg q8-12h / **Same dose for CRRT[†]**	650 mg q24h	HEMO: Dose AD*; CAPD: Dose for CrCl <10	Marked tissue accumulation
ANTITUBERCULOUS ANTIBIOTICS (Excellent review: Nephron 64:169, 1993)								
Ethambutol	4/7-15	15-25 mg per kg q24h	I	q24h	q24-36h / **Same dose for CRRT[†]**	q48h	HEMO: Dose AD*; CAPD: Dose for CrCl <10	25 mg per kg 4-6 hr prior to 3 times per wk dialysis. Streptomycin instead of ethambutol in renal failure
Isoniazid	0.7-4/8-17	5 mg per kg q24h (max. 300 mg)	D	100%	100% / **Same dose for CRRT[†]**	50%	HEMO: Dose AD*; CAPD: Dose for CrCl <10	
Pyrazinamide	9/26	25 mg per kg q24h (max. dose 2.5 gm q24h)	D	100%	100% / **Same dose for CRRT[†]**	12-25 mg per kg q24h	HEMO: 40 mg/kg 24 hrs before each 3x/week dialysis; CAPD: No reduction	
Rifampin	1.5-5/1.8-11	600 mg per day	D	600 mg q24h	300-600 mg q24h / **Same dose for CRRT[†]**	300-600 mg q24h	HEMO: No adjustment; CAPD: Dose for CrCl <10	Biologically active metabolite

[†] CRRT = continuous renal replacement therapy. * AD = after dialysis. * AD refers to timing of dose. CAPD = Continuous ambulatory peritoneal dialysis.
Supplement is to replace drug lost via dialysis; extra drug beyond continuation of regimen used for CrCl <10 mL per min.

TABLE 17A (6)

ANTIMICROBIAL	HALF-LIFE (NORMAL/ESRD) hr	DOSE FOR NORMAL RENAL FUNCTION§	METHOD (see footnote)	ADJUSTMENT FOR RENAL FAILURE — Estimated creatinine clearance (CrCl), mL/min			HEMODIALYSIS, CAPD (see footnote)	COMMENTS & DOSAGE FOR CRRT[‡]
				>50-90	10-50	<10		
ANTIVIRAL AGENTS	For **ANTIRETROVIRALS** See C/D 40:1559, 2005							
Acyclovir, IV	2-4/20	5-12.4 mg per kg q8h	D&I	100% q8h	100% q12-24h	50% q24h	HEMO: Dose AD* CAPD: Dose for CrCl <10	Rapid IV infusion can cause ↑ Cr. CRRT dose 5-10 mg/kg q24h
Adefovir	7.5/15	10 mg po q24h	I	10 mg q24h	10 mg q48-72h	q72h†	HEMO: 10 mg q week AD* CAPD: No data; CRRT: Dose ?
Amantadine	12/500	100 mg po bid	I	q12h	q24-48h	q7days	HEMO/CAPD: Dose for CrCl<10	CRRT: Dose for CrCl 10-50
Cidofovir: Complicated dosing—see package insert								
Induction	2.5/unknown	5 mg per kg once per wk for 2 wks	--	5 mg per kg once per wk	0.5-2 mg per kg once per wk	0.5 mg per kg once per wk	No data—avoid	Major toxicity is renal. No efficacy, safety, or pharmacokinetic data in pts with moderate/severe renal disease.
Maintenance	2.5/unknown	5 mg per kg q2wks	--	5 mg per kg q2wks	0.5-2 mg per kg q2wks	0.5 mg per kg q2wks	No data—avoid	
Didanosine tablets[‡]	0.6-1.6/4.5	125-200 mg q12h buffered tabs	D	200 mg q12h	200 mg q24h	<60 kg: 150 mg q24h >60 kg: 100 mg q24h	HEMO: Dose AD* CAPD/CRRT: Dose for CrCl <10	Based on incomplete data. Data are estimates.
		400 mg q24h enteric-coated tabs	D	400 mg q24h	125-200 mg q24h	Do not use EC tabs	HEMO/CAPD: Dose for CrCl <10 CRRT: Dose for CrCl <10	**If <60 kg & CrCl <10 mL min, do not use EC tabs**
Emtricitabine (CAPS)	10/>10	200 mg q24h	I	200 mg q24h	200 mg q48-72h	200 mg q96h	HEMO: Dose for CrCl <10	See package insert for oral solution.
Emtricitabine + Tenofovir	See each drug	1 tab q24h	I	No change	1 tab q48h	1 tab q48h	Do not use	
Entecavir	128-149/?	0.5 mg q24h	D	0.5 mg q24h	0.15-0.25 mg q24h	0.05 mg q24h	HEMO/CAPD 0.05 mg q24h AD*	
Famciclovir	2.3-3.0/10-22	500 mg q8h	D&I	500 mg q8h	500 mg q12-24h	250 mg q24h	HEMO: Dose AD* CAPD: No data	Give dialysis on dialysis days. CRRT: Not applicable

				CrCl as mL per min per kg body weight—ONLY FOR FOSCARNET						
				>1.4	>1.0-1.4	>0.8-1.0	>0.6-0.8	>0.5-0.6	>0.4-0.5	<0.4
Foscarnet (CMV dosage) Dosage adjustment based on est. CrCl (mL per min) div. by pt's kg	Normal half-life (T½) 3 hrs IV; terminal T½ of 18-88 hrs. T½ very long with ESRD	Induction: 60mg/kg q8h IV Maintenance: 90-120 mg per kg per day IV	D&I	60 q8h 120 q24h	45 q8h 90 q24h	50 q12h 65 q24h	40 q12h 105 q48h	60 q24h 80 q48h	50 q24h 65 q48h	Do not use Do not use

HEMO: Dose AD* CAPD: No data — See package insert for further details.

---

[1] Ref: Transplantation 80:1086, 2005
[2] Ref: for NRTIs and NNRTIs: Kidney International 60:821, 2001
[‡] **CRRT = continuous renal replacement therapy.** * **AD = after dialysis.** "Dose AD" refers to timing of dose. **CAPD = Continuous ambulatory peritoneal dialysis.**
Supplement is to replace drug lost via dialysis; extra drug lost for CrCl <10 mL. per min.

184

TABLE 17A (7)

ANTIMICROBIAL	HALF-LIFE (NORMAL/ ESRD) hr	DOSE FOR NORMAL RENAL FUNCTION§	METHOD * (see footnote)	ADJUSTMENT FOR RENAL FAILURE — Estimated creatinine clearance (CrCl), mL/min >50-90	10-50	<10	HEMODIALYSIS, CAPD* (see footnote)	COMMENTS & DOSAGE FOR CRRT†
ANTIVIRAL AGENTS For ANTIRETROVIRALS see old 40:1559, 2005, (continued)								
Ganciclovir	3.6/30	IV: Induction 5 mg per kg q12h IV / Maintenance 5 mg per kg q24h IV po: 1.0 gm tid po	D&I	Induction 5 mg per kg q12h / 2.5-5.0 mg per kg q24h / 0.5-1 gm tid po	1.25-2.5 mg per kg q24h / 0.6-1.25 mg per kg q24h / 0.5-1.0 gm q24h	1.25 mg per kg 3 times per wk / 0.625 mg per kg 3 times per wk / 0.5 gm 3 times per week	HEMO: Dose AD* / CAPD: Dose for CrCl <10 / HEMO: 0.6 mg per kg AD* / CAPD: Dose for CrCl <10 / HEMO: 0.5 gm AD*	
Lamivudine†	5-7/15-35	300 mg po q24h	D&I	300 mg po q24h	50-150 mg q24h	25-50 mg q24h	HEMO: Dose AD*. CAPD. Dose for CrCl<10. CRRT: 100 mg 1st days, then 50 mg/day	
Oseltamivir, therapy	6-10/>20	75 mg po bid – treatment	I	75 mg q12h	30-50: 75 mg bid / <30: 75 mg qod	No data	HEMO: 30 mg non-dialysis days; CAPD: 30 mg 1-2x/week	
Ribavirin	Use with caution in patients with creatinine clearance <50 mL per min.							
Rimantadine	13-65/Prolonged	100 mg bid po	D	100 mg bid po	100 mg q24h-bid	100 mg q24h	HEMO/CAPD: No data	Use with caution, little data
Stavudine, po†	1-1.4/5.5-8	30-40 mg q12h	D&I	100%	50% q12-24h	≥60 kg 20 mg per day / <60 kg 15 mg per day	HEMO: Dose as for CrCl <10 AD* / CAPD: No data / CRRT: Full dose	
Telbivudine	40-49/No data	600 mg po daily	I	600 mg q24h	30-49: 600 mg q48H / <30: 600 mg q72h	600 mg q96h	HEMO: As for CrCl <10 AD	
Tenofovir, po	17/?	300 mg q24h	D&I	300 mg q24h	30-49: 300 mg q48h / 10-29: 300 mg 2x/wk	No data	HEMO: 300 mg q7d or after 12 hrs of HEMO ‡	
Valacyclovir	2.5-3.3/14	1.0 gm q8h	D&I	1.0 gm q8h	1.0 gm q12-24h / Same dose for CRRT†	0.5 gm q24h	HEMO: Dose AD* / CAPD: Dose for CrCl <10	CAHV dose: As for CrCl 10-50
Valganciclovir	4/67	900 mg po bid	D&I	900 mg po bid	450 mg q24h to 450 mg every other day	DO NOT USE	See package insert	
Zalcitabine†	2.0/>8	0.75 mg q8h	D&I	0.75 mg q8h	0.75 mg q12h / Same dose for CRRT†	0.75 mg q24h	HEMO: Dose AD* / CAPD: No data	CRRT dose: As for CrCl 10-50
Zidovudine†	1.1-1.4/1.4-3	300 mg q12h	D&I	300 mg q12h	300 mg q12h / Same dose for CRRT†	100 mg q8h	HEMO: Dose AD* / CAPD: Dose for CrCl <10 AD	CRRT: Dose for CrCl <10

[1] Ref. for NRTIs and NNRTIs: Kidney International 60:821, 2001

[2] Acute renal failure and Fanconi syndrome reported. † **AD** = after dialysis. "**Dose AD**" refers to timing of dose. **CAPD** = Continuous ambulatory peritoneal dialysis.

‡ **CRRT** = continuous renal replacement therapy. extra drug beyond continuation of regimen used for CrCl <10 mL per min.

Supplement is to replace drug lost via dialysis; extra drug beyond continuation of regimen used for CrCl <10 mL per min.

TABLE 17B – NO DOSAGE ADJUSTMENT WITH RENAL INSUFFICIENCY BY CATEGORY*

Antibacterials		Antifungals	Anti-TBc	Antivirals	
Azithromycin	Linezolid	Andulafngin	Rifabutin	Abacavir	Lopinavir
Ceftriaxone	Minocycline	Caspofungin	Rifapentine	Atazanavir	Nelfinavir
Chloramphenicol	Moxifloxacin	Itraconazole oral solution		Darunavir	Nevirapine
Ciprofloxacin XL	Nafcillin	Ketoconazole		Delavirdine	Raltegravir
Clindamycin	Pyrimethamine	Micafungin		Efavirenz	Ribavirin
Dirithromycin	Rifaximin	Voriconazole, **po only**		Enfuvirtide[1]	Saquinavir
Doxycycline	Tigecycline			Fosamprenavir	Tipranavir
				Indinavir	

[1]Enfuvirtide: Not studied in patients with CrCl <35 mL/min. DO NOT USE

TABLE 18 – ANTIMICROBIALS AND HEPATIC DISEASE DOSAGE ADJUSTMENT*

The following alphabetical list indicates antibacterials excreted/metabolized by the liver **wherein a dosage adjustment may be indicated** in the presence of hepatic disease. Space precludes details; consult the PDR or package inserts for details. List is **not** all-inclusive.

Antibacterials		Antifungals	Antivirals[§]	
Ceftriaxone	Nafcillin	Caspofungin	Abacavir	Indinavir
Chloramphenicol	Rifabutin	Itraconazole	Atazanavir	Lopinavir/ritonavir
Clindamycin	Rifampin	Voriconazole	Darunavir	Nelfinavir
Fusidic acid	Synercid**		Delavirdine	Nevirapine
Isoniazid	Tigecycline		Efavirenz	Rimantadine
Metronidazole	Tinidazole		Enfuvirtide	Ritonavir
			Fosamprenavir	

[§] Ref. on antiretrovirals: *CID 40:174, 2005*   ** Quinupristin/dalfopristin

TABLE 19 – TREATMENT OF CAPD PERITONITIS IN ADULTS*
(*Periton Dial Intl 20:396, 2000*)[2]

EMPIRIC Intraperitoneal Therapy:[3] Culture Results Pending

Drug		Residual Urine Output	
		<100 mL per day	>100 mL per day
Cefazolin +	Can mix in same bag	1 gm per bag, q24h	20 mg per kg BW per bag, q24h
Ceftazidime		1 gm per bag, q24h	20 mg per kg BW per bag, q24h

Drug Doses for SPECIFIC Intraperitoneal Therapy—Culture Results Known. NOTE: Few po drugs indicated

Drug	Intermittent Dosing (once per day)		Continuous Dosing (per liter exchange)	
	Anuric	Non-Anuric	Anuric	Non-Anuric
Gentamicin	0.6mg per kg	↑ dose 25%	MD 8mg	↑ MD by 25%
Cefazolin	15mg per kg	20mg per kg	LD 500mg, MD 125mg	LD 500mg, ↑ MD 25%
Ceftazidime	1000–1500mg	ND	LD 250mg, MD 125mg	ND
Ampicillin	250–500mg po bid	ND	250–500mg po bid	ND
Ciprofloxacin	500mg po bid	ND	LD 50mg, MD 25mg	ND
Vancomycin	15–30mg per kg q5–7 days	↑ dose 25%	MD 30–50mg per L	↑ MD 25%
Metronidazole	250mg po bid	ND	250mg po bid	ND
Amphotericin B	NA	NA	MD 1.5mg	NA
Fluconazole	200mg q24h	ND	200mg q24h	ND
Itraconazole	100mg q12h	100mg q12h	100mg q12h	100mg q12h
Amp-sulbactam	2gm q12h	ND	LD 1.0gm, MD 100mg	ND
TMP-SMX	320/1600mg po q1–2 days	ND	LD 320/1600mg po, MD 80/400mg po q24h	ND

CAPD = continuous ambulatory peritoneal dialysis

[1] Ref. for NRTIs and NNRTIs: *Kidney International 60:821, 2001*
[2] **All doses IP unless indicated otherwise.**
   LD = loading dose, **MD** = maintenance dose, **ND** = no data; **NA** = not applicable—dose as normal renal function.
   Anuric = <100 mL per day, **non-anuric** = >100 mL per day
[3] **Does not provide treatment for MRSA.** If Gram-positive cocci on Gram stain, include vancomycin.
* *See page 2 for other abbreviations*

TABLE 20A – RECOMMENDED CHILDHOOD & ADOLESCENT IMMUNIZATION SCHEDULE: UNITED STATES (INCLUDES SCHEDULE FOR AGES 7-18), 2007 *(MMWR 55 Nos. 51&52: Q2–Q3, 2007)*

Recommended Immunization Schedule for Persons Aged 0–6 Years

Range of Recommended Ages		Catch-up Immunization		Certain High-risk Groups	

AGE ► VACCINE ▼	Birth	1 mo	2 mos	4 mos	6 mos	12 mos	15 mos	18 mos	19-23 mos	2-3 yrs	4-6 yrs
Hepatitis B[1]	HepB	HepB		see footnote 1		HepB				HepB Series	
Rotavirus[2]			Rota	Rota	Rota						
Diphtheria, Tetanus, Pertussis[3]			DTaP	DTaP	DTaP		DTaP				DTaP
Haemophilus influenzae type b[4]			Hib	Hib	Hib[4]	Hib			Hib		
Pneumococcal[5]			PCV	PCV	PCV	PCV				PCV	
										PPV	
Inactivated Poliovirus			IPV	IPV		IPV					IPV
Influenza[6]						Influenza (Yearly)					
Measles, Mumps, Rubella[7]						MMR					MMR
Varicella[8]						Varicella					Varicella
Hepatitis A[9]						HepA (2doses)				HepA Series	
Meningococcal[10]										MPSV4	

This schedule indicates the recommended ages for routine administration of currently licensed childhood vaccines, as of December 1, 2006, for children aged 0–6 years. Additional information is available at **http://www.cdc.gov/nip/recs/child-schedule.htm**. Any dose not administered at the recommended age should be administered at any subsequent visit, when indicated and feasible. Additional vaccines may be licensed and recommended during the year. Licensed combination vaccines may be used whenever any components of the combination are indicated and other components of the vaccine are not contraindicated and if approved by the Food and Drug Administration for that dose of the series. Providers should consult the respective Advisory Committee on Immunization Practices statement for detailed recommendations. Clinically significant adverse events that follow immunization should be reported to the Vaccine Adverse Event Reporting System (VAERS). Guidance about how to obtain and complete a VAERS form is available at **http://www.vaers.hhs.gov** or by telephone, **800-822-7967.**

1. Hepatitis B vaccine (HepB). *(Minimum age: birth)*
At birth:
- Administer monovalent HepB to all newborns before hospital discharge.
- If mother is hepatitis surface antigen (HBsAg)-positive, administer HepB and 0.5 mL of hepatitis B immune globulin (HBIG) within 12 hours of birth.
- If mother's HBsAg status is unknown, administer HepB within 12 hours of birth. Determine the HBsAg status as soon as possible and if HBsAg-positive, administer HBIG (no later than age 1 week).
- If mother is HBsAg-negative, the birth dose can only be delayed with physician's order and mothers' negative HBsAg laboratory report documented in the infant's medical record.

After the birth dose:
- The HepB series should be completed with either monovalent HepB or a combination vaccine containing HepB. The second dose should be administered at age 1–2 months. The final dose should be administered at age ≥24 weeks. Infants born to HBsAg-positive mothers should be tested for HBsAg and antibody to HBsAg after completion of ≥3 doses of a licensed HepB series, at age 9–18 months (generally at the next well-child visit).

4-month dose:
- It is permissible to administer 4 doses of HepB when combination vaccines are administered after the birth dose. If monovalent HepB is used for doses after the birth dose, a dose at age 4 months is not needed.

2. Rotavirus vaccine (Rota). *(Minimum age: 6 weeks)*
- Administer the first dose at age 6–12 weeks. Do not start the series later than age 12 weeks.
- Administer the final dose in the series by age 32 weeks. Do not administer a dose later than age 32 weeks.
- Data on safety and efficacy outside of these age ranges are insufficient.

TABLE 20A (2)

3. Diphtheria and tetanus toxoids and acellular pertussis vaccine (DTaP). *(Minimum age: 6 weeks)*
- The fourth dose of DTaP may be administered as early as age 12 months, provided 6 months have elapsed since the third dose.
- Administer the final dose in the series at age 4–6 years.

4. *Haemophilus influenzae* type b conjugate vaccine (Hib). *(Minimum age: 6 weeks)*
- If PRP-OMP (PedvaxHIB® or ComVax® [Merck]) is administered at ages 2 and 4 months, a dose at age 6 months is not required.
- TriHiBit® (DTaP/Hib) combination products should not be used for primary immunization but can be used as boosters following any Hib vaccine in children aged ≥12 months.

5. Pneumococcal vaccine. *(Minimum age: 6 weeks for pneumococcal conjugate vaccine [PCV]; 2 years for pneumococcal polysaccharide vaccine [PPV])*
- Administer PCV at ages 24–59 months in certain high-risk groups. Administer PPV to children aged ≥2 years in certain high-risk groups. See MMWR 2000;49 (No. RR-9):1–35.

6. Influenza vaccine. *(Minimum age: 6 months for trivalent inactivated influenza vaccine [TIV]; 5 years for live, attenuated influenza vaccine [LAIV])*
- All children aged 6–59 months and close contacts of all children aged 0–59 months are recommended to receive influenza vaccine.
- Influenza vaccine is recommended annually for children aged ≥59 months with certain risk factors, health-care workers, and other persons (including household members) in close contact with persons in groups at high risk. See MMWR 2006;55(No. RR-10):1–41.
- For healthy persons aged 5–49 years, LAIV may be used as an alternative to TIV.
- Children receiving TIV should receive 0.25 mL if aged 6–35 months or 0.5 mL if aged ≥3 years.
- Children aged <9 years who are receiving influenza vaccine for the first time should receive 2 doses (separated by ≥4 weeks for TIV and ≥6 weeks for LAIV).

7. Measles, mumps, and rubella vaccine (MMR). *(Minimum age: 12 months)*
- Administer the second dose of MMR at age 4–6 years. MMR may be administered before age 4–6 years, provided ≥4 weeks have elapsed since the first dose and both doses are administered at age ≥12 months.

8. Varicella vaccine. *(Minimum age: 12 months)*
- Administer the second dose of varicella vaccine at age 4–6 years. Varicella vaccine may be administered before age 4–6 years, provided that ≥3 months have elapsed since the first dose and both doses are administered at age ≥12 months. If second dose was administered ≥28 days following the first dose, the second dose does not need to be repeated.

9. Hepatitis A vaccine (HepA). *(Minimum age: 12 months)*
- HepA is recommended for all children aged 1 year (i.e., aged 12–23 months). The 2 doses in the series should be administered at least 6 months apart.
- Children not fully vaccinated by age 2 years can be vaccinated at subsequent visits.
- HepA is recommended for certain other groups of children, including in areas where vaccination programs target older children. See MMWR 2006;55(No. RR-7):1–23.

10. Meningococcal polysaccharide vaccine (MPSV4). *(Minimum age: 2 years)*
- Administer MPSV4 to children aged 2–10 years with terminal complement deficiencies or anatomic or functional asplenia and certain other high-risk groups. See MMWR 2005;54(No. RR-7):1–21.

Recommended Immunization Schedule for Persons Aged 7–18 Years

Range of Recommended Ages		Catch-up Immunization		Certain High-risk Groups	

AGE ► / VACCINE ▼	7-10 yrs	11-12 yrs	13-14 yrs	15 yrs	16-18 yrs
Tetanus, Diphtheria, Pertussis	see footnote 1	Tdap	Tdap		
Human Papillomavirus	see footnote 2	HPV (3 doses)	HPV Series		
Meningococcal	MPSV4	MCV4	MCV4	MCV4	
Pneumococcal		PPV			
Influenza		Influenza (Yearly)			
Hepatitis A		HepA Series			
Hepatitis B		HepB Series			
Inactivated Poliovirus		IPV Series			
Measles, Mumps, Rubella		MMR Series			
Varicella		Varicella Series			

This schedule indicates the recommended ages for routine administration of currently licensed childhood vaccines, as of December 1, 2006, for children aged 7–18 years. Additional information is available at http://www.cdc.gov/nip/recs/child-schedule.htm. Any dose not administered at the recommended age should be administered at any subsequent visit, when indicated and feasible. Additional vaccines may be licensed and

188

TABLE 20A (3)

recommended during the year. Licensed combination vaccines may be used whenever any components of the combination are indicated and other components of the vaccine are not contraindicated and if approved by the Food and Drug Administration for that dose of the series. Providers should consult the respective Advisory Committee on Immunization Practices statement for detailed recommendations. Clinically significant adverse events that follow immunization should be reported to the Vaccine Adverse Event Reporting System (VAERS). Guidance about how to obtain and complete a VAERS form is available at **http://www.vaers.hhs.gov** or by telephone, **800-822-7967.**

1. Tetanus and diphtheria toxoids and acellular pertussis vaccine (Tdap). *(Minimum age: 10 years for BOOSTRIX® and 11 years for ADACEL™)*
- Administer at age 11–12 years for those who have completed the recommended childhood DTP/DTaP vaccination series and have not received a tetanus and diphtheria toxoids vaccine (Td) booster dose.
- Adolescents aged 13–18 years who missed the 11–12 year Td/Tdap booster dose should also receive a single dose of Tdap if they have completed the recommended childhood DTP/DTaP vaccination series.

2. Human papillomavirus vaccine (HPV). *(Minimum age: 9 years)*
- Administer the first dose of the HPV vaccine series to females at age 11–12 years.
- Administer the second dose 2 months after the first dose and the third dose 6 months after the first dose.
- Administer the HPV vaccine series to females at age 13–18 years if not previously vaccinated.

3. Meningococcal vaccine. *(Minimum age: 11 years for meningococcal conjugate vaccine [MCV4]; 2 years for meningococcal polysaccharide vaccine [MPSV4])*
- Administer MCV4 at age 11–12 years and to previously unvaccinated adolescents at high school entry (at approximately age 15 years).
- Administer MCV4 to previously unvaccinated college freshmen living in dormitories; MPSV4 is an acceptable alternative.
- Vaccination against invasive meningococcal disease is recommended for children and adolescents aged ≥2 years with terminal complement deficiencies or anatomic or functional asplenia and certain other high-risk groups. See *MMWR* 2005;54(No. RR-7):1–21. Use MPSV4 for children aged 2–10 years and MCV4 or MPSV4 for older children.

4. Pneumococcal polysaccharide vaccine (PPV). *(Minimum age: 2 years)*
- Administer for certain high-risk groups. See *MMWR* 1997;46(No. RR-8):1–24, and *MMWR* 2000;49(No. RR-9):1–35.

5. Influenza vaccine. *(Minimum age: 6 months for trivalent inactivated influenza vaccine [TIV]; 5 years for live, attenuated influenza vaccine [LAIV])*
- Influenza vaccine is recommended annually for persons with certain risk factors, health-care workers, and other persons (including household members) in close contact with persons in groups at high risk. See *MMWR* 2006;55 (No. RR-10):1–41.
- For healthy persons aged 5–49 years, LAIV may be used as an alternative to TIV.
- Children aged <9 years who are receiving influenza vaccine for the first time should receive 2 doses (separated by ≥4 weeks for TIV and ≥6 weeks for LAIV).

6. Hepatitis A vaccine (HepA). *(Minimum age: 12 months)*
- The 2 doses in the series should be administered at least 6 months apart.
- HepA is recommended for certain other groups of children, including in areas where vaccination programs target older children. See *MMWR* 2006;55 (No. RR-7):1–23.

7. Hepatitis B vaccine (HepB). *(Minimum age: birth)*
- Administer the 3-dose series to those who were not previously vaccinated.
- A 2-dose series of Recombivax HB® is licensed for children aged 11–15 years.

8. Inactivated poliovirus vaccine (IPV). *(Minimum age: 6 weeks)*
- For children who received an all-IPV or all-oral poliovirus (OPV) series, a fourth dose is not necessary if the third dose was administered at age ≥4 years.
- If both OPV and IPV were administered as part of a series, a total of 4 doses should be administered, regardless of the child's current age.

9. Measles, mumps, and rubella vaccine (MMR). *(Minimum age: 12 months)*
- If not previously vaccinated, administer 2 doses of MMR during any visit, with ≥4 weeks between the doses.

10. Varicella vaccine. *(Minimum age: 12 months)*
- Administer 2 doses of varicella vaccine to persons without evidence of immunity.
- Administer 2 doses of varicella vaccine to persons aged <13 years at least 3 months apart. Do not repeat the second dose, if administered ≥28 days after the first dose.
- Administer 2 doses of varicella vaccine to persons aged ≥13 years at least 4 weeks apart.

TABLE 20B – CATCH-UP IMMUNIZATION SCHEDULE FOR PERSONS AGED 4 MONTHS–18 YEARS WHO START LATE OR WHO ARE ≥1 MONTH BEHIND — UNITED STATES, 2007

The table below provides catch-up schedules and minimum intervals between doses for children whose vaccinations have been delayed. A vaccine series does not need to be restarted, regardless of the time that has elapsed between doses. Use the section appropriate for the child's age.

Vaccine	Minimum Age for Dose 1	CATCH-UP SCHEDULE FOR PERSONS AGED 4 MONTHS–6 YEARS			
		Minimum Interval Between Doses			
		Dose 1 to Dose 2	Dose 2 to Dose 3	Dose 3 to Dose 4	Dose 4 to Dose 5
Hepatitis B[1]	Birth	4 weeks	8 weeks (and 16 weeks after first dose)		
Rotavirus[2]	6 weeks	4 weeks	4 weeks		
Diphtheria, Tetanus, Pertussis[3]	6 weeks	4 weeks	4 weeks	6 months	6 months[3]
Haemophilus influenzae type b[4]	6 weeks	4 weeks if first dose administered at age <12 months 8 weeks (as final dose) if first dose administered at age 12–14 months No further doses needed if first dose administered at age ≥15 months	4 weeks[4] if current age <12 months 8 weeks (as final dose)[4] if current age ≥12 months and second dose administered at age <15 months No further doses needed if previous dose administered at age ≥15 months	8 weeks (as final dose) This dose only necessary for children aged 12 months–5 years who received 3 doses before age 12 months	
Pneumococcal[5]	6 weeks	4 weeks if first dose administered at age <12 months and current age <24 months 8 weeks (as final dose) if first dose administered at age ≥12 months or current age 24–59 months No further doses needed for healthy children if first dose administered at age ≥24 months	4 weeks if current age <12 months 8 weeks (as final dose) if current age ≥12 months No further doses needed for healthy children if previous dose administered at age ≥24 months	8 weeks (as final dose) This dose only necessary for children aged 12 months–5 years who received 3 doses before age 12 months	
Inactivated Poliovirus[6]	6 weeks	4 weeks	4 weeks	4 weeks[6]	
Measles, Mumps, Rubella[7]	12 months	4 weeks			
Varicella[8]	12 months	3 months			
Hepatitis A[9]	12 months	6 months			
		CATCH-UP SCHEDULE FOR PERSONS AGED 7–18 YEARS			
Tetanus, Diphtheria/ Tetanus, Diphtheria, Pertussis[10]	7 years[10]	4 weeks	8 weeks if first dose administered at age <12 months 6 months if first dose administered at age ≥12 months	6 months if first dose administered at age <12 months	

TABLE 20B (2)

CATCH-UP SCHEDULE FOR PERSONS AGED 7-18 YEARS (continued)			12 weeks	
Human Papillomavirus[11] (Minimum age: 9 years)	9 years			
Hepatitis A[9] (Minimum age: 12 months)	12 months	6 months		
Hepatitis B[1] (Minimum age: 6 weeks)	Birth	4 weeks	8 weeks (and 16 weeks after first dose)	
Inactivated Poliovirus[6] (Minimum age: 6 weeks)	6 weeks	4 weeks	4 weeks	4 weeks[6]
Measles, Mumps, Rubella[3] (Minimum age: 12 months)	12 months	4 weeks		
Varicella[3] (Minimum age: 12 months)	12 months	4 weeks if first dose administered at ≥13 years / 3 months if first dose administered at age <13 years		

1. **Hepatitis B vaccine (HepB).** *(Minimum age: birth)*
- Administer the 3-dose series to those who were not previously vaccinated.
- A 2-dose series of Recombivax HB® is licensed for children aged 11-15 years.

2. **Rotavirus vaccine (Rota).** *(Minimum age: 6 weeks)*
Do not start the series later than age 12 weeks.
- Administer the final dose in the series by age 32 weeks. Do not administer a dose later than age 32 weeks.
- Data on safety and efficacy outside of these age ranges are insufficient.

3. **Diphtheria and tetanus toxoids and acellular pertussis vaccine (DTaP).** *(Minimum age: 6 weeks)*
- The fifth dose is not necessary if the fourth dose was administered at age ≥4 years.
- DTaP is not indicated for persons aged ≥7 years.

4. **Haemophilus influenzae type b conjugate vaccine (Hib).** *(Minimum age: 6 weeks)*
- Vaccine is not generally recommended for children aged ≥5 years.
- If current age <12 months and the first 2 doses were PRP-OMP (PedvaxHIB® or ComVax® [Merck]), the third (and final) dose should be administered at age 12-15 months and at least 8 weeks after the second dose.
- If first dose was administered at age 7-11 months, administer 2 doses separated by 4 weeks plus a booster at age 12-15 months.

5. **Pneumococcal conjugate vaccine (PCV).** *(Minimum age: 6 weeks)*
- Vaccine is not generally recommended for children aged ≥5 years.

6. **Inactivated poliovirus vaccine (IPV).** *(Minimum age: 6 weeks)*
- For children who received an all-IPV or all-oral poliovirus (OPV) series, a fourth dose is not necessary if third dose was administered at age ≥4 years.
- If both OPV and IPV were administered as part of a series, a total of 4 doses should be administered, regardless of the child's current age.

7. **Measles, mumps, and rubella vaccine (MMR).** *(Minimum age: 12 months)*
- The second dose of MMR is recommended routinely at age 4-6 years, but may be administered earlier if desired.
- If not previously vaccinated, administer 2 doses of MMR during any visit with ≥4 weeks between the doses.

8. **Varicella vaccine.** *(Minimum age: 12 months)*
- The second dose of varicella vaccine is recommended routinely at age 4-6 years but may be administered earlier if desired.
- Do not repeat the second dose in persons aged <13 years if administered ≥28 days after the first dose.

9. **Hepatitis A vaccine (HepA).** *(Minimum age: 12 months)*
- HepA is recommended for certain groups of children, including in areas where vaccination programs target older children. See *MMWR* 2006;55(No. RR-7):1-23

10. **Tetanus and diphtheria toxoids vaccine (Td) and tetanus and diphtheria toxoids and acellular pertussis vaccine (Tdap).** *(Minimum ages: 7 years for Td, 10 years for BOOSTRIX®, and 11 years for ADACEL™)*
- Tdap should be substituted for a single dose of Td in the primary catch-up series or as a booster if age appropriate; use Td for other doses.
- A 5-year interval from the last Td dose is encouraged when Tdap is used as a booster dose. A booster (fourth) dose is needed if any of the previous doses were administered at age <12 months. Refer to ACIP recommendations for further information. See *MMWR* 2006;55(No. RR-3).

11. **Human papillomavirus vaccine (HPV).** *(Minimum age: 9 years)*
- Administer the HPV vaccine series to females at age 13-18 years if not previously vaccinated.

Table 20C - ADULT IMMUNIZATION IN THE UNITED STATES
(MMWR 56 No.41:Q1–Q4, 2007) (Travelers: see Med Lett 38:17, 1006)

**Recommended Adult Immunization Schedule, by vaccine and age group —United States,
October 2007–September 2008**

Vaccine	Age group (years)		
	19–49	50–64	≥65
Tetanus, diphtheria, pertussis (Td/Tdap)[1]*	1 dose booster every 10 years		
	Substitute 1 dose of Tdap for Td		
Human papillomavirus (HPV)[2]*	3 doses (females) (0, 2, 6 mos)		
Measles, mumps, rubella (MMR)[3]*	1 or 2 doses	1 dose	
Varicella[4]*	2 doses (0, 4–8 weeks)		
Influenza[5]*	1 dose annually	1 dose annually	
Pneumococcal (polysaccharide)[6,7]	1–2 doses		1 dose
Hepatitis A[8]*	2 doses (0, 6–12 mos, or 0, 6–18 mos)		
Hepatitis B[9]*	3 doses (0, 1–2, 4–6 mos)		
Meningococcal[10]	1 or more doses		
Zoster[11]			1 dose

* Covered by the Vaccine Injury Compensation Program.

▇▇▇ For all persons in this category who meet the age requirements and who lack evidence of immunity (e.g., lack documentation of vaccination or have no evidence of prior infection)

▨▨▨ Recommended if some other risk factor is present (e.g., on the basis of medical, occupational, lifestyle, or other indications).

**NOTE: These recommendations must be read along with the footnotes.
Approved by the Advisory Committee on Immunization Practices (ACIP), the American Academy of Family Physicians, the American College of Obstetricians and Gynecologists, and the American College of Physicians. Complete statements from ACIP are available at http://www.cdc.gov/vaccines/pubs/acip-list.htm.**

1. Tetanus, diphtheria, and acellular pertussis (Td/Tdap) vaccination
Tdap should replace a single dose of Td for adults aged <65 years who have not previously received a dose of Tdap. Only one of two Tdap products (Adacel® [Sanofi Pasteur]) is licensed for use in adults.
Adults with uncertain histories of a complete primary vaccination series with tetanus and diphtheria toxoid-containing vaccines should begin or complete a primary vaccination series. A primary series for adults is 3 doses of tetanus and diphtheria toxoid-containing vaccines; administer the first 2 doses at least 4 weeks apart and the third dose 6–12 months after the second. However, Tdap can substitute for any one of the doses of Td in the 3-dose primary series. The booster dose of tetanus and diphtheria toxoid-containing vaccine should be administered to adults who have completed a primary series and if the last vaccination was received ≥10 years previously. Tdap or Td vaccine may be used, as indicated.
If the person is pregnant and received the last Td vaccination ≥10 years previously, administer Td during the second or third trimester; if the person received the last Td vaccination in <10 years, administer Tdap during the immediate postpartum period. A one-time administration of 1 dose of Tdap with an interval as short as 2 years from a previous Td vaccination is recommended for postpartum women, close contacts of infants aged <12 months, and all health-care workers with direct patient contact. In certain situations, Td can be deferred during pregnancy and Tdap substituted in the immediate postpartum period, or Tdap can be administered instead of Td to a pregnant woman after an informed discussion with the woman.
Consult the ACIP statement for recommendations for administering Td as prophylaxis in wound management.

2. Human papillomavirus (HPV) vaccination
HPV vaccination is recommended for all females aged ≤26 years who have not completed the vaccine series. History of genital warts, abnormal Papanicolaou test, or positive HPV DNA test is not evidence of prior infection with all known HPV types; HPV vaccination is still recommended for these persons.
Ideally, vaccine should be administered before potential exposure to HPV through sexual activity; however, females who are sexually active should still be vaccinated. Sexually active females who have not been infected with any of the HPV vaccine types receive the full benefit of the vaccination. Vaccination is less beneficial from females who have already been infected with one or more of the HPV vaccine types. A complete series consists of 3 doses. The second dose should be administered 2 months after the first dose; the third dose should be administered 6 months after the first dose.
Although HPV vaccination is not specifically recommended for females with the medical indications described in Figure 2, "Vaccines that might be indicated for adults based on medical and other indications," it is not a live-virus vaccine and can be administered. However, immune response and vaccine efficacy might be less than in persons who do not have the medical indications described or who are immunocompetent.

TABLE 20C (2)

3. Measles, mumps, rubella (MMR) vaccination

Measles component: adults born before 1957 can be considered immune to measles. Adults born during or after 1957 should receive ≥1 dose of MMR unless they have a medical contraindication, documentation of ≥1 dose, history of measles based on health-care provider diagnosis, or laboratory evidence of immunity.

A second dose of MMR is recommended for adults who 1) have been recently exposed to measles or are in an outbreak setting; 2) have been previously vaccinated with killed measles vaccine; 3) have been vaccinated with an unknown type of measles vaccine during 1963–1967; 4) are students in postsecondary educational institutions; 5) work in a health-care facility; or 6) plan to travel internationally.

Mumps component: adults born before 1957 can generally be considered immune to mumps. Adults born during or after 1957 should receive 1 dose of MMR unless they have a medical contraindication, history of mumps based on health-care provider diagnosis, or laboratory evidence of immunity.

A second dose of MMR is recommended for adults who 1) are in an age group that is affected during a mumps outbreak; 2) are students in postsecondary educational institutions; 3) work in a health-care facility; or 4) plan to travel internationally. For unvaccinated healthcare workers born before 1957 who do not have other evidence of mumps immunity, consider administering 1 dose on a routine basis and strongly consider administering a second dose during an outbreak.

Rubella component: administer 1 dose of MMR vaccine to women whose rubella vaccination history is unreliable or who lack laboratory evidence of immunity. For women of childbearing age, regardless of birth year, routinely determine rubella immunity and counsel women regarding congenital rubella syndrome. Women who do not have evidence of immunity should receive MMR vaccine on completion or termination of pregnancy and before discharge from the health-care facility.

4. Varicella vaccination

All adults without evidence of immunity to varicella should receive 2 doses of single-antigen varicella vaccine unless they have a medical contraindication. Special consideration should be given to those who 1) have close contact with persons at high risk for severe disease (e.g., health-care personnel and family contacts of immunocompromised persons) or 2) are at high risk for exposure or transmission (e.g., teachers; child care employees; residents and staff members of institutional settings, including correctional institutions; college students; military personnel; adolescents and adults living in households with children; nonpregnant women of childbearing age; and international travelers).

Evidence of immunity to varicella in adults includes any of the following: 1) documentation of 2 doses of varicella vaccine at least 4 weeks apart; 2) U.S.-born before 1980 (although for health-care personnel and pregnant women, birth before 1980 should not be considered evidence of immunity); 3) history of varicella based on diagnosis or verification of varicella by a health-care provider (for a patient reporting a history of or presenting with an atypical case, a mild case, or both, health-care providers should seek either an epidemiologic link with a typical varicella case or to a laboratory-confirmed case or evidence of laboratory confirmation, if it was performed at the time of acute disease); 4) history of herpes zoster based on health-care provider diagnosis; or 5) laboratory evidence of immunity or laboratory confirmation of disease. Assess pregnant women for evidence of varicella immunity. Women who do not have evidence of immunity should receive the first dose of varicella vaccine upon completion or termination of pregnancy and before discharge from the health-care facility. The second dose should be administered 4–8 weeks after the first dose.

5. Influenza vaccination

Medical indications: chronic disorders of the cardiovascular or pulmonary systems, including asthma; chronic metabolic diseases, including diabetes mellitus, renal or hepatic dysfunction, hemoglobinopathies, or immunosuppression (including immunosuppression caused by medications or human immunodeficiency virus [HIV]); any condition that compromises respiratory function or the handling of respiratory secretions or that can increase the risk of aspiration (e.g., cognitive dysfunction, spinal cord injury, or seizure disorder or other neuromuscular disorder); and pregnancy during the influenza season. No data exist on the risk for severe or complicated influenza disease among persons with asplenia; however, influenza is a risk factor for secondary bacterial infections that can cause severe disease among persons with asplenia.

Occupational indications: health-care personnel and employees of long-term–care and assisted-living facilities. *Other indications:* residents of nursing homes and other long-term–care and assisted-living facilities; persons likely to transmit influenza to persons at high risk (e.g., in-home household contacts and caregivers of children aged 0–59 months, or persons of all ages with high-risk conditions); and anyone who would like to be vaccinated. Healthy, nonpregnant adults aged ≤49 years without high-risk medical conditions who are not contacts of severely immunocompromised persons in special care units can receive either intranasally administered live, attenuated influenza vaccine (FluMist®) or inactivated vaccine. Other persons should receive the inactivated vaccine.

6. Pneumococcal polysaccharide vaccination

Medical indications: chronic pulmonary disease (excluding asthma); chronic cardiovascular diseases; diabetes mellitus; chronic liver diseases, including liver disease as a result of alcohol abuse (e.g., cirrhosis); chronic alcoholism, chronic renal failure, or nephrotic syndrome; functional or anatomic asplenia (e.g., sickle cell disease or splenectomy [if elective splenectomy is planned, vaccinate at least 2 weeks before surgery]); immunosuppressive conditions; and cochlear implants and cerebrospinal fluid leaks. Vaccinate as close to HIV diagnosis as possible.

Other indications: Alaska Natives and certain American Indian populations and residents of nursing homes or other long-term–care facilities.

7. Revaccination with pneumococcal polysaccharide vaccine

One-time revaccination after 5 years for persons with chronic renal syndrome; functional or anatomic asplenia (e.g., sickle cell disease or splenectomy); or immunosuppressive conditions. For persons aged ≥65 years, one-time revaccination if they were vaccinated ≥5 years previously and were aged <65 years at the time of primary vaccination.

8. Hepatitis A vaccination

Medical indications: persons with chronic liver disease and persons who receive clotting factor concentrates.

Behavioral indications: men who have sex with men and persons who use illegal drugs.

Occupational indications: persons working with hepatitis A virus (HAV)-infected primates or with HAV in a research laboratory setting.

TABLE 20C (3)

Other indications: persons traveling to or working in countries that have high or intermediate endemicity of hepatitis A (a list of countries is available at http://wwwn.cdc.gov/travel/contentdiseases.aspx) and any person seeking protection from HAV infection.

Single-antigen vaccine formulations should be administered in a 2-dose schedule at either 0 and 6–12 months (Havrix®), or 0 and 6–18 months (Vaqta®). If the combined hepatitis A and hepatitis B vaccine (Twinrix®) is used, administer 3 doses at 0, 1, and 6 months.

9. Hepatitis B vaccination

Medical indications: persons with end-stage renal disease, including patients receiving hemodialysis; persons seeking evaluation or treatment for a sexually transmitted disease (STD); persons with HIV infection; and persons with chronic liver disease.

Occupational indications: health-care personnel and public-safety workers who are exposed to blood or other potentially infectious body fluids.

Behavioral indications: sexually active persons who are not in a long-term, mutually monogamous relationship (e.g., persons with more than one sex partner during the previous 6 months); current or recent injection-drug users; and men who have sex with men.

Other indications: household contacts and sex partners of persons with chronic hepatitis B virus (HBV) infection; clients and staff members of institutions for persons with developmental disabilities; international travelers to countries with high or intermediate prevalence of chronic HBV infection (a list of countries is available at http://wwwn.cdc.gov/travel/contentdiseases.aspx); and any adult seeking protection from HBV infection.

Settings where hepatitis B vaccination is recommended for all adults: STD treatment facilities; HIV testing and treatment facilities; facilities providing drug-abuse treatment and prevention services; health-care settings targeting services to injection-drug users or men who have sex with men; correctional facilities; end-stage renal disease programs and facilities for chronic hemodialysis patients; and institutions and nonresidential day care facilities for persons with developmental disabilities.

Special formulation indications: for adult patients receiving hemodialysis and other immunocompromised adults. 1 dose of 40 μg/mL (Recombivax HB®) or 2 doses of 20 μg/mL (Engerix-B®) administered simultaneously.

10. Meningococcal vaccination

Medical indications: adults with anatomic or functional asplenia or terminal complement component deficiencies.

Other indications: first-year college students living in dormitories; microbiologists who are routinely exposed to isolates of *Neisseria meningitidis*; military recruits; and persons who travel to or live in countries in which meningococcal disease is hyperendemic or epidemic (e.g., the "meningitis belt" of sub-Saharan Africa during the dry season [December–June]), particularly if their contact with local populations will be prolonged. Vaccination is required by the government of Saudi Arabia for all travelers to Mecca during the annual Hajj.

Meningococcal conjugate vaccine is preferred for adults with any of the preceding indications who are aged ≤55 years, although meningococcal polysaccharide vaccine (MPSV4) is an acceptable alternative. Revaccination after 3–5 years might be indicated for adults previously vaccinated with MPSV4 who remain at increased risk for infection (e.g., persons residing in areas in which disease is epidemic).

11. Herpes zoster vaccination

A single dose of zoster vaccine is recommended for adults aged ≥60 years regardless of whether they report a prior episode of herpes zoster. Persons with chronic medical conditions may be vaccinated unless a contraindication or precaution exists for their condition.

12. Selected conditions for which *Haemophilus influenzae* type b (Hib) vaccine may be used

Hib conjugate vaccines are licensed for children aged 6 weeks–71 months. No efficacy data are available on which to base a recommendation concerning use of Hib vaccine for older children and adults with the chronic conditions associated with an increased risk for Hib disease. However, studies suggest good immunogenicity in patients who have sickle cell disease, leukemia, or HIV infection or who have had splenectomies; administering vaccine to these patients is not contraindicated.

13. Immunocompromising conditions

Inactivated vaccines generally are acceptable (e.g., pneumococcal, meningococcal, and influenza [trivalent inactivated influenza vaccine]) and live vaccines generally are avoided in persons with immune deficiencies or immune suppressive conditions. Information on specific conditions is available at http://www.cdc.gov/vaccines/pubs/acip-list.htm.

This schedule indicates the recommended age groups and medical indications for routine administration of currently licensed vaccines for persons aged ≥19 years, as of October 1, 2007. Licensed combination vaccines may be used whenever any components of the combination are indicated and when the vaccine's other components are not contraindicated. For detailed recommendations on all vaccines, including those used primarily for travelers or those issued during the year, consult the manufacturers' package inserts and the complete statements from the Advisory Committee on Immunization Practices (available at http://www.cdc.gov/vaccines/pubs/acip.htm).

Report all clinically significant postvaccination reactions to the Vaccine Adverse Event Reporting System (VAERS). Reporting forms and instructions on filing a VAERS report are available at http://www.vaers.hhs.gov or by telephone, 800-822-7967.

Information on how to file a Vaccine Injury Compensation Program claim is available at http://www.hrsa.gov/vaccinecompensation or by telephone, 800-338-2382. To file a claim for vaccine injury, contact the U.S. Court of Federal Claims, 717 Madison Place, N.W., Washington, D.C. 20005; telephone, 202-357-6400.

Use of trade names and commercial sources is for identification only and does not imply endorsement by the U.S. Department of Health and Human Services.

194

TABLE 20C (4)

Vaccines that might be indicated for adults based on medical and other indications — United States, October 2007– September 2008

Vaccine	Pregnancy	Immuno-compromising conditions (excluding human immunodeficiency virus [HIV]), medications, radiation[13]	HIV infection[1,12,13] CD4+ T lymphocyte count <200 cells/µL	HIV infection[1,12,13] CD4+ T lymphocyte count ≥200 cells/µL	Diabetes, heart disease, chronic pulmonary disease, chronic alcoholism	Asplenia[12] (including elective splenectomy and terminal complement component deficiencies)	Chronic liver disease	Kidney failure, end-stage renal disease, receipt of hemodialysis	Health-care personnel
Tetanus, diphtheria, pertussis (Td/Tdap)*,[11]	1 dose Td booster every 10 yrs								
	Substitute 1 dose of Tdap for Td								
Human papillomavirus (HPV)*	3 doses for females through age 26 yrs (0, 2, 6 mos)								
Measles, mumps, rubella (MMR)*	Contraindicated		Contraindicated	1 or 2 doses					
Varicella*	Contraindicated		Contraindicated	2 doses (0, 4-8 wks)					
Influenza*	1 dose TIV annually				1 dose TIV annually	1-2 doses			1 dose TIV or LAIV annually
Pneumococcal (polysaccharide)[6,7]				1-2 doses					
Hepatitis A*				2 doses (0, 6-12 mos, or 0, 6-18 mos)					
Hepatitis B*				3 doses (0, 1-2, 4-6 mos)					
Meningococcal[9]*				1 or more doses					
Zoster[11]	Contraindicated				1 dose				

* Covered by the Vaccine Injury Compensation Program.

For all persons in this category who meet the age requirements and who lack evidence of immunity (e.g., lack documentation of vaccination or have no evidence of prior infection)

Recommended if some other risk factor is present (e.g., on the basis of medical, occupational, lifestyle, or other indications)

TABLE 20D – ANTI-TETANUS PROPHYLAXIS, WOUND CLASSIFICATION, IMMUNIZATION

WOUND CLASSIFICATION			IMMUNIZATION SCHEDULE				
Clinical Features	Tetanus Prone	Non-Tetanus Prone	History of Tetanus Immunization	Dirty, Tetanus-Prone Wound		Clean, Non-Tetanus Prone Wound	
				Td[1,2]	TIG	Td	TIG
Age of wound	> 6 hours	≤ 6 hours					
Configuration	Stellate, avulsion	Linear	Unknown or < 3 doses	Yes	Yes	Yes	No
Depth	> 1 cm	≤ 1 cm	3 or more doses	No[3]	No	No[4]	No

Mechanism of injury	Missile, crush, burn, frostbite	Sharp surface (glass, knife)	[1] Td = Tetanus & diphtheria toxoids adsorbed (adult)
			   TIG = Tetanus immune globulin (human)
			[2] Yes if wound >24hr old.
			   For children <7yr, DPT (DT if pertussis vaccine
			   contraindicated);			

Devitalized tissue	Present	Absent					
Contaminants (dirt, saliva, etc.)	Present	Absent	For persons ≥7yr, Td preferred to tetanus toxoid alone. [3] Yes if >5 years since last booster [4] Yes if >10 years since last booster			
(From ACS Bull. 69:22,23, 1984, No. 10)			*[From MMWR 39:37, 1990; MMWR 46(SS-2):15, 1997]*				

TABLE 20E –RABIES POST-EXPOSURE PROPHYLAXIS
All wounds should be cleaned immediately & thoroughly with soap & water. This has been shown
to protect 90% of experimental animals![1]

Post-Exposure Prophylaxis Guide, United States, 2000
(CID 30:4, 2000; NEJM 351:2626, 2004; MMWR 56:RR-3, 2007)

Animal Type	Evaluation & Disposition of Animal	Recommendations for Prophylaxis
Dogs, cats, ferrets	Healthy & available for 10-day observation	Don't start unless animal develops sx, then immediately begin HRIG + HDCV or RVA
	Rabid or suspected rabid	Immediate vaccination
	Unknown (escaped)	Consult public health officials
Skunks, raccoons, bats,[*] foxes, coyotes, most carnivores	Regard as rabid	Immediate vaccination
Livestock, rodents, rabbits; includes hares, squirrels, hamsters, guinea pigs, gerbils, chipmunks, rats, mice, woodchucks		Almost never require anti-rabies rx. Consult public health officials.

[*] Most recent cases of human rabies in U.S. due to contact (not bites) with silver-haired bats or rarely big brown bats (*MMWR 46:770, 1997; AnIM 128:922, 1998*). For more detail, see *CID 30:4, 2000; JAVMA 219:1687, 2001; CID 37:96, 2003 (travel medicine advisory); Ln 363:959, 2004; EID 11:1921, 2005; MMWR 55 (RR-5), 2006.*

Post-Exposure Rabies Immunization Schedule
IF NOT PREVIOUSLY VACCINATED

Treatment	Regimen[2]
Local wound cleaning	**All post-exposure treatment should begin with immediate, thorough cleaning of all wounds with soap & water.**
Human rabies immune globulin (HRIG)	20 units per kg body weight given once on day 0. If anatomically feasible, the full dose should be infiltrated around the wound(s), the rest should be administered IM in the gluteal area. HRIG should **not** be administered in the **same syringe, or** into the **same anatomical site** as vaccine, or more than 7 days after the initiation of vaccine. Because HRIG may partially suppress active production of antibody, no more than the recommended dose should be given.[3]
Vaccine	Human diploid cell vaccine (HDCV), rabies vaccine adsorbed (RVA), or purified chick embryo cell vaccine (PCEC) 1.0 mL **IM (deltoid area[4])**, one each days 0, 3, 7, 14, & 28.

IF PREVIOUSLY VACCINATED[5]

Treatment	Regimen[2]
Local wound cleaning	All post-exposure treatment should begin with immediate, thorough cleaning of all wounds with soap & water.
HRIG	HRIG should **not** be administered
Vaccine	HDCV, RVA or PCEC, 1.0 mL **IM (deltoid area[4])**, one each on days 0 & 3

CORRECT VACCINE ADMINISTRATION SITES

Age Group	Administration Site
Children & adults	**DELTOID[4]** only (**NEVER** in gluteus)
Infants & young children	Outer aspect of thigh (anterolateral thigh) may be used (**NEVER** in gluteus)

[1] From *MMWR 48:RR-1, 1999; CID 30:4, 2000;* B.T. Matyas, Mass. Dept. of Public Health
[2] These regimens are applicable for all age groups, including children.
[3] In most reported post-exposure treatment failures, only identified deficiency was failure to infiltrate wound(s) with HRIG (*CID 22:228, 1996*). However, several failures reported from SE Asia in patients in whom WHO protocol followed (*CID 28:143, 1999*).
[4] The **deltoid** area is the **only** acceptable site of vaccination for adults & older children. For infants & young children, outer aspect of the thigh (anterolateral thigh) may be used. Vaccine should **NEVER** be administered in gluteal area.
[5] Any person with a history of pre-exposure vaccination with HDCV, RVA, PCEC; prior post-exposure prophylaxis with HDCV, RVA, PCEC; or previous vaccination with any other type of rabies vaccine & a documented history of antibody response to the prior vaccination

TABLE 21 SELECTED DIRECTORY OF RESOURCES

ORGANIZATION	PHONE/FAX	WEBSITE(S)
ANTIPARASITIC DRUGS & PARASITOLOGY INFORMATION *(CID 37:694, 2003)*		
CDC Drug Line	Weekdays: 404-639-3670	www.cdc.gov/ncidod/srp/drugs/drug-service.html
	Evenings, weekends, holidays: 404-639-2888	
DPDx: Lab ID of parasites		www.dpd.cdc.gov/dpdx/default.htm
Gorgas Course Tropical Medicine		http://info.dom.uab.edu/gorgas
Malaria	daytime: 770-488-7788	www.cdc.gov/malaria
	other: 770-488-7100	
Panorama Compound. Pharm.	800-247-9767/818-787-7256	www.uniquerx.com
World Health Organization (WHO)		www.who.org
Parasites & Health		www.dpd.cdc.gov/dpdx/HTML/Para_Health.htm
BIOTERRORISM		
Centers for Disease Control & Prevention	770-488-7100	www.bt.cdc.gov
Infectious Diseases Society of America	703-299-0200	www.idsociety.org
Johns Hopkins Center Civilian Biodefense		www.jhsph.edu
Center for Biosecurity of the Univ. of Pittsburgh Med. Center		www.upmc-biosecurity.org
US Army Medical Research Institute of Inf. Dis.		www.usamriid.army.mil
HEPATITIS B		
ACT-HBV		www.act-hbv.com
HEPATITIS C *(CID 35:754, 2002)*		
CDC		www.cdc.gov/ncidod/diseases/hepatitis/C
Individual		http://hepatitis-central.com
Medscape		www.medscape.com
HIV		
General		
HIV InSite		http://hivinsite.ucsf.edu
Johns Hopkins AIDS Service		www.hopkins-aids.edu
Drug Interactions		
Johns Hopkins AIDS Service		www.hopkins-aids.edu
Liverpool HIV Pharm. Group		www.hiv-druginteractions.org
Other		http://AIDS.medscape.com
Prophylaxis/Treatment of Opportunistic Infections; HIV Treatment		www.aidsinfo.nih.gov
IMMUNIZATIONS *(CID 36:355, 2003)*		
CDC, Natl. Immunization Program	404-639-8200	www.cdc.gov/vaccines/
FDA, Vaccine Adverse Events	800-822-7967	www.fda.gov/cber/vaers/vaers.htm
National Network Immunization Info.	877-341-6644	www.immunizationinfo.org
Influenza vaccine, CDC	404-639-8200	www.cdc.gov/vaccines/
Institute for Vaccine Safety		www.vaccinesafety.edu
OCCUPATIONAL EXPOSURE, BLOOD-BORNE PATHOGENS (HIV, HEPATITIS B & C)		
National Clinicians' Post-Exposure Hotline	888-448-4911	www.ucsf.edu/hivcntr
Q-T$_c$ INTERVAL PROLONGATION BY DRUGS		www.qtdrugs.org
SEXUALLY TRANSMITTED DISEASES		www.cdc.gov/std/treatment/TOC2002TG.htm
		Slides: http://www.phac-aspc.gc.ca/slm-maa/slides/index.html
TRAVELERS' INFO: Immunizations, Malaria Prophylaxis, More		
Amer. Soc. Trop. Med. & Hyg.		www.astmh.org
CDC, general	877-394-8747/888-232-3299	http://wwwn.cdc.gov/travel/default.asp
CDC, Malaria:		www.cdc.gov/malaria
Prophylaxis		http://wwwn.cdc.gov/travel/default.asp
Treatment	770-488-7788	www.who.int/health_topics/malaria
MD Travel Health		www.mdtravelhealth.com
Pan American Health Organization		www.paho.org
World Health Organization (WHO)		www.who.int/home-page
VACCINE & IMMUNIZATION RESOURCES *(CID 36:355, 2003)*		
American Academy of Pediatrics		www.cispimmunize.org
CDC, National Immunization Program		www.cdc.gov/vaccines/
National Network for Immunization Information		www.immunizationinfo.org

TABLE 22A – ANTI-INFECTIVE DRUG-DRUG INTERACTIONS
Importance: ± = theory/anecdotal; + = of probable importance; ++ = of definite importance

ANTI-INFECTIVE AGENT (A)	OTHER DRUG (B)	EFFECT	IMPORT
Amantadine (Symmetrel)	Alcohol	↑ CNS effects	+
	Anticholinergic and anti-Parkinson agents (ex. Artane, scopolamine)	↑ effect of B: dry mouth, ataxia, blurred vision, slurred speech, toxic psychosis	+
	Trimethoprim	↑ levels of A & B	+
	Digoxin	↑ levels of B	±
Aminoglycosides—parenteral (amikacin, gentamicin, kanamycin, netilmicin, sisomicin, streptomycin, tobramycin)	Amphotericin B	↑ nephrotoxicity	++
	Cis platinum (Platinol)	nephro & ototoxicity	+
	Cyclosporine	↑ nephrotoxicity	+
	Neuromuscular blocking agents	apnea or respiratory paralysis	+
	Loop diuretics (e.g., furosemide)	↑ ototoxicity	++
	NSAIDs	↑ nephrotoxicity	+
	Non-polarizing muscle relaxants	↑ apnea	+
	Radiographic contrast	↑ nephrotoxicity	+
	Vancomycin	↑ nephrotoxicity	+
Aminoglycosides—oral (kanamycin, neomycin)	**Oral anticoagulants (dicumarol, phenindione, warfarin)**	↑ prothrombin time	+
Amphotericin B and ampho B lipid formulations	Antineoplastic drugs	↑ nephrotoxicity risk	+
	Digitalis	toxicity of B if K⁺ ↓	+
	Nephrotoxic drugs: aminoglyco- sides, cidofovir, cyclosporine, fos- carnet, pentamidine	↑ nephrotoxicity of A	++
Ampicillin, amoxicillin	Allopurinol	↑ frequency of rash	++
Fosamprenavir	Antiretrovirals—see Table 22B & Table 22C		
	Contraceptives, oral	↓ levels of A & B; use other contraception	++
	Lovastatin/simvastatin	↑ levels of B—avoid	++
	Methadone	↓ levels of A & B	++
	Rifabutin	↑ levels of B (↓ dose by 50–75%)	++
	Rifampin	↓ levels of A—avoid	++
Atazanavir	See protease inhibitors and Table 22B & Table 22C		
Atovaquone	Rifampin (perhaps rifabutin)	↓ serum levels of A; ↑ levels of B	+
	Metoclopramide	↓ levels of A	+
	Tetracycline	↓ levels of A	++

Azole Antifungal Agents¹ [Flu = fluconazole, Itr = itraconazole, Ket = ketoconazole, Posa = posaconazole Vor = voriconazole, + = occurs, blank space = either studied & no interaction OR no data found (may be in pharm. co. databases)]

Flu	Itr	Ket	Posa	Vor			
+	+				Amitriptyline	↑ levels of B	+
+	+	+		+	Calcium channel blockers	↑ levels of B	++
	+	+			Carbamazepine (vori contraind)	↓ levels of A	++
+	+	+	+	+	Cyclosporine	↑ levels of B, ↑ risk of nephrotoxicity	+
	+				Didanosine	↓ absorption of A	+
+	+			+	Efavirenz	↓ levels of A, ↑ levels of B	++ (avoid)
	+	+	+	+	H₂ blockers, antacids, sucralfate	↓ absorption of A	+
+	+	+	+	+	Hydantoins (phenytoin, Dilantin)	↑ levels of B, ↓ levels of A	++
+	+	+			Isoniazid	↓ levels of A	+
			+	+	Lovastatin/simvastatin	Rhabdomyolysis reported; ↑ levels of B	++
					Methadone	↑ levels of B	+
+	+	+	+	+	Midazolam/triazolam, po	↑ levels of B	++
+	+	+	+	+	Oral anticoagulants	↑ effect of B	++
+	+	+			Oral hypoglycemics	↑ levels of B	++
			+	+	Pimozide	↑ levels of B—avoid	++
	+	+	+		Protease inhibitors	↑ levels of B	++
	+	+	+		Proton pump inhibitors	↓ absorption of A, ↑ levels of B	++
+	+	+	+	+	Rifampin/rifabutin (vori contraindi- cated)	↑ levels of B, ↓ serum levels of A	++
				+	Sirolimus (vori contraindicated)	↑ levels of B	++
+		+	+	+	Tacrolimus	↑ levels of B with toxicity	++
+	+				Theophyllines	↑ levels of B	+
	+	+	+		Trazodone	↑ levels of B	++
+					Zidovudine	↑ levels of B	+
Caspofungin					Cyclosporine	↑ levels of A	++
					Tacrolimus	↓ levels of B	++
					Carbamazepine, dexamethasone, efavirenz, nevirapine, phenytoin, rifamycin	↓ levels of A; ↑ dose of caspofungin to 70 mg/d	++

¹ Major interactions given; unusual or minor interactions manifest as toxicity of non-azole drug due to ↑ serum levels: Caffeine (Flu), digoxin (Itr), felodipine (Itr), fluoxetine (Itr), indinavir (Ket), lovastatin/simvastatin, quinidine (Ket), tricyclics (Flu), vincristine (Itr), and ↓ effectiveness of oral contraceptives.

TABLE 22A (2)

ANTI-INFECTIVE AGENT (A)	OTHER DRUG (B)	EFFECT	IMPORT
Cephalosporins with methyl-tetrathiozolethiol side-chain	Oral anticoagulants (dicumarol, warfarin), heparin, thrombolytic agents, platelet aggregation inhibitors	↑ effects of B, bleeding	+
Chloramphenicol	Hydantoins	↑ toxicity of B, nystagmus, ataxia	++
	Iron salts, Vitamin B12	↓ response to B	++
	Protease inhibitors—HIV	↑ levels of A & B	++
Clindamycin (Cleocin)	Kaolin	↓ absorption of A	+
	Muscle relaxants, e.g., atracurium, baclofen, diazepam	↑ frequency/duration of respiratory paralysis	+
Cycloserine	Ethanol	↑ frequency of seizures	+
	INH, ethionamide	↑ frequency of drowsiness/dizziness	+
Dapsone	Didanosine	↓ absorption of A	+
	Oral contraceptives	↓ effectiveness of B	+
	Pyrimethamine	↑ in marrow toxicity	+
	Rifampin/Rifabutin	↓ serum levels of A	+
	Trimethoprim	↑ levels of A & B (methemoglobinemia)	+
	Zidovudine	May ↑ marrow toxicity	+
Daptomycin	HMG-CoA inhibitors (statins)	DC statin while on dapto	++
Delavirdine (Rescriptor)	See non-nucleoside reverse transcriptase inhibitors (NNRTIs) and Table 22C		
Didanosine (ddI) (Videx)	Allopurinol	↑ levels of A—**AVOID**	++
	Cisplatin, dapsone, INH, metronidazole, nitrofurantoin, stavudine, vincristine, zalcitabine	↑ risk of peripheral neuropathy	+
	Ethanol, lamivudine, pentamidine	↑ risk of pancreatitis	+
	Fluoroquinolones	↓ absorption 2° to chelation	+
	Drugs that need low pH for absorption: dapsone, indinavir, itra/ketoconazole, pyrimethamine, rifampin, trimethoprim	↓ absorption	+
	Methadone	↓ levels of A	++
	Ribavirin	↑ levels ddI metabolite—**avoid**	++
	Tenofovir	↑ levels of A **(reduce dose of A)**	++
Doripenem	Probenecid	↑ levels of A	++
	Valproic acid	↓ levels of B	++
Doxycycline	Aluminum, bismuth, iron, Mg⁺⁺	↓ absorption of A	+
	Barbiturates, hydantoins	↓ serum t½ of A	+
	Carbamazepine (Tegretol)	↓ serum t½ of A	+
	Digoxin	↑ serum levels of B	+
	Warfarin	↑ activity of B	++
Efavirenz (Sustiva)	See non-nucleoside reverse transcriptase inhibitors (NNRTIs) and Table 22C		
Ertapenem (Invanz)	Probenecid	↑ levels of A	+
Ethambutol (Myambutol)	Aluminum salts (includes didanosine buffer)	↓ absorption of A & B	+

Fluoroquinolones (**Cipro** = ciprofloxacin; **Gati** = gatifloxacin; **Gemi** = gemifloxacin; **Levo** = levofloxacin; **Moxi** = moxifloxacin; **Oflox** = ofloxacin)
NOTE: Blank space = either studied and no interaction OR no data found (pharm. co. may have data)

Cipro	Gati	Gemi	Levo	Moxi	Oflox		EFFECT	IMPORT
+	+	+	+			Antiarrhythmics (procainamide, amiodarone)	↑ Q-T interval (torsade)	++
+	+	+	+	+	+	Insulin, oral hypoglycemics	↑ & ↓ blood sugar	++
+						Caffeine	↑ levels of B	+
+				+		Cimetidine	↑ levels of A	+
+		+			+	Cyclosporine	↑ levels of B	±
+	+	+			+	Didanosine	↓ absorption of A	++
+	+	+	+	+	+	Cations: Al+++, Ca++, Fe++, Mg++, Zn++ (antacids, vitamins, dairy products), citrate/citric acid	↓ absorption of A (some variability between drugs)	++
+						Foscarnet	↑ risk of seizures	+
+					+	Methadone	↑ levels of B	++
+		+			+	NSAIDs	↑ risk CNS stimulation/seizures	++
+						Phenytoin	↑ or ↓ levels of B	++
+	+	+			+	Probenecid	↓ renal clearance of A	+
+						Rasagiline	↑ levels of B	++
				+		Rifampin	↓ levels of A (CID 45:1001, 2007)	++
+	+	+	+		+	Sucralfate	↓ absorption of A	++
+						Theophylline	↑ levels of B	++
+						Thyroid hormone	↓ levels of B	++
+						Tizanidine	↑ levels of B	++
+		+			+	Warfarin	↑ prothrombin time	++
Foscarnet (Foscavir)						Ciprofloxacin	↑ risk of seizures	+
						Nephrotoxic drugs: aminoglycosides, ampho B, cis-platinum, cyclosporine	↑ risk of nephrotoxicity	+
						Pentamidine IV	↑ risk of severe hypocalcemia	++

200

TABLE 22A (3)

ANTI-INFECTIVE AGENT (A)	OTHER DRUG (B)	EFFECT	IMPORT
Ganciclovir (Cytovene) & **Valganciclovir** (Valcyte)	Imipenem	↑ risk of seizures reported	+
	Probenecid	↑ levels of A	+
	Zidovudine	↓ levels of A, ↑ levels of B	+
Gentamicin	*See Aminoglycosides—parenteral*		
Indinavir	*See protease inhibitors and Table 22B & Table 22C*		
Isoniazid	**Alcohol, rifampin**	**↑ risk of hepatic injury**	++
	Aluminum salts	↓ absorption (take fasting)	++
	Carbamazepine, phenytoin	↑ levels of B with nausea, vomiting, nystagmus, ataxia	++
	Itraconazole, ketoconazole	↓ levels of B	+
	Oral hypoglycemics	↓ effects of B	+
Lamivudine	Zalcitabine	**Mutual interference—do not combine**	++
Linezolid (Zyvox)	Adrenergic agents	Risk of hypertension	++
	Aged, fermented, pickled or smoked foods —↑ tyramine	Risk of hypertension	+
	Rasagiline (MAO inhibitor)	Risk of serotonin syndrome	+
	Rifampin	↓ levels of A	++
	Serotonergic drugs (SSRIs)	Risk of serotonin syndrome	++
Lopinavir	*See protease inhibitors*		

Macrolides *[Ery = erythromycin, Azi = azithromycin, Clr = clarithromycin; Dir = dirithromycin; + = occurs, blank space = either studied and no interaction OR no data (pharm. co. may have data)]*

Ery	Dir	Azi	Clr			
+	+		+	Carbamazepine	↑ serum levels of B, nystagmus, nausea, vomiting, ataxia	++ (avoid w/ erythro)
+			+	Cimetidine, **ritonavir**	↑ levels of B	+
+			+	Clozapine	↑ serum levels of B, CNS toxicity	+
			+	Colchicine	**↑ levels of B (potent, fatal)**	++ (avoid)
+				Corticosteroids	↑ effects of B	+
+	+	+	+	Cyclosporine	↑ serum levels of B with toxicity	+
+	+	+	+	Digoxin, digitoxin	↑ serum levels of B (10% of cases)	+
			+	Efavirenz	↓ levels of A	++
+	+		+	Ergot alkaloids	↑ levels of B	++
+	+		+	Lovastatin/simvastatin	↑ levels of B; rhabdomyolysis	++
+			+	Midazolam, triazolam	↑ levels of B, ↑ sedative effects	+
+	+		+	Phenytoin	↑ levels of B	+
+		+	+	Pimozide	**↑ Q-T interval**	++
+			+	Rifampin, rifabutin	↓ levels of A	+
+	+		+	Tacrolimus	↑ levels of B	++
+			+	Theophylline	↑ serum levels of B with nausea, vomiting, seizures, apnea	++
+	+		+	Valproic acid	↑ levels of B	+
+	+		+	Warfarin	May ↑ prothrombin time	+
			+	Zidovudine	↓ levels of B	+

ANTI-INFECTIVE AGENT (A)	OTHER DRUG (B)	EFFECT	IMPORT
Maraviroc	Clarithromycin	↑ serum levels of A	++
	Delavirdine	↑ levels of A	++
	Itaconazole/ketoconazole	↑ levels of A	++
	Nefazodone	↑ levels of A	++
	Protease Inhibitors (not tipranavir/ritonavir)	↑ levels of A	++
	Anticonvulsants: carbamazepine, phenobarbital, phenytoin	↓ levels of A	++
	Efavirenz	↓ levels of A	++
	Rifampin	↓ levels of A	++
Mefloquine	β-adrenergic blockers, calcium channel blockers, quinidine, quinine	↑ arrhythmias	+
	Divalproex, valproic acid	↓ level of B with seizures	++
	Halofantrine	Q-T prolongation	++ (avoid)
Methenamine mandelate or hippurate	Acetazolamide, sodium bicarbonate, thiazide diuretics	↓ antibacterial effect 2° to ↑ urine pH	++
Metronidazole Tinidazole	Alcohol	Disulfiram-like reaction	+
	Cyclosporin	↑ levels of B	++
	Disulfiram (Antabuse)	Acute toxic psychosis	+
	Lithium	↑ levels of B	++
	Oral anticoagulants	↑ anticoagulant effect	++
	Phenobarbital, hydantoins	↑ levels of B	++
Micafungin	Nifedipine	↑ levels of B	+
	Sirolimus	↑ levels of B	+
Nelfinavir	*See protease inhibitors and Table 22B & Table 22C*		
Nevirapine (Viramune)	*See non-nucleoside reverse transcriptase inhibitors (NNRTIs) and Table 22C*		
Nitrofurantoin	Antacids	↓ absorption of A	+

TABLE 22A (4)

ANTI-INFECTIVE AGENT (A)	OTHER DRUG (B)	EFFECT	IMPORT

Non-nucleoside reverse transcriptase inhibitors (NNRTIs): For interactions with protease inhibitors, see Table 22C.
Del = delavirdine, Efa = efavirenz, Nev = nevirapine

Del	Efa	Nev	Co-administration contraindicated:		
+			Anticonvulsants: carbamazepine, phenobarbital, phenytoin		++
+			Antimycobacterials: rifabutin, rifampin		++
+			Antipsychotics: pimozide		++
+	+	+	Benzodiazepines: alprazolam, midazolam, triazolam		++
+	+		Ergotamine		++
+	+		HMG-CoA inhibitors (statins): lovastatin, simvastatin, atorvastatin, pravastatin		++
+			St. John's wort		++
			Dose change needed:		
+			Amphetamines	↑ levels of B—**caution**	++
+		+	Antiarrhythmics: amiodarone, lidocaine, others	↓ or ↑ levels of B—**caution**	++
+	+	+	Anticonvulsants: carbamazepine, phenobarbital, phenytoin	↓ levels of A and/or B	++
+	+	+	Antifungals: itraconazole, ketoconazole, voriconazole	Potential ↓ levels of B, ↑ levels of A	++ (avoid)
		+	Antirejection drugs: cyclosporine, rapamycin, sirolimus, tacrolimus	↑ levels of B	++
+		+	Calcium channel blockers	↑ levels of B	++
+		+	Clarithromycin	↑ levels of B metabolite	++
+			Cyclosporine	↑ levels of B	++
+			Dexamethasone	↓ levels of A	++
+	+	+	Sildenafil, vardenafil, tadalafil	↓ levels of B	++
+		+	Fentanyl, methadone	↓ levels of B	++
+			Gastric acid suppression: antacids, H-2 blockers, proton pump inhibitors	↓ levels of A	++
	+	+	Methadone, fentanyl	↓ levels of B	++
	+	+	Oral contraceptives	↓ or ↑ levels of B	++
+	+	+	Protease inhibitors—see Table 22C		
+	+	+	**Rifabutin, rifampin**	↑ or ↓ levels of rifabutin; ↓ levels of A—**caution**	++
+	+	+	St. John's wort	↓ levels of B	++
			Warfarin	↑ levels of B	++

Pentamidine, IV	Amphotericin B	↑ risk of nephrotoxicity	+
	Foscarnet	↑ risk of hypocalcemia	+
	Pancreatitis-assoc drugs, eg, alcohol, valproic acid	↑ risk of pancreatitis	+

Piperacillin	Cefoxitin	Antagonism vs pseudomonas	++
Pip-tuzobactam	Methotrexate	↑ levels of B	++
Primaquine	Chloroquine, dapsone, INH, probenecid, quinine, sulfonamides, TMP/SMX, others	↑ **risk of hemolysis in G6PD-deficient patients**	++

Protease Inhibitors—Anti-HIV Drugs. (*Atazan* = atazanavir; *Darun* = darunavir; *Fosampren* = fosamprenavir; *Indin* = indinavir; *Lopin* = lopinavir; *Nelfin* = nelfinavir; *Saquin* = saquinavir; *Tipran* = tipranavir). For interactions with antiretrovirals, see Table 22B & Table 22C. *Only a partial list—check package insert*
Also see http://aidsinfo.nih.gov

Atazan	Darun	Fosampren	Indin	Lopin	Nelfin	Saquin	Tipran		EFFECT	IMPORT
								Analgesics:		
							+	1. Alfentanil, fentanyl, hydrocodone, tramadol	↑ levels of B	+
	+			+			+	2. Codeine, hydromorphone, morphine, methadone	↓ levels of B (JAIDS 41:563, 2006)	+
+	+	+	+	+	+			**Anti-arrhythmics: amiodarone, lidocaine, mexiletine, flecainide**	↑ levels of B; do not co-administer	++
+	+	+	+	+	+		+	**Anticonvulsants: carbamazepine, clonazepam, phenobarbital**	↓ levels of A, ↑ levels of B	++
+	+	+		+				Antidepressants, all tricyclic	↑ levels of B	++
+	+						+	Antidepressants, all other	↑ levels of B; do not use pimozide	++
	+							Antidepressants: SSRIs	↓ levels of B - avoid	++
+	+	+	+	+	+		+	**Benzodiazepines, e.g., diazepam, midazolam, triazolam**	↑ **levels of B—do not use**	++
+	+			+		+		Calcium channel blockers (all)	↑ levels of B	++
+	+			+	+	+		Clarithro, erythro	↑ levels of B if renal impairment	+
+	+			+	+		+	Contraceptives, oral	↑ levels of B	++
	+			+				Corticosteroids: prednisone, dexamethasone	↓ levels of A, ↑ levels of B	+
+	+	+	+	+	+		+	Cyclosporine	↑ levels of B, monitor levels	+
+	+	+	+	+	+		+	Ergot derivatives	↑ **levels of B—do not use**	++
	+		+		+			Erythromycin, clarithromycin	↑ levels of A & B	++
			+		+			Grapefruit juice (>200 mL/day)	↓ indinavir ↑ saquinavir levels	++
+	+	+	+	+		+		H2 receptor antagonists	↓ levels of A	++

TABLE 22A (5)

ANTI-INFECTIVE AGENT (A)								OTHER DRUG (B)	EFFECT	IMPORT
Atazan	Darun	Fosampren	Indin	Lopin	Nelfin	Saquin	Tipran	**Protease Inhibitors** *(continued)* Also see http://aidsinfo.nih.gov		
+	+	+	+	+	+	+	+	**HMG-CoA reductase inhibitors (statins): lovastatin, simvastatin**	↑ levels of B—do not use	+ +
+								Irinotecan	↓ levels of B—do not use	+ +
	+	+	+	+	+	+	+	Ketoconazole, itraconazole, ? vori	↑ levels of A, ↑ levels of B	+
			+			+		Metronidazole	Poss. disulfiram reaction, alcohol	+
			+					Phenytoin (*JAIDS 36:1034, 2004*)	↓ levels of A & B	+ +
+	+	+	+	+	+		+	**Pimozide**	↑ levels of B—do not use	+ +
+	+	+	+	+	+		+	Proton pump inhibitors	↓ levels of A	+ +
+	+	+	+	+	+	+	+	Rifampin, rifabutin	↓ levels of A, ↑ levels of B **(avoid)**	+ + (avoid)
+	+	+	+	+	+	+	+	Sildenafil (Viagra), tadalafil, vardenafil	Varies, some ↑ & some ↓ levels of B	+ +
+	+	+	+	+	+	+	+	**St. John's wort**	↓ levels of A—do not use	+ +
+	+	+	+	+	+	+	+	Sirolimus, tacrolimus	↑ levels of B	+ +
+								Tenofovir	↓ levels of A—add ritonavir	+ +
	+		+	+				Theophylline	↓ levels of B	+
							+	Warfarin	↑ levels of B	+

ANTI-INFECTIVE AGENT (A)	OTHER DRUG (B)	EFFECT	IMPORT
Pyrazinamide	INH, rifampin	May ↑ risk of hepatotoxicity	±
Pyrimethamine	Lorazepam	↑ risk of hepatotoxicity	+
	Sulfonamides, TMP/SMX	↑ risk of marrow suppression	+
	Zidovudine	↑ risk of marrow suppression	+
Quinine	Digoxin	↑ digoxin levels; ↑ toxicity	+ +
	Mefloquine	↑ arrhythmias	+
	Oral anticoagulants	↑ prothrombin time	+ +
Quinupristin- dalfopristin (Synercid)	Anti-HIV drugs: NNRTIs & PIs	↑ levels of B	+ +
	Antineoplastic: vincristine, docetaxel, paclitaxel	↑ levels of B	+ +
	Calcium channel blockers	↑ levels of B	+ +
	Carbamazepine	↑ levels of B	+ +
	Cyclosporine, tacrolimus	↑ levels of B	+ +
	Lidocaine	↑ levels of B	+ +
	Methylprednisolone	↑ levels of B	+ +
	Midazolam, diazepam	↑ levels of B	+ +
	Statins	↑ levels of B	+ +
Ribavirin	Didanosine	↑ levels of B → toxicity—**avoid**	+ +
	Stavudine	↓ levels of B	+ +
	Zidovudine	↓ levels of B	+ +
Rifamycins (rifampin, rifabutin) *See footnote for less severe or less common interactions* Ref.: *ArIM 162:985, 2002* **The following is a partial list of drugs with rifampin-induced ↑ metabolism and hence lower than anticipated serum levels:** ACE inhibitors, dapsone, diazepam, digoxin, diltiazem, doxycycline, fluconazole, fluvastatin, haloperidol, moxifloxacin, nifedipine, progestins, triazolam, tricyclics, voriconazole, zidovudine	Al OH, ketoconazole, PZA	↓ levels of A	+
	Atovaquone	↑ levels of A, ↓ levels of B	+
	Beta adrenergic blockers (metoprolol, propranolol)	↓ effect of B	+
	Caspofungin	↓ levels of B—increase dose	+ +
	Clarithromycin	↑ levels of A, ↓ levels of B	+ +
	Corticosteroids	replacement requirement of B	+ +
	Cyclosporine	↓ effect of B	+ +
	Delavirdine	↑ levels of A, ↓ levels of B—avoid	+ +
	Digoxin	↓ levels of B	+ +
	Disopyramide	↓ levels of B	+ +
	Fluconazole	↑ levels of A[1]	+ +
	Amprenavir, indinavir, nelfinavir, ritonavir	↑ levels of A (↓ dose of A), ↓ levels of B	+ +
	INH	Converts INH to toxic hydrazine	+ +
	Itraconazole[1], ketoconazole	↓ levels of B, ↑ levels of A[1]	+ +
	Linezolid	↓ levels of B	+ +
	Methadone	↓ serum levels (withdrawal)	+
	Nevirapine	↓ levels of B—avoid	+ +
	Oral anticoagulants	Suboptimal anticoagulation	+ +
	Oral contraceptives	↓ effectiveness; spotting, pregnancy	+
	Phenytoin	↓ levels of B	+
	Protease inhibitors	↑ levels of A, ↓ levels of B—**CAUTION**	+ +
	Quinidine	↓ effect of B	+
	Sulfonylureas	↓ hypoglycemic effect	+
	Tacrolimus	↓ levels of B	+ +
	Theophylline	↑ levels of B	+

[1] Up to 4wk may be required after RIF discontinued to achieve detectable serum itra levels; ↑ levels assoc with uveitis or polymyolysis

TABLE 22A (6)

ANTI-INFECTIVE AGENT (A)	OTHER DRUG (B)	EFFECT	IMPORT
Rifamycins *(continued)*			
	TMP/SMX	↓ levels of A	+
	Tocainide	↓ effect of B	+
Rimantadine	*See Amantadine*		
Ritonavir	*See protease inhibitors and Table 22B & Table 22C*		
Saquinavir	*See protease inhibitors and Table 22B & Table 22C*		
Stavudine	Dapsone, INH	May ↑ risk of peripheral neuropathy	±
	Ribavirin	↓ levels of A—**avoid**	++
	Zidovudine	Mutual interference—do not combine	++
Sulfonamides	Cyclosporine	↓ cyclosporine levels	+
	Methotrexate	↑ antifolate activity	+
	Oral anticoagulants	↑ prothrombin time; bleeding	+
	Phenobarbital, rifampin	↓ levels of A	+
	Phenytoin	↑ levels of B; nystagmus, ataxia	+
	Sulfonylureas	↑ hypoglycemic effect	+
Telithromycin (Ketek)	Carbamazine	↓ levels of A	++
	Digoxin	↑ levels of B—do digoxin levels	++
	Ergot alkaloids	↑ **levels of B—avoid**	++
	Itraconazole; ketoconazole	↑ levels of A; no dose change	+
	Metoprolol	↑ levels of B	++
	Midazolam	↑ levels of B	++
	Oral anticoagulants	↑ prothrombin time	+
	Phenobarb, phenytoin	↓ levels of A	++
	Pimozide	↑ **levels of B; QT prolongation—AVOID**	++
	Rifampin	↓ **levels of A—avoid**	++
	Simvastatin	↑ levels of B (↑ risk of myopathy)	++
	Sotalol	↓ levels of B	++
	Theophylline	↑ levels of B	++
Tenofovir	Atazanavir	↓ levels of B—add ritonavir	++
	Didanosine (ddI)	↑ **levels of B (reduce dose)**	++
Terbinafine	Cimetidine	↑ levels of A	+
	Phenobarbital, rifampin	↓ levels of A	+
Tetracyclines	*See Doxycycline, plus:*		
	Atovaquone	↓ levels of B	+
	Digoxin	↑ toxicity of B (may persist several months—up to 10% pts)	++
	Methoxyflurane	↑ toxicity; polyuria, renal failure	+
	Sucralfate	↓ absorption of A (separate by ≥2 hrs)	+
Thiabendazole	Theophyllines	↑ serum theophylline, nausea	+
Tigecycline	Oral contraceptives	↓ levels of B	++
Tinidazole (Tindamax)	*See Metronidazole—similar entity, expect similar interactions*		
Tobramycin	*See Aminoglycosides*		
Trimethoprim	Amantadine, dapsone, digoxin, methotrexate, procainamide, zidovudine	↑ serum levels of B	++
	Potassium-sparing diuretics	↑ serum K+	++
	Thiazide diuretics	↓ serum Na+	+
Trimethoprim-Sulfamethoxazole	Azathioprine	Reports of leukopenia	+
	Cyclosporine	↓ levels of B, ↑ serum creatinine	+
	Loperamide	↑ levels of B	+
	Methotrexate	Enhanced marrow suppression	++
	Oral contraceptives, pimozide, and 6-mercaptopurine	↓ effect of B	+
	Phenytoin	↑ levels of B	+
	Rifampin	↑ levels of B	+
	Warfarin	↑ activity of B	+
Valganciclovir (Valcyte)	*See Ganciclovir*		
Vancomycin	Aminoglycosides	↑ frequency of nephrotoxicity	++
Zalcitabine (ddC) (HIVID)	Valproic acid, pentamidine (IV), alcohol, lamivudine	↑ pancreatitis risk	+
	Cisplatin, INH, metronidazole, vincristine, nitrofurantoin, d4T, dapsone	↑ risk of peripheral neuropathy	+
Zidovudine (ZDV) (Retrovir)	Atovaquone, fluconazole, methadone	↑ levels of A	+
	Clarithromycin	↓ levels of A	±
	Indomethacin	↑ levels of ZDV toxic metabolite	+
	Nelfinavir	↓ levels of A	++
	Probenecid, TMP/SMX	↑ levels of A	+
	Rifampin/rifabutin	↓ levels of A	++
	Stavudine	**Interference—DO NOT COMBINE!**	++
	Valproic Acid	↑ levels of A	++

TABLE 22B – DRUG-DRUG INTERACTIONS BETWEEN PROTEASE INHIBITORS
(Adapted from Guidelines for the Use of Antiretroviral Agents in HIV-infected Adults & Adolescents; see www.aidsinfo.nih.gov)

NAME (Abbreviation, Trade Name)	Atazanavir (ATV, Reyataz)	Darunavir (DRV, Prezista)	Fosamprenavir (FOS-APV, Lexiva)	Indinavir (IDV, Crixivan)	Lopinavir/Ritonavir (LP/R, Kaletra)	Nelfinavir (NFV, Viracept)	Saquinavir (SQV, Invirase)	Tipranavir (TPV)
Atazanavir (ATV, Reyataz)		ATV 300 mg once daily with (DRV 600 mg + ritonavir 100 mg bid)	**Do not co-administer; risk of additive ↑ in indirect bilirubin**		RTV 100mg ↑ ATV AUC↑ 238%		SQV (Invirase) 1600mg + ATV 300mg + RTV 100mg, all q24h	
DARUNAVIR (DRV, Prezista)	ATV 300 mg once daily with (DRV 600 mg + ritonavir 100 mg bid)		No data	Dose unclear	**DO NOT co-administer.** Doses not established	No data	**DO NOT co-administer.** Doses not established	No data
FOSAMPRENAVIR (FOS-APV, Lexiva)	**Do not co-administer; risk of additive ↑ in bilirubin**	No data			↓ serum conc; both drugs; **do not co-administer**		Insufficient data	FosAPV levels ↓. **Do not co-administer**
Indinavir (IDV, Crixivan)	**Do not co-administer; risk of additive ↑ in bilirubin**	Dose unclear	↓ serum conc. both drugs; **do not co-administer**		IDV AUC↑. IDV dose 600mg q12h	↑ IDV & NFV levels. Dose: IDV 1200mg q12h; NFV 1250mg q12h	SQV levels ↑ 4-7 fold. Dose: Insufficient data	No data
Lopinavir/Ritonavir (LP/R, Kaletra)	RTV 100mg ↑ ATV AUC↑ 238%	**DO NOT co-administer.** Doses not established	↓ serum conc. both drugs; **do not co-administer**	IDV AUC↑; IDV dose 600mg q12h		Dose: LP/R 533/133mg q12h; NFV 1000mg q12h	SQV levels ↑. Dose: SQV 1000mg b.i.d. LP/R standard	LPV levels ↓. **Do not co-administer**
Nelfinavir (NFV, Viracept)		No data		↑ IDV & NFV levels. Dose: IDV 1200mg q12h; NFV 1250mg q12h	LP levels ↓; NFV levels ↑ Dose LP/R 533/133mg q12h; NFV 1000mg q12h		Dose SQV 1200mg b.i.d. NFV 1250mg b.i.d.	No data
Saquinavir (SQV, Fortovase/ Invirase)	SQV (Invirase) 1600mg + ATV 300mg + RTV 100mg, all q24h	**DO NOT co-administer.** Doses not established	SQV (Invirase) 1000mg q12h + RTV 100-200mg q12h + FOS-APV 700mg q12h	SQV levels ↑ 4-7 fold. Dose: Insufficient data	SQV levels ↑. Dose: SQV 1000mg b.i.d, LP/R-standard	Dose SQV 1200mg b.i.d, NFV 1250 mg b.i.d.		SQV↓. **Do not co-administer**
Tipranavir (TPV)	No data	No data	Fos-APV levels ↓. **Do not co-administer**	No data	LPV levels ↓. **Do not co-administer**	No data	SQV ↓ **Do not co-administer**	

† AUC = area under the curve

TABLE 22C – DRUG-DRUG INTERACTIONS BETWEEN NON-NUCLEOSIDE REVERSE TRANSCRIPTASE INHIBITORS (NNRTIS) AND PROTEASE INHIBITORS
(Adapted from Guidelines for the Use of Antiretroviral Agents in HIV-infected Adults & Adolescents; see www.aidsinfo.nih.gov)

NAME (Abbreviation, Trade Name)	Atazanavir (ATV, Reyataz)	DARUNAVIR (DRV, Prezista)	Fosamprenavir (FOS-APV, Lexiva)	Indinavir (IDV, Crixivan)	Lopinavir/Ritonavir (LP/R, Kaletra)	Nelfinavir (NFV, Viracept)	Saquinavir—softgel (SQV, Invirase)	Tipranavir (TPV)
Delavirdine (DLV, Rescriptor)	No data	No data	Co-administration not recommended	IDV levels ↑ 40%. Dose: IDV 600mg q8h; DLV standard	Expect LP levels to ↑. No dose data	NFV levels ↑ 2X. DLV levels ↓ 50%. Dose: No data	SQV levels ↑ 5X. Dose: SQV 800mg q8h; DLV standard	No data
Efavirenz (EFZ, Sustiva)	ATV AUC ↓ 74%. Dose: EFZ standard; ATA/RTV 300/100mg q24h with food	Standard doses of both drugs	FOS-APV levels ↓. Dose: EFZ standard; FOS-APV 1400mg + RTV 300mg q24h or 700mg FOS-APV + 100mg RTV q12h	Levels: IDV ↓ 31%. Dose: IDV 1000mg q8h; EFZ standard	Level of LP ↓ 40%. Dose: LP/R 533/133 mg q12h, EFZ standard	Standard doses	Level: SQV ↓ 62%. Dose: SQV softgel 400mg + RTV 400mg q12h	No dose change necessary
Nevirapine (NVP, Viramune)	No data	Standard doses of both drugs	No data	IDV levels ↓ 28%. Dose: IDV 1000mg q8h or combine with RTV, NVP standard	LP levels ↓ 53%. Dose: LP/R 533/133 standard	Standard doses	Dose: SQV softgel + RTV 400/400mg, both q12h	No data

TABLE 23 – LIST OF GENERIC AND COMMON TRADE NAMES

GENERIC NAME: TRADE NAMES	GENERIC NAME: TRADE NAMES	GENERIC NAME: TRADE NAMES
Abacavir: Ziagen	Drotrecogin alfa: Xigris	Nystatin: Mycostatin
Abacavir+Lamivudine: Epzicom	Efavirenz: Sustiva	Ofloxacin: Floxin
Abacavir+Lamivudine+Zodovudine: Trizivir	Efavirenz/Emtricitabine/Tenofovir: Atripla	Oseltamivir: Tamiflu
Acyclovir: Zovirax	Emtricitabine: Emtriva	Oxacillin: Prostaphlin
Adefovir: Hepsera	Emtricitabine + tenofovir: Truvada	Palivizumab: Synagis
Albendazole: Albenza	Enfuvirtide (T-20): Fuzeon	Paromomycin: Humatin
Amantadine: Symmetrel	Entecavir: Baraclude	Pentamidine: NebuPent, Pentam 300
Amikacin: Amikin	Ertapenem: Invanz	Piperacillin: Pipracil
Amoxicillin: Amoxil, Polymox	Erythromycin(s): Ilotycin	Piperacillin/tazobactam: Zosyn
Amox./clav.: Augmentin, Augmentin ES-600; Augmentin XR	Ethyl succinate: Pediamycin	Piperazine: Antepar
	Glucoheptonate: Erythrocin	Podophyllotoxin: Condylox
Amphotericin B: Fungizone	Estolate: Ilosone	Posaconazole: Noxafil
Ampho B-liposomal: AmBisome	Erythro/sulfisoxazole: Pediazole	Praziquantel: Biltricide
Ampho B-cholesteryl complex: Amphotec	Ethambutol: Myambutol	Primaquine: Primachine
	Ethionamide: Trecator	Proguanil: Paludrine
Ampho B-lipid complex: Abelcet	Famciclovir: Famvir	Pyrantel pamoate: Antiminth
Ampicillin: Omnipen, Polycillin	Fluconazole: Diflucan	Pyrimethamine: Daraprim
Ampicillin/sulbactam: Unasyn	Flucytosine: Ancobon	Pyrimethamine/sulfadoxine: Fansidar
Atazanavir: Reyataz	Fosamprenavir: Lexiva	Quinupristin/dalfopristin: Synercid
Atovaquone: Mepron	Foscarnet: Foscavir	Raltegravir: Isentress
Atovaquone + proguanil: Malarone	Fosfomycin: Monurol	Retapamulin: Altabax
Azithromycin: Zithromax	Ganciclovir: Cytovene	Ribavirin: Virazole, Rebetol
Azithromycin ER: Zmax	Gatifloxacin: Tequin	Rifabutin: Mycobutin
Aztreonam: Azactam	Gemifloxacin: Factive	Rifampin: Rifadin, Rimactane
Caspofungin: Cancidas	Gentamicin: Garamycin	Rifapentine: Priftin
Cefaclor: Ceclor, Ceclor CD	Griseofulvin: Fulvicin	Rifaximin: Xifaxan
Cefadroxil: Duricef	Halofantrine: Halfan	Rimantadine: Flumadine
Cefazolin: Ancef, Kefzol	Idoxuridine: Dendrid, Stoxil	Ritonavir: Norvir
Cefdinir: Omnicef	INH + RIF: Rifamate	Saquinavir: Invirase, Fortovase
Cefditoren pivoxil: Spectracef	INH + RIF + PZA: Rifater	Spectinomycin: Trobicin
Cefepime: Maxipime	Interferon alfa: Intron A	Stavudine: Zerit
Cefixime^NUS: Suprax	Interferon, pegylated: PEG-Intron, Pegasys	Stibogluconate: Pentostam
Cefoperazone-sulbactam: Sulperazon^NUS	Interferon + ribavirin: Rebetron	Silver sulfadiazine: Silvadene
	Imipenem + cilastatin: Primaxin, Tienam	Sulfamethoxazole: Gantanol
Cefotaxime: Claforan	Imiquimod: Aldara	Sulfasalazine: Azulfidine
Cefotetan: Cefotan	Indinavir: Crixivan	Sulfisoxazole: Gantrisin
Cefoxitin: Mefoxin	Itraconazole: Sporanox	Telbivudine: Tyzeka
Cefpodoxime proxetil: Vantin	Iodoquinol: Yodoxin	Telithromycin: Ketek
Cefprozil: Cefzil	Ivermectin: Stromectol	Tenofovir: Viread
Ceftazidime: Fortaz, Tazicef, Tazidime	Kanamycin: Kantrex	Terbinafine: Lamisil
Ceftibuten: Cedax	Ketoconazole: Nizoral	Thalidomide: ThalomidThiabendazole: Mintezol
Ceftizoxime: Cefizox	Lamivudine: Epivir, Epivir-HBV	
Ceftriaxone: Rocephin	Lamivudine + abacavir: Epzicom	Ticarcillin: Ticar
Cefuroxime: Zinacef, Kefurox, Ceftin	Levofloxacin: Levaquin	Tigecycline: Tygacil
Cephalexin: Keflex	Linezolid: Zyvox	Tinidazole: Tindamax
Cephradine: Anspor, Velosef	Lomefloxacin: Maxaquin	Tipranavir: Aptivus
Chloroquine: Aralen	Lopinavir/ritonavir: Kaletra	Tobramycin: Nebcin
Cidofovir: Vistide	Loracarbef: Lorabid	Tretinoin: Retin A
Ciprofloxacin: Cipro, Cipro XR	Mafenide: Sulfamylon	Trifluridine: Viroptic
Clarithromycin: Biaxin, Biaxin XL	Maraviroc: Selzentry	Trimethoprim: Proloprim, Trimpex
Clindamycin: Cleocin	Mebendazole: Vermox	Trimethoprim/sulfamethoxazole: Bactrim, Septra
Clofazimine: Lamprene	Mefloquine: Lariam	
Clotrimazole: Lotrimin, Mycelex	Meropenem: Merrem	Valacyclovir: Valtrex
Cloxacillin: Tegopen	Mesalamine: Asacol, Pentasa	Valganciclovir: Valcyte
Colistimethate: Coly-Mycin M	Methenamine: Hiprex, Mandelamine	Vancomycin: Vancocin
Cycloserine: Seromycin	Metronidazole: Flagyl	Voriconazole: Vfend
Dalbavancin: Zeven	Micafungin: Mycamine	Zalcitabine: HIVID
Daptomycin: Cubicin	Minocycline: Minocin	Zanamivir: Relenza
Darunavir: Prezista	Moxifloxacin: Avelox	Zidovudine (ZDV): Retrovir
Delavirdine: Rescriptor	Mupirocin: Bactroban	Zidovudine + 3TC: Combivir
Dicloxacillin: Dynapen	Nafcillin: Unipen	Zidovudine + 3TC + abacavir: Trizivir
Didanosine: Videx	Nelfinavir: Viracept	
Diethylcarbamazine: Hetrazan	Nevirapine: Viramune	
Diloxanide furoate: Furamide	Nitazoxanide: Alinia	
Dirithromycin: Dynabac	Nitrofurantoin: Macrobid, Macrodantin	
Doxycycline: Vibramycin		

TABLE 23 (2)
LIST OF COMMON TRADE AND GENERIC NAMES

TRADE NAME: GENERIC NAME	TRADE NAME: GENERIC NAME	TRADE NAME: GENERIC NAME
Abelcet: Ampho B-lipid complex	Garamycin: Gentamicin	Retin A: Tretinoin
Albenza: Albendazole	Halfan: Halofantrine	Retrovir: Zidovudine (ZDV)
Aldara: Imiquimod	Hepsera: Adefovir	Reyataz: Atazanavir
Alinia: Nitazoxanide	Herplex: Idoxuridine	Rifadin: Rifampin
Altabax: Retapamulin	Hiprex: Methenamine hippurate	Rifamate: INH + RIF
AmBisome: Ampho B-liposomal	HIVID: Zalcitabine	Rifater: INH + RIF + PZA
Amikin: Amikacin	Humatin: Paromomycin	Rimactane: Rifampin
Amoxil: Amoxicillin	Ilosone: Erythromycin estolate	Rocephin: Ceftriaxone
Amphotec: Ampho B-cholesteryl complex	Ilotycin: Erythromycin	Selzentry: Maraviroc
Ancef: Cefazolin	Intron A: Interferon alfa	Septra: Trimethoprim/sulfa
Ancobon: Flucytosine	Invanz: Ertapenem	Seromycin: Cycloserine
Anspor: Cephradine	Invirase: Saquinavir	Silvadene: Silver sulfadiazine
Antepar: Piperazine	Isentress: Raltegravir	Spectracef: Cefditoren pivoxil
Antiminth: Pyrantel pamoate	Kantrex: Kanamycin	Sporanox: Itraconazole
Aptivus: Tipranavir	Kaletra: Lopinavir/ritonavir	Stoxil: Idoxuridine
Aralen: Chloroquine	Keflex: Cephalexin	Stromectol: Ivermectin
Asacol: Mesalamine	Kefurox: Cefuroxime	Sulfamylon: Mafenide
Atripla: Efavirenz/emtricitabine/tenofovir	Ketek: Telithromycin	Sulperazon^NUS: Cefoperazone-sulbactam
Augmentin, Augmentin ES-600 Augmentin XR: Amox./clav.	Lamisil: Terbinafine	Suprax: Cefixime^NUS
Avelox: Moxifloxacin	Lamprene: Clofazimine	Sustiva: Efavirenz
Azactam: Aztreonam	Lariam: Mefloquine	Symmetrel: Amantadine
Azulfidine: Sulfasalazine	Levaquin: Levofloxacin	Synagis: Palivizumab
Bactroban: Mupirocin	Lexiva: Fosamprenavir	Synercid: Quinupristin/dalfopristin
Bactrim: Trimethoprim/sulfamethoxazole	Lorabid: Loracarbef	Tamiflu: Oseltamivir
Baraclude: Entecavir	Macrodantin, Macrobid: Nitrofurantoin	Tazicef: Ceftazidime
Biaxin, Biaxin XL: Clarithromycin	Malarone: Atovaquone + proguanil	Tegopen: Cloxacillin
Biltricide: Praziquantel	Mandelamine: Methenamine mandel.	Tequin: Gatifloxacin
Cancidas: Caspofungin	Maxaquin: Lomefloxacin	Thalomid: Thalidomide
Ceclor, Ceclor CD: Cefaclor	Maxipime: Cefepime	Ticar: Ticarcillin
Cedax: Ceftibuten	Mefoxin: Cefoxitin	Tienam: Imipenem
Cefizox: Ceftizoxime	Mepron: Atovaquone	Timentin: Ticarcillin-clavulanic acid
Cefotan: Cefotetan	Merrem: Meropenem	Tinactin: Tolnaftate
Ceftin: Cefuroxime axetil	Minocin: Minocycline	Tindamax: Tinidazole
Cefzil: Cefprozil	Mintezol: Thiabendazole	Trecator SC: Ethionamide
Cipro, Cipro XR: Ciprofloxacin & extended release	Monocid: Cefonicid	Trizivir: Abacavir + ZDV + 3TC
Claforan: Cefotaxime	Monurol: Fosfomycin	Trobicin: Spectinomycin
Coly-Mycin M: Colistimethate	Myambutol: Ethambutol	Truvada: Emtricitabine + tenofovir
Combivir: ZDV + 3TC	Mycamine: Micafungin	Tygacil: Tigecycline
Crixivan: Indinavir	Mycobutin: Rifabutin	Tyzeka: Telbivudine
Cubicin: Daptomycin	Mycostatin: Nystatin	Unasyn: Ampicillin/sulbactam
Cytovene: Ganciclovir	Nafcil: Nafcillin	Unipen: Nafcillin
Daraprim: Pyrimethamine	Nebcin: Tobramycin	Valcyte: Valganciclovir
Diflucan: Fluconazole	NebuPent: Pentamidine	Valtrex: Valacyclovir
Duricef: Cefadroxil	Nizoral: Ketoconazole	Vancocin: Vancomycin
Dynapen: Dicloxacillin	Norvir: Ritonavir	Vantin: Cefpodoxime proxetil
Emtriva: Emtricitabine	Noxafil: Posaconazole	Velosef: Cephradine
Epivir, Epivir-HBV: Lamivudine	Omnicef: Cefdinir	Vermox: Mebendazole
Epzicom: Lamivudine + abacavir	Omnipen: Ampicillin	Vfend: Voriconazole
Factive: Gemifloxacin	Pediamycin: Erythro. ethyl succinate	Vibramycin: Doxycycline
Famvir: Famciclovir	Pediazole: Erythro. ethyl succinate + sulfisoxazole	Videx: Didanosine
Fansidar: Pyrimethamine + sulfadoxine	Pegasys, PEG-Intron: Interferon, pegylated	Viracept: Nelfinavir
Flagyl: Metronidazole	Pentam 300: Pentamidine	Viramune: Nevirapine
Floxin: Ofloxacin	Pentasa: Mesalamine	Virazole: Ribavirin
Flumadine: Rimantadine	Pipracil: Piperacillin	Viread: Tenofovir
Fortaz: Ceftazidime	Polymox: Amoxicillin	Vistide: Cidofovir
Fortovase: Saquinavir	Polycillin: Ampicillin	Xifaxan: Rifaximin
Fulvicin: Griseofulvin	Prezista: Darunavir	Xigris: Drotrecogin alfa
Fungizone: Amphotericin B	Priftin: Rifapentine	Yodoxin: Iodoquinol
Furadantin: Nitrofurantoin	Primaxin: Imipenem + cilastatin	Zerit: Stavudine
Fuzeon: Enfuvirtide (T-20)	Proloprim: Trimethoprim	Zeven: Dalbavancin
Gantanol: Sulfamethoxazole	Prostaphlin: Oxacillin	Ziagen: Abacavir
Gantrisin: Sulfisoxazole	Rebetol: Ribavirin	Zinacef: Cefuroxime
	Rebetron: Interferon + ribavirin	Zithromax: Azithromycin
	Relenza: Zanamivir	Zmax: Azithromycin ER
	Rescriptor: Delavirdine	Zovirax: Acyclovir
		Zosyn: Piperacillin/tazobactam
		Zyvox: Linezolid

208

INDEX OF MAJOR ENTITIES

PAGES (page numbers bold if major focus)

A

Abacavir 74, 78, **154**, **155**, 156, 157, 164, **161**, 185, 206, 207
Abacavir/Lamivudine 153
Abortion, prophylaxis/septic **22**, 56, **169**
Acanthamoeba 153
Acinetobacter 7, 19, 37, 42, 45, 61, 66, 68, 70, 72
Acne rosacea and vulgaris **45**, **46**, 132, 147
Actinomycosis 12, 61, 66, 68, 70, **94**
Activated Protein C (Drotrecogin) 56
Acyclovir 6, 11, 12, 13, 24, 43, 47, 48, 55, 74, 78, 140, 141, 142, 143, **147**, 148, 151, 175, 183, 206, 207
Adefovir 74, 78, **137**, 148, 151, 183, 206, 207
Adenovirus 11, 32, 34, 40, 135, 151
Adverse reactions
  Antibacterials 80
  Antifungals 105
  Antimycobacterials 120
  Antiparasitic drugs 132, 134
  Antiretroviral drugs 164
  Antiviral drugs 147, 148
Aeromonas hydrophila 15, 49, 61, 66, 68, 69
AIDS 6, **9**, 13, **17**, 18, 21, 24, 32, **40**, 41, 46, 51, 55, 64, 92, **97**, **98**, **99**, 100, 102, 103, 107, 111, 116, 117, 118, 121, 123, 126, 127, 131, 136, 137, 138, 141, 142, 143, 147, 148, **152**, 165, 173, 197
Albendazole 74, 78, 124, 128, 129, 130, 131, **132**, 206, 207
Allergic bronchopulmonary aspergillosis 94
Amantadine 40, 74, **149**, 151, 183, 198, 203, 206, 207
Amebiasis 15, 17, 32, 123
Amebic meningoencephalitis **124**
Amikacin 48, 61, 62, 69, 74, 76, 80, **93**, 102, 118, 119, 121, 177, 178, 198, 206, 207
Aminoglycosides, single daily dose 93, 178
Amnionitis, septic abortion 22
Amoxicillin 9, 10, 18, 20, 31, 33, 34, 35, 37, 38, 39, 45, 46, 52, 59, 61, 62, 63, 65, 72, 75, 80, 85, 94, 167, 169, 177, 181, 198, 206, 207
Amoxicillin-clavulanate 9, 10, 12, 13, 14, 19, 30, 33, 35, 37, 38, 41, 43, 45, 46, 47, 48, 49, 50, 55, 61, 62, 63, 75, 80, 85, 95, 116, 167, 169, 177
Amphotericin B, ampho B 12, 13, 27, 51, 56, 58, 74, 77, 93, 94, 95, 96, 97, **98**, 99, 101, 102, 103, **105**, 106, 124, 147, 175, 182, 185, 198, 199, 201, 206, 207
  lipid ampho B preps 13, 56, 77, 94, 95, 97, 99, 102, **105**, 124, 175, 182, 198
Ampicillin 6, 7, 8, 16, 17, 19, 25, 26, 27, 31, 32, 33, 34, 37, 38, 42, 53, 54, 59, 61, 62, 63, 65, 71, 72, 75, 80, **85**, 94, 167, 177, 181, 185, 198, 206, 207
Ampicillin-sulbactam 13, 14, 19, 22, 23, 24, 26, 27, 31, 32, 40, 41, 42, 44, 47, 49, 55, 58, 61, 62, 65, 71, 72, 75, 80, **85**, 177, 185
Anaplasma (Ehrlichia) 52, 62
Angiostrongylus 9
Anidulafungin 28, 74, 77, 95, 96, 97, 106, 185
Anisakiasis **128**
Anthrax 35, **38**, 46, 47, 50, 59, 61
Antifungals 94
Antimony compounds 132
Antiretroviral Drugs & Therapy/Antiviral Drugs 135, 152
Aphthous stomatitis 41, 54, 98, 122
Appendicitis 17, **42**
Arcanobacterium haemolyticum 43, 61
Arthritis, septic 15, 20, **28**, 29, 52, 54, 64, 88, 132, 142
  reactive (Reiter's) 24, **28**
Ascariasis **128**
Aspergilloma 94

Aspergillosis 12, 13, 27, 37, 45, 56, 57, 58, 85, **94**, **95**, 97, 106, 107, 108, 109, 175
Aspergillus flavus 109
Aspergillus fumigatus 109
Aspergillus terreus 109
Aspiration pneumonia **39**
Asplenia 46, 51, 56, 124, 167
Atabrine **132**
Atazanavir 74, 78, 153, 154, 158, 160, **165**, 174, 185, 198, 201, 203, 204, 205, 206, 207
Atazanavir + ritonavir 153
Athlete's foot (Tinea pedis) 48, **101**
Atovaquone, atovaquone + proguanil 51, 74, 78, 79, 124, 125, 126, 127, **132**, 176, 198, 202, 203, 206, 207
Atripla 153
Azithromycin 9, 11, 15, 16, 17, 20, 21, 30, 32, 33, 34, 35, 36, 37, 38, 40, 41, 43, 44, 46, 48, 49, 51, 52, 53, 54, 59, 61, 62, 63, 64, 69, 72, 74, 79, 83, 88, 117, 118, 119, 124, 127, 167, 177, 185, 200, 206, 207
Azole antifungals 91, **94**
AZT (zidovudine) 74, 79, 147, 164, 173, 174, 184, 198, 199, 200, 202, 203, 206, 207
Aztreonam 4, 14, 19, 38, 42, 54, 56, 58, 61, 62, 63, 65, 72, 74, 76, 80, **86**, 87, 177, 181, 206, 207

B

Babesia, babesiosis **51**, 52, **124**, 167
Bacillary angiomatosis 46, **51**, 61
Bacillus anthracis (anthrax) 35, 38, 46, 47, 50, 59, 61
Bacillus cereus, subtilis **13**, 61
Bacitracin 61
Bacterial endocarditis 18, 25, 26, 27, 51, 64, 88, 171
Bacterial peritonitis 15, 19, 23, 31, 42, 50, 51, 55, 98, 106, 169, 170
Bacterial vaginosis **23**, 62
Bacteriuria, asymptomatic **31**, 64, 167, 170
Bacteroides species 5, 6, 14, **19**, 22, 23, 32, 35, 40, 42, 46, 47, 48, 50, 58, 61, 66, 68, 70
Balanitis **23**, **24**, 28
Balantidium coli **123**
Bartonella henselae, quintana 5, 27, 32, 40, 41, 46, **51**, 61
Baylisascariasis 128
BCG 110, **117**
Bell's palsy **139**
Benzathine penicillin, Bicillin 21, 22, 43, 48, 54, 61, 75, 85
Benznidazole 128, **132**
Biliary sepsis **14**, 19, 55
Biloma, post-transplant 32
Biological weapons 59, 197
Bites 24, **46**, **47**, 49, 53, 142, 146, 196
Bithionol 130, **134**
BK virus, post-renal transplant 151
Blastocystis hominis **123**
Blastomyces dermatitidis 95, 109
Blastomycosis 50, **95**, 103
Blepharitis **11**
Boils (furunculosis) **47**, **49**
Bordetella pertussis (whooping cough) 32, 61, 195
Borrelia burgdorferi, B. garinii, B. afzelii 29, 52, 61
Borrelia recurrentis 52
Botulism (food-borne, infant, wound) **57**, **59**
Brain abscess **6**, 10, 44, 62, 103, 127
Breast infection (mastitis, abscess) 5
Bronchitis, bronchiolitis 32, 33, 34, 35, 88, 144
Bronchopneumonia **33**
Brucellosis 29, **53**, 61, 64, 70
Brugia malayi 129
Buccal cellulitis 41

Bold numbers indicate major considerations. Antibiotic selection often depends on modifying circumstances and alternative agents.

PAGES (page numbers bold if major focus)

Burkholderia (Pseudomonas) cepacia **39**, 61, 66, 68, 70
Burkholderia pseudomallei (melioidosis) **37**, 51, **61**
Burns **48**, 56, 58, 195
Bursitis, septic **29**
Buruli ulcer 119

C
Calymmatobacterium granulomatis **21**
Campylobacter jejuni, fetus 15, 17, 28, 61, 72
Canaliculitis 12
Candida albicans 18, 23, 43
Candida albicans, glabrata, krusei, lusitaniae 18, 23, 43, **96**, **97**, 98, 106, 108, 109, 175
Candidemia, candidiasis 12, 13, 14, 18, 23, 24, 27, 32, 41, 43, 48, 49, 51, 55, 56, 58, **96**, **97**, 98, 106, 107, 108, 109, 175
CAPD peritonitis 43, 98, 185
Capillariasis 128
Capnocytophaga ochracea, canimorsus **46**, 56, 61
Capreomycin 74, 112, **121**
Carbapenems 61, 76, 80, 86
Caspofungin 51, 56, 58, 74, 77, 95, 96, 97, 98, 99, **106**, 185, 198, 206, 207
Cat bite **46**
Catfish sting **46**
Cat-scratch disease 6, 32, 40, 41, 46, 51
Cavernous sinus thrombosis **57**
CDC Drug Service 123, 132
Cefaclor, Cefaclor–ER 9, 67, 75, 81, **87**, 177, 206, 207
Cefadroxil 67, 75, 81, **87**, 177, 206, 207
Cefazolin 4, 12, 13, 25, 26, 41, 48, 56, 61, 67, 75, 81, **86**, 167, 168, 169, 170, 177, 179, 185, 206, 207
Cefdinir 9, 10, 35, 45, 67, 75, 81, **87**, 177, 206, 207
Cefditoren pivoxil 35, 67, 75, 81, **87**, 206, 207
Cefepime 4, 7, 8, 9, 10, 28, 37, 42, 45, 56, 63, 67, 72, 76, 81, **87**, 177, 179, 206, 207
Cefixime 16, 18, 20, 62, 67, 75, 81, 87, 167, 177
Cefoperazone–sulbactam 86
Cefotaxime 6, 7, 8, 10, 13, 16, 20, 29, 33, 34, 45, 42, 44, 49, 52, 53, 54, 61, 62, 63, 67, 72, 75, 81, **86**, 87, 177, 179, 206, 207
Cefotetan 19, 23, 41, 42, 58, 61, 67, 75, 81, **86**, 168, 169, 179, 206, 207
Cefoxitin 19, 20, 22, 23, 32, 40, 42, 44, 47, 58, 61, 62, 67, 75, 81, **86**, 87, 118, 168, 169, 177, 179, 201, 206, 207
Cefpirome **87**
Cefpodoxime proxetil 9, 10, 20, 35, 45, 62, 72, 75, 81, **87**, 177, 206, 207
Cefprozil 9, 10, 35, 45, 67, 75, 81, **87**, 177, 206, 207
Ceftazidime 4, 6, 7, 8, 9, 10, 12, 13, 17, 29, 37, 39, 43, 45, 49, 56, 61, 63, 67, 72, 75, 81, 86, 87, 177, 179, 185, 206, 207
Ceftibuten 9, 67, 75, 81, **87**, 177, 206, 207
Ceftizoxime 20, 29, 67, 76, 81, **86**, 168, 177, 179, 206, 207
Ceftobiprole 14, 48, 49, 50, 67, 71, 73, 76, 81, 87, 179
Ceftriaxone 6, 7, 8, 10, 11, 13, 14, 16, 17, 18, 20, 21, 22, 23, 24, 25, 27, 29, 34, 35, 36, 39, 40, 41, 42, 43, 44, 47, 52, 53, 54, 55, 56, 57, 61, 62, 64, 67, 72, 76, 81, **87**, 94, 167, 169, 177, 185, 206, 207
Cefuroxime 9, 10, 34, 35, 41, 46, 52, 61, 62, 67, 72, 75, 81, **86**, 87, 168, 169, 177, 179, 206, 207
Cefuroxime axetil 9, 10, 46, 52, 61, 67, 75, 81, **87**, 207
Cellulitis (erysipelas) 13, 41, 46, 48, 57, 64
Cephalexin 5, 46, 49, 62, 67, 75, 81, **87**, 177, 206, 207
Cephalosporins, overall/generations 67, 75, 76, 86, 87
Cephradine 206, 207
Cervicitis **20**, **22**, 64
Cestodes (tapeworms) **130**, **131**, 134
Chagas disease 128, 176

PAGES (page numbers bold if major focus)

Chancroid **20**, 41, 62
Chickenpox 12, 13, 57, 139, 142, 143, 186, 191
Chlamydia trachomatis 11, 20, 21, 22, 24, 28, 30, 33, 34, 43, 61, 66, 167
Chlamydophila (Chlamydia) pneumoniae 32, 33, 34, 35, 61, 66
Chloramphenicol 7, 8, 16, 21, 37, 39, 44, 53, 54, 59, 61, 62, 63, 64, 69, 71, 72, 74, 77, 83, **88**, 94, 177, 185, 199
Chloroquine 74, 125, 126, **132**, 133, 201, 206, 207
Cholangitis **14**, 31, 168
Cholecystitis 14, 168
Cholera 15, 17, 63
Chromoblastomycosis **98**, 107
Chryseobacterium/Flavobacterium 61
Cidofovir 60, 74, 135, 139, 144, 146, **147**, 151, 183, 198, 206, 207
Ciprofloxacin 4, 8, 9, 10, 12, 14, 15, 16, 17, 18, 19, 20, 21, 24, 26, 27, 28, 29, 30, 31, 32, 39, 42, 46, 47, 48, 49, 50, 51, 53, 54, 55, 56, 59, 60, 61, 62, 63, 64, 65, 72, 74, 76, 83, **90**, 112, 113, 118, 119, **121**, 123, 168, 170, 177, 179, 185, 199, 206, 207
Citrobacter 61, 66, 68
Clarithromycin 9, 18, 32, 33, 34, 35, 37, 38, 39, 43, 44, 46, 48, 49, 51, 56, 57, 59, 61, 62, 72, 74, 76, 79, 83, **88**, 116, 117, 118, 119, 120, 122, 124, 127, 167, 177, 180, 200, 201, 202, 203, 206, 207
Clindamycin 4, 10, 13, 16, 17, 19, 22, 23, 27, 38, 40, 41, 42, 43, 44, 46, 47, 48, 49, 50, 51, 56, 57, 58, 59, 61, 62, 63, 69, 71, 72, 74, 76, 79, 83, **88**, 94, 124, 125, 126, 127, 167, 169, 177, 185, 199, 206, 207
Clofazimine 74, 103, 118, 119, 120, **122**, 206, 207
Clonorchis sinensis **130**
Clostridial myonecrosis **41**, 49, 64
Clostridium difficile colitis 15, **16**, 61, 66, 68, 70, 86, 87, 88
Clostridium perfringens 22, 41, 49, 61, 66, 68
Clotrimazole 23, 24, 97, 206
Cloxacillin 65, 75, 85, 206, 207
CMV 13, 18, 33, 138, 139, 147, 148, 151, 151, 198
CMV retinitis 13, 139, 147
Coccidioides immitis 98, 109, 175
Coccidioidomycosis 9, 39, 49, 98, 99, 107
Colistin 7, 37, 61, 69, 74, 77, 83, 199
Colitis, antibiotic-associated 85, 88, 121
Combivir 153, 154, 155, 157
Conjunctivitis (all types) 6, **11**, **12**, **13**, 20, 28, 54, 141, 150
Contaminated traumatic wound **41**
Corneal laceration 12
Coronavirus 40, **135**
Corticosteroids and meningitis **6**, **7**, **8**
Corynebacterium jeikeium 58, 61, 65, 67, 69
Coxiella burnetii 27, **35**, **61**
Coxsackievirus 43
"Crabs" (Phthirus pubis) 21, 131
Creeping eruption 128
Crohn's disease 18
Cryptococcosis 8, 9, 24, **99**, 103, 107, 109
Cryptococcus neoformans 9, 24, 109
Cryptosporidium 15, 17, 93, **123**
C-Section 22, 169
CSF 6, 7, 8, 9, 18, 21, 38, 51, 52, 59, 75, 76, 79, 88, 101, 106, 107, 114, 122, 127, 135, 136, 139, 140, 141, 147, 169
Cycloserine 74, 112, 116, 119, **122**, 199, 206, 207
Cyclospora **15**, 17, **123**
Cyclosporine 89, 93, 106, 182, 198, 199, 200, 201, 202, 203
Cystic fibrosis 35, 36, **39**, 93, 94
Cysticercosis **134**
Cystitis **30**, 64, 85, 135

PAGES (page numbers bold if major focus)

Cytomegalovirus   13, 18, 33, 138, 139, 147, 148, 151, 175, 183

D

d4T (stavudine)   74, 79, **164**, 174, 184, 199, 202, 203, 206, 207
Dacryocystitis   13
Dalbavancin   58, 63, 69, 71, 73, 74, 77, 83, **88**, 206, 207
Dandruff (seborrheic dermatitis)   **48**, 173
Dapsone   47, 74, 78, 119, 120, **122**, 126, 127, **133**, 199, 201, 203
Daptomycin   4, 28, 50, 58, 63, 69, 71, 73, 74, 77, 79, 83, 91, 180, 199, 206, 207
Darunavir   74, 78, 160, 165, 185, 201, 204, 205, 206, 207
ddC (zalcitabine)   74, 79, **164**, 184, 199, 200, 203, 206, 207
ddI (didanosine)   74, 79, **164**, 183, 198, 199, 202, 203, 206, 207
Decubitus ulcer   48
Dehydroemetine   **132**
Delavirdine   74, 78, 158, **164**, 185, 199, 201, 202, 205, 206, 207
Dematiaceous molds   109
Dengue   **136**
Dermatophytosis   **100**, **101**
Desensitization
   penicillin   74
   TMP-SMX   **92**
Diabetic foot   5, **14**, 48
Dialysis: Hemo- and peritoneal   43, 98, 170, **178**, **180**, **181**, **182**, **183**
Diarrhea   **15**, 17, 53, 64, 80, 82, 83, 85, 86, 87, 88, 91, 106, 107, 119, 122, 123, 124, 132, 133, 134, 135, 144, 146, 147, 148, 150, 161, 164, 165, 166, 173
Dicloxacillin   5, 9, 29, 46, 47, 48, 49, 65, 75, 80, **85**, 177, 206, 207
Didanosine (ddI)   74, 79, **164**, 183, 198, 199, 202, 203, 206, 207
Didanosine (ddI)   156
Didanosine + (emtricitabine or lamivudine)   153
Dientamoeba fragilis   123
Diethylcarbamazine   129, **134**, 206
Diiodohydroxyquin   123
Diloxanide   123, 206
Diphtheria; C. diphtheriae   43, 44, 61, 64, 186, 195
Dipylidium caninum   128, 130
Dirithromycin   43, 62, 63, 69, 76, 185, 200, 206
Dirofilariasis (heartworms)   129
Disulfiram reactions   88, 106, 121, 132, 200, 202
Diverticulitis   15, 19, 42
Dog bite (also see Rabies)   **46**
Donovanosis   **21**
Doripenem   14, 19, 22, 31, 32, 37, 42, 45, 49, 50, 55, 65, 74, 76, 80, 86, 179, 199
"DOT" bacteroides (non-fragilis bacteroides)   61
Doxycycline   6, 11, 17, 18, 20, 21, 22, 23, 24, 27, 30, 33, 34, 35, 37, 38, 39, 43, 44, 46, 47, 49, 51, 52, 53, 57, 59, 60, 61, 62, 63, 64, 69, 71, 73, 77, 83, **89**, 94, 118, 119, 123, 125, 126, 129, 167, 169, 177, 185, 199, 203, 206, 207
Dracunculus (guinea worm)   **128**
Drotrecogin alfa (activated protein C)   56, 206, 207
Drug-drug interactions   35, 81, 82, 84, 88, 89, 92, 106, 107, 108, 117, 121, 132, 148, 165, 166, 197, 198, 199, 200, 201, 202, 203, 204, 205
Duodenal ulcer (Helicobacter pylori)   18, 62, 64
Dysentery, bacillary   64, 123

E

Ear Infections   **9**, **10**, 64
Ebola/Marburg virus   135
EBV (Epstein-Barr virus)   **40**, **139**

PAGES (page numbers bold if major focus)

Echinocandin   96, 109
Echinocandin   109
Echinococcosis   130
Efavirenz   153, 154, 157, 159, 160, 205, 206, 207
Efavirenz (Sustiva)   74, 78, 116, **165**, 174, 185, 198, 199, 200, 201, 206, 207
Eflornithine   74, 127, **133**
Ehrlichiosis, monocytic & granulocytic   51, 52, 53, 62, 124
Eikenella   27, 44, 47, **62**
Elephantiasis (filariasis)   129
Empyema, lung   39
Empyema, subdural   6
Emtricitabine   74, 79, 153, 156, 157, 164, 183, 206, 207
Encephalitis   **6**, 41, 51, 52, 127, 128, **140**, 142
Encephalitozoon   124
Endocarditis
   Native valve   25, 26, 27, 64
   Prosthetic valve   27, 71
Endomyometritis   19, **22**, 42
Endophthalmitis   **13**, 97
Endotoxin shock (septic shock)   **56**
Enfuvirtide   162, 185
Enfuvirtide (T20, fusion inhibitor)   74, 79, **166**, 185, 206, 207
Entamoeba histolytica   15, 17, 18, 32, 123
Entecavir   74, 78, 137, 148, 151, 183, 206, 207
Enteric fever   54
Enterobacter   10, 48, 54, 62, 65, 67, 69, 86, 87
Enterobius vermicularis   **128**
Enterococci   6, 13, 14, 19, 24, **25**, **26**, 27, 30, 31, 32, 41, 42, 48, 55, 62, 64, 65, 67, 69, 86
   Drug-resistant   **26**, 65, 71, 86
   Vancomycin-resistant   **26**, 32, 62, **69**, 70, 71
Enterococcus faecalis   **26**, 30, 48, 62, 65, 67, 69, **71**
Enterococcus faecium   26, 62, 65, 69, 71, 86
Enterocolitis, pseudomembranous or neutropenic   15, **17**, 64, 87
Enterocytozoon bieneusi   17, 124
Enterovirus   6, 42, 43, **135**
Epididymitis   **24**, 53
Epiglottitis   44, 62
Epstein-Barr virus (infectious mono)   **40**, **139**
Ertapenem   19, 31, 36, 42, **65**, 74, 76, **80**, **86**, 177, 179, 199, 206, 207
Erysipelas   13, 48, 57
Erysipelothrix   **62**
Erythema multiforme   **48**, 87, 164
Erythema nodosum   **49**, 120, 122
Erythrasma   **49**, 101
Erythromycin   4, 11, 15, 20, 21, 22, 32, 33, 34, 35, 38, 41, 43, 44, 46, 47, 48, 49, 50, 51, 52, 54, 59, 61, 62, 63, 69, 72, 73, 74, 76, 79, 83, **88**, 93, 94, 119, 167, 169, 177, 180, 200, 201, 206, 207
Escherichia coli   5, 6, 8, 15, 16, **17**, 30, 31, 42, 45, 48, 54, 62, 65, 67, 69, 123
   O157 H7   15, 16
   enterotoxigenic (traveler's diarrhea)   15
Etanercept   18, 29
Ethambutol   74, 78, 111, 112, 113, 114, 115, 116, 117, 118, 119, **120**, 182, 199, 206, 207
Ethionamide   74, 112, 114, 116, 120, **122**, 182, 199, 206, 207
Extended-spectrum β-lactamases (ESBL)   37, 42, 62
Extended-spectrum (β-lactamases (ESBL)   62, 72
Extended-spectrum (-lactamases (ESBL)   72
Eyeworm (Onchocerca volvulus)   129

F

Famciclovir   12, 24, 74, 78, 140, 141, 142, 143, **148**, 151, 183, 206, 207
Fansidar (pyrimethamine sulfadoxine)   133, 134, 206, 207

PAGES (page numbers bold if major focus)

Fasciola buski, hepatica **130**
Fever blisters (cold sores) **141**
Filariasis **129**, 134
Fitzhugh-Curtis syndrome 22
Flucloxacillin **85**
Fluconazole 23, 27, 28, 32, 45, 51, 55, 74, 77, 94, 95, 96, 97, 98, 99, 100, 101, 106, **107**, 109, 124, 175, 182, 185, 198, 202, 203, 206, 207
Flucytosine 74, 77, 97, 99, **106**, 109, 124, 182, 206, 207
Fluke infestation (Trematodes) 130
Fluoroquinolones 10, 11, 14, 15, 16, 17, 18, 21, 24, 28, 30, 31, 33, 34, 35, 37, 38, 39, 40, 42, 43, 44, 45, 46, 47, 54, 56, 59, 61, 62, 63, 64, 65, 71, 72, 79, 88, **90**, 113, 118, 119, 121, 199
Folliculitis; hot tub folliculitis 49, 50
Fomivirsen 139
Foot, diabetic 5, 14, 48
Fosamprenavir 74, 79, 153, 154, 160, 165, 174, 185, 201, 204, 205, 206, 207
Fosamprenavir + ritonavir 153
Foscarnet 74, 78, 138, 139, 141, 143, **147**, 151, 183, 198, 199, 201, 206
Fosfomycin 30, 63, 69, 71, 74, 77, **91**, 206, 207
Fournier's gangrene **50**
Francisella tularensis 35, 38, 40, 41, 50, **53**, 60, 62, 64, 70
Fumagillin 124, 133
Furunculosis **47**, **49**
Fusariosis 101, 107
Fusarium sp. 108, 109
Fusidic acid 4, 49, 63, 69, 71, 92, 185
Fusobacterium necrophorum 12, 44, 45, 46

G

G6PD deficiency 30, 47, 91, 92, 122, 125, 126, 132, 133, 201
Ganciclovir 55, 74, 78, 138, 139, 142, **147**, 151, 175, 184, 200, 206, 207
Gancyclovir 203
Gardnerella vaginalis **23**, 62
Gas gangrene **41**, 50, 56, 64
Gastric ulcer, gastritis (H. pylori) **18**, 62, 64
Gastroenteritis 15, 16, 17, 144
Gatifloxacin 8, 11, 31, 35, 36, 39, 42, 45, 59, 63, 65, 71, 74, 76, 83, **90**, 119, 179, 199, 206, 207
Gemifloxacin 30, 33, 35, 38, 45, 62, 63, 65, 72, 74, 76, 83, 90, 119, 199, 206, 207
Genital herpes 6, 24, **140**, **141**
Gentamicin 6, 7, 8, 11, 12, 17, 23, 25, 26, 27, 31, 33, 51, 53, 56, 59, 60, 61, 62, 63, 64, 69, 71, 73, 74, 76, 80, **93**, 169, 170, 177, 178, 185, 198, 200, 206, 207
Giardiasis 15, 17, **123**, 133
Gnathostoma 9, 129
Gonococcal arthritis, disseminated GC 28, 29, 64
Gonococcal ophthalmia 11
Gonorrhea 11, **20**, 22, 23, 24, 28, 29, 62, 65, 67, 69, 167
Granuloma inguinale 21
Griseofulvin 100, 101, **106**, 206, 207
Group B strep, including neonatal 4, 6, 22, 24, 28, 33, 48, **54**, 63, **167**

H

HACEK acronym; infective endocarditis **27**
Haemophilus aphrophilus, H. ducreyi 20, **27**, 64
Haemophilus influenzae 5, 7, **8**, 9, **10**, 11, 13, 28, 32, 33, 35, 37, 39, 40, 41, 44, 54, 56, 57, 62, 64
Hafnia 63
Hantavirus pulmonary syndrome **40**, 129, 135
Headache 158, 160
Heartworms (dirofilariasis) 129
Helicobacter pylori 18, 62, 64
Hemodialysis 58, 88, **178**, **181**

PAGES (page numbers bold if major focus)

Hemolytic uremic syndrome **15**, 16, 30, 148
Hemophilus aphrophilus, H. ducreyi 66, 68, 70
Hemophilus influenzae 65, 67, 69, **167**, 186
Hemorrhagic bullae (Vibrio skin infection) 49
Hemorrhagic fevers 59, 135, 136
Hepatic abscess **32**, **123**
Hepatic disease/drug dosage adjustment 185
Hepatitis A, B & C 29, 32, 121, 136, 137, 148, 149, 151, 164, 165, 167, 172, 174, 175, 186, 191, 197, 206, 207
Hepatitis B occupational exposure 172
Hepatitis B prophylaxis 136, **172**, 186, 187, 197
Herpes infections 6, 11, 12, 13, 17, 20, 21, 24, 30, 41, 43, 49, 55, 138, 139, 140, 141, 143, 148, 151, 175
  mucocutaneous **141**, **142**
Herpes simiae 47, **142**
Herpes simplex 6, 11, 12, 13, 18, 21, 24, 41, 43, **139**, **140**, **141**, 151, 175
Herpes zoster 49, 143
Heterophyes (intestinal fluke) 130
HHV-6, HHV-7, HHV-8 infections **139**
Hidradenitis suppurativa 48
Histoplasma capsulatum 101, 102, 109
Histoplasmosis 9, 39, 40, **101**, **102**, 107, 109
HIV 6, 9, 13, 17, 18, 20, 21, 39, 40, 41, 43, 46, 51, 78, 79, 99, 100, 103, 106, 110, 111, 115, 116, 117, 118, 119, 121, 123, 124, 126, 135, 136, 137, 138, 139, 141, 142, 143, 147, 148, 149, **152**, **164**, **165**, 167, 172, 173, 174, 197, 199, 201, 202, 204, 205
  Prophylaxis: needlestick & sexual 173
Hoignes syndrome (reaction to procaine) 85
Hookworm 128
Hordeolum (stye) 11
Hot tub folliculitis **50**
Hymenolepis **130**
Hyperalimentation, sepsis **58**

I

Imidazoles, topical **107**
Imipenem 9, 10, 14, 19, 22, 26, 31, 32, 37, 40, 42, 45, 47, 48, 49, 50, 55, 56, 58, 61, 62, 63, 65, 72, 74, 76, 80, **86**, 102, 118, 177, 179, 200, 206, 207
Imiquimod 150, 206, 207
Immune globulin, IV (IVIG) 6, 54, 56, 57, 136
Immunizations. See Table 20, children & adults 7, 41, 143, 144, 186, 191, 195, 197
Impetigo 49
Inclusion conjunctivitis 11
Indinavir 74, 79, 116, 161, 165, 185, 199, 200, 201, 202, 204, 205, 206, 207
Infectious mononucleosis (see EBV) 43, 139, 173
Inflammatory bowel disease 18, 49, 132
Infliximab 18, 29, 102, 142
Influenza A 40, 98, **144**, 149, 150, 151, 191, 197
INH (isoniazid) 74, 78, 110, 111, 112, 113, 114, 115, 116, 117, 119, **121**, 122, 182, 185, 198, 199, 200, 201, 202, 203, 206, 207
Integrase Inhibitor 166
Interferon-gamma 110
Interferons 61, 99, 110, 135, 136, 137, 146, **148**, **149**, 150, 151, 206, 207
Iodoquinol 123, **132**, 206, 207
Isepamicin 74, **93**, 178
Isospora belli 17, **123**
Isotretinoin **46**
Itraconazole 23, 74, 77, 94, 95, 97, 98, 99, 100, 101, 103, **107**, 109, 124, 175, 182, 185, 198, 199, 200, 201, 202, 203, 206, 207
IV line infection & prophylaxis 13, 57, 58, 74
Ivermectin 74, 78, 128, 129, 131, **134**, 206, 207

J

Jock itch (T. cruris) 101

PAGES (page numbers bold if major focus)

K

Kala-azar	133
Kaletra	161, 204, 205
Kanamycin	62, 76, 80, **93**, 112, 119, 178, 198, 206, 207
Kaposi's sarcoma	40, 139
Katayama fever	130
Kawasaki syndrome	**54**, 135
Keratitis	11, 12, 124, 141
Ketoconazole	9, 48, 74, 97, 100, 101, 103, **107**, 124, 185, 198, 199, 200, 201, 202, 203, 206, 207
Kikuchi-Fujimoto (necrotizing lymphadenitis)	**40**
Klebsiella species	10, 31, 32, 37, 39, 42, 54, 62, 65, 67, 69, **72**

L

Lactobacillus sp.	58, **62**
Lamivudine	154, 155, 157
Lamivudine (3TC)	74, 79, 137, 148, 151, **164**, 174, 184, 199, 200, 203, 206, 207
Larva migrans	**128**
Laryngitis	44
Lassa fever, Ebola	59, **135**
Legionnaire's disease/Legionella sp.	27, 35, 36, 37, 40, 62, 64, 66, 68, 70
Leishmaniasis	41, 50, **124**, 133
Lemierre's disease (jugular vein phlebitis)	44
Leprosy	**120**, 122, 129
Leptospirosis	6, 32, **53**, 62, 89
Leuconostoc	58, **62**
Leukemia	55, 85, 95, 111
Levofloxacin	4, 11, 12, 13, 14, 15, 16, 17, 19, 20, 24, 28, 29, 30, 31, 32, 33, 35, 36, 37, 38, 39, 40, 42, 45, 46, 48, 49, 50, 52, 55, 56, 59, 61, 62, 63, 65, 71, 72, 76, 83, **90**, 112, 113, 119, 170, 180, 199, 206, 207
Lice	
body, head, pubic, & scabies	21, 27, 51, **131**, 134
Lincomycin	**88**
Lindane	131
Line sepsis	13, **57**, **58**, 74
Linezolid	4, 5, 8, 14, 26, 29, 32, 33, 34, 36, 38, 43, 49, 50, 54, 55, 58, 62, 63, 69, 71, 73, 74, 77, 79, 80, **89**, 102, 113, 116, 118, 119, 171, 180, 185, 200, 206, 207
Listeria monocytogenes	6, 7, 8, 9, 12, 16, 33, 54, 62, 64, 65, 67, 69
Liver abscess	32, 123
Liver disease/drug dosage adjustment	**185**
Loa loa	129
Lobomycosis	103
Lomefloxacin	199, 206, 207
Lopinavir	154, 161, 204, 205
Lopinavir/ritonavir	153, 155
Lopinavir/ritonavir & lopinavir	74, 79, 116, **165**, 174, 185, 200, 201, 206, 207
Loracarbef	9, 67, 75, **87**, 177, 206, 207
Ludwig's angina	41, 44
Lung abscess, putrid	**39**, 64
Lyme disease	8, **28**, **29**, 40, 51, **52**, 64
Lymphadenitis	40, 41, 46, 51
Lymphangitis, nodular	**41**
Lymphedema (congenital = Milroy's disease)	**48**
Lymphogranuloma venereum	21, 41, 110

M

MAC, MAI (Mycobacterium avium-intracellulare complex)	**117**, **118**, 119
Macrolide antibiotics	9, 10, 34, 35, 37, 38, 43, 48, 63, 69, 72, 74, 76, 83, 88, 119, 177, 180, 200
Madura foot	**102**, 103
Malacoplakia (pyelonephritis variant)	31
Malaria	79, 89, 123, **125**, **126**, 132, 133, 167, 197
Malarone (atovaquone + proguanil)	125, 126, **132**
Malassezia furfur (Tinea versicolor)	48, 58, **101**

PAGES (page numbers bold if major focus)

Malathion	131
Mansonella	**129**
Maraviroc	74, 79, 163, 166, 200, 206, 207
Mastitis	5
Mastoiditis	**10**
Measles, measles vaccine	87, **144**, 186, 191
Mebendazole	74, 128, 129, **134**, 206, 207
Mefloquine	74, 78, 125, 126, **133**, 200, 202, 206, 207
Meibomianitis	11
Melarsoprol	127, 128, **133**
Meleney's gangrene	**50**
Melioidosis (Burkholderia pseudomallei)	**37**, 51, **61**
Meningitis	
Aseptic	6, 9, 91, 92, 135, 136
Bacterial (acute and chronic)	6, **7**, **8**, 52, 62, 72, 87, 88, 114, 177
eosinophilic	9
Meningococci	6, 7, 8, 13, 28, 54, 55, 56, 62, 64, 65, 67, 69, 77, 89, 167
Meningococcus, meningitis	**6**, **7**, **8**, 13, 28, 56, 62, 64, 65, 67, 69
Prophylaxis	**8**
Meropenem	7, 8, 9, 10, 14, 19, 22, 31, 32, 37, 40, 42, 45, 48, 49, 50, 55, 56, 58, 61, 62, 63, 65, 72, 74, 76, 80, **86**, 177, 179, 206, 207
Mesalamine	18, 206, 207
Metagonimus	130
Metapneumovirus	40, 144
Methenamine mandelate & hippurate	**91**, 200, 206, 207
Methicillin	26, 27, 34, 62, 63, 65, 71
Methicillin-resistant Staph. aureus (MRSA)	4, 5, 6, 7, 11, 13, 14, 24, 26, 27, 28, 29, 31, 33, 36, 37, 38, 39, 40, 41, 45, 47, 48, 49, 50, 51, 54, 55, 56, 58, 63, 65, 67, 69, 71, 73, 144, 168
Metronidazole	5, 6, 13, 14, 15, 17, 18, 19, 20, 23, 32, 39, 41, 42, 44, 46, 47, 48, 50, 55, 57, 58, 61, 62, 69, 74, 77, 78, 83, **91**, 123, 128, 132, 167, 169, 177, 180, 185, 199, 200, 202, 203, 206, 207
Micafungin	28, 74, 77, 95, 96, 97, 106, 185, 200, 206, 207
Miconazole	23, 97, **107**
Microsporidia	17, 124
Miltefosine	133
Minocycline	14, 46, 47, 49, 50, 58, 61, 62, 63, 69, 71, 73, 77, 89, 102, 118, 119, 120, 185, 206, 207
Mollaret's recurrent meningitis	141
Monkey bite	**47**, 135, 142, 144
Monkey pox	144
Monobactams	80, **86**
Mononeuritis multiplex	138
Moraxella catarrhalis	9, 10, 13, 33, 35, 36, 38, 44, 62, 65, 67, 69
Morganella species	62, 66, 67
Moxifloxacin	7, 8, 11, 17, 19, 30, 33, 35, 36, 37, 38, 39, 40, 42, 45, 46, 48, 56, 59, 62, 63, 65, 71, 72, 74, 76, 83, **90**, 113, 118, 119, 120, 185, 199, 206, 207
MRSA	4, 5, 6, 7, 11, 13, 14, 24, 26, 27, 28, 29, 31, 33, 36, 37, 38, 39, 40, 41, 45, 47, 48, 49, 50, 51, 54, 55, 56, 58, 63, 65, 67, 69, 71, 73, 144, 168
Mucormycosis	45, 57, **102**
Multidrug-resistant TB	**112**, 113
Mumps	42, 186, 191
Mupirocin	47, 49, 92, 168, 206, 207
Mycobacteria	9, 29, 34, 39, 40, 41, 42, 50, 70, 89, 110, **111**, 112, **113**, **116**, 117, **118**, 119, 120
Mycobacterium abscessus, M. bovis, M. celatum, M.chelonae, M. genavense, M. gordonae, M. haemophilum, M. kansasii, M. marinum, M. scrofulaceum, M. simiae, M. ulcerans, M. xenopi, M. leprae	**25**, 29, 40, 41, 47, 89, 117, **118**, **119**, **120**, **142**

PAGES (page numbers bold if major focus)

Mycobacterium tuberculosis 8, 9, 29, 34, 39, 40, 49,
110, 111, 112, 113, 116, 117
Directly observed therapy (DOT)   111, **112**, 116
Drug-resistant   **117**
Pulmonary   39, 40, **112**, **113**
Mycoplasma
genitalium   20
pneumoniae   32, 33, 35, 43, 62, 66, 70
Myiasis   131
Myositis   41, 57

N

Naegleria fowleri   124
Nafcillin   4, 5, 6, 10, 13, 25, 26, 27, 28, 29, 31, 38, 39, 40,
41, 42, 45, 47, 48, 50, 51, 56, 62, 63, 65, 73, 75, 80, 85,
177, 185, 206, 207
Necrotizing enterocolitis   **15**, 167
Necrotizing fasciitis   41, 48, 50, 57
Needlestick
HIV, Hepatitis B & C   173
Needlestick,HIV, Hepatitis B & C   **172**, **174**
Neisseria
gonorrhoeae 11, 20, 22, 23, 24, 28, 29, 62, 65, 67, 69,
167
meningitidis   7, 8, 13, 28, 56, **62**, 64, 65, 67, 69
Nelfinavir 74, 79, 116, 161, **165**, 185, 200, 201, 202, 203,
204, 205, 206, 207
Nematodes (roundworms)   **128**, **129**, 134
Neomycin   9, 12, 76, **93**, 132, 169, 198
Neonatal sepsis   54, 167
Netilmicin   25, 74, 80, 93, 178, 198
Neurocysticercosis   130, 131
Neurosyphilis   **21**
Neutropenia   17, 36, 37, 45, 48, 54, 55, 56, 57, 58, **80**,
81, **83**, 85, 88, 89, 94, 95, 96, 98, 102, 105, 106, 124,
133, 147
Nevirapine   74, 79, 155, 159, 165, 174, 185, 198, 200,
201, 202, 205, 206, 207
Nifurtimox   128, **133**, 176
Nitazoxanide   74, 78, 123, 128, 133, 146, 206, 207
Nitrofurantoin   30, 63, 69, 71, 74, 91, 170, 180, 199, 200,
203, 206, 207
Nocardia brasiliensis, asteroides   62, 89, **102**, **103**
Nocardiosis   6, 41, 62, 89, **102**, **103**
Norovirus (Norwalk-like virus)   15, 144
Novobiocin   63
Nursing (breast milk) & antibiotics   5, 22
Nystatin   12, 23, 97, **107**, 206, 207

O

Ofloxacin   9, 20, 30, 61, 62, 65, 74, 76, 83, **90**, 111, 112,
118, 119, 120, **122**, 199, 206, 207
Onchocerciasis   129, 134
Onychomycosis   14, 100, 107
Ophthalmia neonatorum   **11**
Opisthorchis (liver fluke)   130
Orbital cellulitis   **13**
Orchitis   24
Organ transplantation, infection & prophylaxis   175
Oseltamivir   40, 74, 78, 79, **144**, **150**, 151, 184, 206, 207
Osteomyelitis
Chronic   5, 64
Contiguous (post-operative, post-nail puncture)   **4**, **5**
Hematogenous   5, 64
Osteonecrosis of the jaw   **5**
Spinal implant   **5**
Vertebral   **4**, 51
Otitis externa—chronic, malignant, & swimmer's ear   **9**
Otitis media   6, **9**, **10**, 64, 88, 92
Oxacillin   4, 5, 6, 10, 25, 26, 27, 28, 29, 31, 38, 39, 40, 41,
42, 45, 47, 48, 49, 50, 51, 55, 56, 62, 63, 65, 73, 75, 80,
85, 177, 206, 207

PAGES (page numbers bold if major focus)

P

Palivizumab   32, **150**, 206, 207
Pancreatitis   156, 157
Pancreatitis, pancreatic abscess   **41**, 54, 87, 89, 133,
164, 165, 199, 201, 203
Papillomavirus   **145**
Papovavirus/Polyoma virus   **145**
Paracoccidioidomycosis   **103**
Paragonimus   130
Parapharyngeal space infection   41, 44
Parasitic infections   123, 132, 134
Paromomycin   93, 123, 132, 206, 207
Paronychia   24, 97, 165
Parotitis   **42**
Parvovirus B19   29, **145**
PAS (para-aminosalicylic acid)   **122**
Pasteurella multocida   46, 62, 66, 68
Pegylated interferon   135, 137, 148, 149, 151, 206, 207
Peliosis hepatis   **32**, **51**
Pelvic inflammatory disease (PID)   **22**, **23**, 46, 64
Pelvic suppurative phlebitis   22, **58**
Penciclovir   140, 141, 148
Penicillin allergy   7, 8, 21, 22, 25, 26, 42, 43, 44, 45, 47,
48, 49, 52, 74, 85, 86, 87, 94
Penicillin desensitization   74
Penicillin G   6, 7, 8, 12, 17, 18, 21, 22, 25, 26, 29, 35, 38,
41, 43, 44, 46, 48, 50, 52, 53, 54, 56, 57, 59, 61, 62, 63,
65, 71, 72, 75, 80, **85**, 94, 167, 169, 177, 181
Penicillin V   14, 18, 43, 44, 46, 48, 54, 65, 75, **85**, 94, 167,
177
Penicilliosis   **103**
Pentamidine   40, 74, 124, 126, 127, **133**, 147, 182, 198,
199, 201, 203, 206, 207
Peptostreptococcus   5, 63, **66**, **68**, **70**
Pericarditis   **28**, 64, 94, 114
Perinephric abscess   **31**
Perirectal abscess   **17**, **19**
Peritoneal dialysis, infection   43, 98, 170, 185
Peritonitis
Bacterial/spontaneous   15, 19, 42, 98
Spontaneous—prevention   42
Pertussis   **32**, 61, 195
Phaeohyphomycosis   **103**
Pharmacodynamics   79
Pharmacokinetics, pharmacology   **75**, **76**, **78**
Pharyngitis/tonsillitis   20, 28, **43**, 54, 64
Phenytoin   202
Phlebitis, septic   10, 22, **44**, 48, **58**
Photosensitivity 46, 80, 81, 83, 84, 89, 90, 92, 106, 108,
121, 132, 134
PID   **22**, **23**, 46, 64
Pinworms   128, 134
Piperacillin 12, 39, 48, 65, 75, 80, **85**, 168, 177, 181, 201,
206, 207
Piperacillin-tazobactam 10, 14, 19, 22, 24, 31, 32, 37, 38,
39, 40, 41, 42, 44, 47, 48, 49, 50, 55, 56, 58, 61, 63, 65,
72, 75, 80, 85, 95, 177
Plague   35, 38, 50, 59, 63
Plesiomonas shigelloides   15, 62
PML (progressive multifocal leukoencephalopathy)   **145**
Pneumococci, drug-resistant   7, 9, 10, 34, 38, 40, **63**,
72
Pneumocystis (carinii) jiroveci   40, 64, 92, 126, 176,
177
Pneumonia
adult   33, 37, 38, 39, 40, 48, 53, 64, 72, 91, 126, 135,
138, 142, 146, 150, 151
community-acquired   **37**, 146
hospital-acquired   **37**
neonatal/infants/children   33, **34**

214

PAGES (page numbers bold if major focus)

Pneumonia, aspiration 39
Pneumonia, chronic 39
Pneumonia, community-acquired 73
Pneumonia, ventilator –acquired 37, 73
Podofilox 145, **150**
Polyenes 109
Polymyxin B, polymyxin E 9, 11, 12, 37, 72, 77, **90**
Polyoma virus 145
Posaconazole 74, 77, 95, 98, 99, 101, 102, 103, 107, 109, 175, 198, 206, 207
PPD (TST) 110, 111
Praziquantel 74, 78, 130, 131, **134**, 206, 207
Pregnancy, antibiotics in 8, 17, 20, 22, 23, 30, 31, 37, 38, 39, 46, 51, 52, 53, 59, 60, 89, 99, 106, 107, 111, 116, 121, 122, 123, 125, 126, 127, 129, 130, 132, 133, 134, 142, 148, 149, 150, 164, 165, 173, 174, 202
Pregnancy, risk from anti-infectives 74
Primaquine 40, 125, 126, **133**, 201, 206
Proctitis 17, 20
Progressive multifocal leukoencephalopathy (PML) **145**
Proguanil, atovaquone-proguanil 74, 125, 126, 132, 206, 207
Prophylaxis 167
Prostatitis, prostatodynia 20, 24, 31, 64
Prosthetic joint infection/prophylaxis 5, 16, 29, 169
Prosthetic valve endocarditis 27, 71, 168
Protease inhibitors 116, 119, **165**, 198, 199, 200, 201, 202, 203
Protein binding 75, 76, 78, 79
Pseudallescheria boydii (Scedosporium sp.) 102, **103**, 107, 109
Pseudomembranous enterocolitis 16, 64, 88
Pseudomonas aeruginosa 4, 5, 7, 8, 9, 10, 12, 13, 14, 17, 19, 24, 27, 29, 31, 32, 33, 36, 37, 38, 39, 40, 42, 43, 45, 48, 49, 50, 63, 66, 68, 70, **72**, 75, 85, 86, 87
Pseudotumor cerebri 89
Puncture wound 50, 173
Pyelonephritis 30, 31, 55, 64, 91
Pyomyositis 41
Pyrantel pamoate 128, 134, 206, 207
Pyrazinamide 74, 78, 111, **112**, **113**, **114**, **115**, **116**, 117, 119, **121**, 182, 202, 206, 207
Pyridoxine 114, 116, 119, 121, 122
Pyrimethamine 74, 78, 123, 127, **133**, 134, 176, 185, 199, 202, 206, 207

Q

Q fever 27, 61
QTc prolongation **88**, **89**, **90**, 107, 126
Quinacrine HCl 123, 132, 133
Quinidine gluconate 74, 126, 133, 200, 202
Quinine 51, 74, 124, 125, 126, 133, 182, 200, 201, 202
Quinolones 79, 83, 168
Quinupristin-dalfopristin 25, 26, 58, 63, 71, 73, 83, **89**, 185, 202, 206, 207

R

Rabies, rabies vaccine 6, 46, 132, 146, 196
Raltegravir 74, 79, 163, 166, 185, 206, 207
Rape victim 167
Rat bite 47
Red neck syndrome & vancomycin **88**
Reiter's syndrome 24, **28**
Relapsing fever 52
Renal failure, dosing 178, 185
Resistant bacteria 65
Resource directory (phone numbers, websites) 197
Respiratory syncytial virus (RSV) 32, 34, 40, 144, 150, 151
Retapamulin 49, 92, 206, 207
Retinitis **13**, 41, 127, 138, 139, **147**
Reverse transcriptase inhibitors **164**

Rheumatic fever 28, 29, 43, 54
Rheumatoid arthritis, septic joint **28**, **29**, 64
Rhinosinusitis 9, 44, 45
Rhinovirus 34, 44, **146**
Rhodococcus equi 63
Ribavirin 32, 59, 74, 78, 135, 137, 144, 146, 149, **150**, 151, 184, 185, 199, 202, 203, 206, 207
Ribavirin + interferon 149
Rickettsial diseases **53**, 54, 63, 70
Rifabutin 74, 111, 112, 113, 114, 116, 117, 118, 119, **122**, 185, 198, 199, 200, 201, 202, 206, 207
Rifampin, Rifamate, Rifater 4, 5, 8, 26, 27, 28, 29, 38, 43, 46, 47, 48, 51, 52, 53, 58, 59, 61, 62, 63, 69, 71, 72, 73, 74, 77, 78, 83, 107, 110, 111, 112, 113, 114, 115, 116, 117, 118, 119, 120, **121**, 124, 177, 182, 185, 198, 199, 200, 201, 202, 203, 206, 207
Rifamycins 116, 202
Rifapentine 112, 115, 116, 119, **122**, 185, 206, 207
Rifaximin 17, 18, 74, 77, 91, 185, 206, 207
Rimantadine 40, 74, 78, **149**, 151, 184, 185, 203, 206, 207
Ringworm 100, 101
Ritonavir 74, 79, 116, 154, 155, 161, **165**, **166**, 174, 185, 200, 201, 202, 203, 204, 205, 206, 207
Rocky Mountain spotted fever 55, 64
Rotavirus 186, 189, 190
Rubella vaccine 29, **191**

S

Salmonellosis, bacteremia 4, **15**, **16**, **17**, 28, 54, 63, 65, 67, 69
Salpingitis 23
Saquinavir 74, 79, 116, 155, 162, **166**, 185, 201, 202, 203, 204, 205, 206, 207
SARS (Severe Acute Resp. Syndrome) 40, 135, 146
SBE (subacute bacterial endocarditis) 25, 26, 27
SBP (spontaneous bacterial peritonitis) 42
Scabies & Norwegian scabies 21, 131, 134
Scedosporium apiospermum (Pseudoallescheria boydii) 109
Scedosporium prolificans 103, 109
Scedosporium sp. (Pseudallescheria boydii) 102, **103**, 107, 109
Schistosomiasis 128, 130, 134
Scrofula **40**
Seborrheic dermatitis (dandruff) 48, 173
"Sepsis" and "septic shock" 14, 46, 48, 49, 50, 54, 55, 56, 57, 117, 168
"Sepsis" and "septic shock" 96
Sepsis, abortion; amnionitis **22**
Sepsis, neonatal **54**
Septata intestinalis 17, 124
Serratia marcescens 63, 65, 67, 69, 87
Serum levels of selected anti-infectives **75**, **76**, **78**
Severe acute respiratory distress syndrome (SARS) 40, 135, 146
Sexual contacts/assaults 11, **20**, 23, 41, 107, 149, **167**, 173, 174
Shigellosis **15**, **16**, **17**, 28, 63, 65, 67, 69
Shingles 49, 143
Sickle cell disease 4, 28, 167
Sinusitis 6, 32, **45**, 64, 88, 94, 102, 103, 150
Skin 154, 156
Smallpox 60, 146
Snake bite, spider bite 47
Sparganosis **131**
Spectinomycin 20, 62, 93, 206, 207
Spiramycin 8, 127, 134
Spirochetosis 17
Splenectomy 46, 51, 56, 124, **167**
Splenic abscess **51**

PAGES (page numbers bold if major focus)

Sporotrichosis **41**, **102**, 104
Spotted fevers 53, 55, 63, 64
Staph. aureus 4, 5, 6, 7, 9, 10, 11, 12, 13, 14, 16, 24,
25, 26, 27, 28, 29, 31, 33, 34, 35, 36, 37, 38, 39, 40, 41,
42, 43, 44, 45, 46, 47, 48, 49, 50, 51, 54, 55, 56, 57, 58,
63, 64, 65, 67, 69, 71, 87, 88, 168
  Community-acquired 14, 50, 63, 71, 73
  Endocarditis 26, 64, 88
Staph. epidermidis 5, 7, 11, 12, 13, 15, 27, 28, 41, 43,
47, 48, 54, 58, 63, 65, 67, 69, 71
Staph. hemolyticus 31, **63**
Staph. lugdunensis 5, 63
Staph. saprophyticus 30, 63
Staph. scalded skin syndrome **50**
Stavudine (d4T) 74, 79, 157, **164**, 174, 184, 199, 202,
203, 206, 207
Stenotrophomonas maltophilia 37, 38, 63, 66, 68, 70
Stevens-Johnson 165
Stevens-Johnson syndrome 165
Stibogluconate 124, **132**, 206
Stomatitis **41**, 54, 97, 98, 122, 141
Streptobacillus moniliformis **47**, 63
Streptococcal toxic shock 48, 50, 56, 57
Streptococci 4, 6, 10, 13, 14, 22, 23, 24, 25, 26, 27, 28,
29, 32, 33, 38, 39, 40, 41, 43, 44, 45, 46, 47, 48, 49, 50,
51, 54, 55, 56, 57, 58, 63, 64, 65, 67, 69, **71**, 76, 86,
119, 167
Streptococcus
  bovis **25**, 117
  group B, prophylaxis **167**
  milleri complex 6, 39, 40, 63, 65
  pneumoniae 7, 8, 9, 10, 11, 12, 13, 28, 34, 36, 38, 39,
  40, 44, 54, 56, 63, 64, 65, 67, 69, **72**, 167, 191
  pyogenes 12, 13, 14, 28, 29, 43, 44, 48, 57, 63
Streptomycin 18, 26, 53, 59, 60, 62, 64, 71, 74, 78, 93,
110, 112, 113, 116, 119, **121**, 178, 182, 198
Strongyloidiasis **128**, 134
Subdural empyema **6**
Sulfadiazine 48, 54, 58, 103, 124, 127, 133, 134, 206,
207
Sulfadoxine + pyrimethamine 74, 133, 134, 206, 207
Sulfasalazine 18, 206, 207
Sulfisoxazole 10, 33, 54, **92**, 102, 177, 206, 207
Sulfonamide desensitization **92**
Sulfonamides 30, 48, 49, 62, 63, 74, 77, 92, 102, 103,
134, 180, 201, 202, 203, 206, 207
Suppurative phlebitis 10
Suramin **128**, **134**
Surgical procedures, prophylaxis 168, 169, 170
Synercid® (quinupristin-dalfopristin) 25, 26, 58, 63, 71,
73, 83, **89**, 185, 202, 206, 207
Syphilis 8, 9, 17, **20**, **21**, **22**, 33, 40, 41, 167

T
Tapeworms
  Taenia saginata, T. solium, D. latum, D. caninum 128,
  130
Teicoplanin 26, 63, 69, 71, **88**, 180
Telavancin 49, 50, 69, 71, 73, 77, 180
Telbivudine 74, 78, 137, 184, 206, 207
Telithromycin 35, 36, 37, 38, 43, 44, 45, 61, 62, 63, 69,
72, 74, 76, 80, **89**, 180, 203, 206, 207
Tenofovir 74, 79, 153, 157, 158, **164**, 183, 184, 199, 202,
203, 206, 207
Tenofovir + Emtricitabine 153
Terbinafine 74, 98, 100, 101, 103, **107**, 109, 182, 203,
206, 207
Tetanus prophylaxis 47, **195**
Tetanus, Clostridium tetani 14, 46, 47, 49, 50, 57, 61,
186, **195**

PAGES (page numbers bold if major focus)

Tetracycline 11, 18, 20, 21, 22, 46, 47, 51, 52, 57, 61, 62,
63, 72, 77, 83, 89, 123, 125, 126, 128, 133, 177, 181,
198
Thalidomide 74, 120, 122, 206, 207
Thiabendazole **134**, 203, 206, 207
Thrombophlebitis
  Jugular vein (Lemierre's) **44**
  Pelvic vein(s) **22**, 58
  Septic (suppurative) **48**, **58**
Thrush 43, **97**, 173
Ticarcillin 12, 39, 65, 75, 80, **86**, 177, 181, 206, 207
Ticarcillin-clavulanate 10, 14, 19, 22, 24, 31, 32, 38, 40,
41, 42, 44, 47, 48, 49, 50, 55, 56, 58, 61, 63, 65, 72, 75,
80, **86**, 177
Tigecycline 19, 42, 48, 50, 69, 71, 72, 74, 77, 83, 89, 185,
203, 206, 207
Tinea capitis, corporis, cruris, pedis, versicolor 48, **100**,
101, 131
Tinidazole 18, 23, 74, 78, 92, 123, 132, 177, 185, 200,
203, 206, 207
Tipranavir 74, 79, **166**, 185, 201, 206, 207
Tobramycin 9, 11, 12, 13, 17, 27, 37, 38, 39, 53, 56, 59,
60, 62, 63, 69, 74, 76, 80, 85, **93**, 118, 177, 178, 198,
203, 206, 207
Tonsillitis 43
Torsades de pointes 88, 90
Toxic shock syndrome (strep., staph., clostridia) 48,
50, 56, **57**
Toxocariasis 129
Toxoplasma gondii, toxoplasmosis 6, 40, **127**, 176
Trachoma **11**
Transplantation, infection 95, 99, 175
  prophylaxis See Table 15E
Traveler's diarrhea **17**, 64, 91
Trematodes (flukes) **130**, 134
Trench fever 51
Trichinosis 129
Trichomoniasis (vaginitis) 20, **23**, 127
Trichostrongylus **128**
Trichuris 128
Tricuspid valve infection, S. aureus 26
Trifluridine 12, 141, **148**, 206
Trimethoprim-sulfamethoxazole 4, 5, 6, 7, 8, 9, 14, 15,
16, 17, 18, 19, 21, 24, 30, 31, 32, 33, 37, 38, 39, 40, 41,
42, 44, 45, 46, 47, 48, 49, 50, 53, 55, 59, 61, 62, 63, 69,
71, 72, 73, 77, 83, 91, 92, 102, 103, 118, 119, 123, 124,
126, 127, 133, 167, 170, 176, 177, 180, 185, 203, 206,
207
Trizivir 156
Truvada 153
Trypanosomiasis **128**, 133, 134, 176
Tuberculosis 8, 9, 18, 29, 34, 39, 40, 49, 103, **110, 111**,
112, **113**, **114, 115**, **116**, 117, 118, 119, 121, 185
  Multidrug-resistant **112, 113**, **114**
  Tuberculin skin test (TST) **110, 111**
Tularemia (Francisella tularensis) 35, 38, 40, 41, 50,
53, **60**, 62, 64, 70
Typhilitis—neutropenic enterocolitis—cecitis **17**
Typhoid fever 15, 16, 54, 64
Typhus group (louse-borne, murine, scrub) 53, 89

U
Ulcerative colitis **18**, 123
Urethral catheter, indwelling 31, **91**
Urethritis, non-gonococcal 20, 22, 64
Urinary tract infection 30, 31, 57, 63, 71, 85, 91, 92,
98, 177

V
Vaccinia, contact 146
Vaginitis **23**, 30, 98
Vaginosis, bacterial 23, 62

216

PAGES (page numbers bold if major focus)

Valacyclovir 12, 24, 74, 78, 140, 141, 142, 143, **148**, 151, 184, 206, 207

Valganciclovir 74, 78, 138, 139, **147**, 151, 175, 184, 200, 203, 206, 207

Vancomycin 4, 5, 6, 7, 8, 10, 12, 13, 14, 15, 16, 25, 26, 27, 28, 29, 33, 34, 36, 37, 38, 39, 40, 41, 43, 45, 48, 49, 50, 51, 54, 55, 56, 57, 58, 61, 62, 63, 69, 71, 72, 73, 74, 77, 79, 83, 86, **88**, 89, 93, 167, 168, 169, 170, 177, 181, 185, 198, 203, 206, 207

Varicella zoster 12, 13, 57, 139, 142, 143, 186, 187, 191

Ventilator-associated pneumonia 37, 38, 150

Ventriculitis, V-P shunt 7, 88

Vibrio cholerae, parahemolyticus, vulnificus **17**, 49, 63, 70

Vincent's angina 44

Viral infections 152

Visceral larval migrans 129

Voriconazole 28, 56, 58, 74, 77, 94, 95, 96, 97, 98, 99, 101, 103, **108**, 109, 175, 182, 185, 198, 201, 202, 206, 207

VRE (vancomycin-resistant enterococci) 26, 32, 86

W

Warts 22, 150

West Nile virus 6, 57, 136, 146

Whipple's disease 8, **18**

Whipworm 128

Whirlpool folliculitis (hot tub folliculitis) 49, **50**

Whitlow, herpetic **24**, 141

Whooping cough 32, 61, 195

Wound infection, post-op, post-trauma 41, 49, 50

Wuchereria bancrofti 129

X

Xanthomonas (Stenotrophomonas) maltophilia 38, 63, 66, 68, 70

Y

Yersinia enterocolitica & pestis **17**, 28, 32, **41**, 49, 59, 63, 66, 68, 70

Z

Zalcitabine 158

Zalcitabine (ddC) 74, 79, **164**, 184, 199, 200, 203, 206, 207

Zanamivir 40, 74, 144, **150**, 151, 206, 207

Zidovudine (ZDV, AZT) 74, 79, 147, 154, 155, 157, 158, 164, 173, 174, 184, 198, 199, 200, 202, 203, 206, 207

Zidovudine/ Lamivudine 153

Zygomycetes 109